HIV AND THE BLOOD SUPPLY

AN ANALYSIS OF CRISIS DECISIONMAKING

Lauren B. Leveton, Harold C. Sox, Jr., and Michael A. Stoto,
Editors

Committee to Study HIV Transmission Through Blood and Blood
Products
Division of Health Promotion and Disease Prevention
INSTITUTE OF MEDICINE

NATIONAL ACADEMY PRESS
Washington, D.C. 1995

National Academy Press 2101 Constitution Avenue, N.W. Washington, D.C. 20418

NOTICE: The project that is the subject of this report was approved by the Governing Board of the National Research Council, whose members are drawn from the councils of the National Academy of Sciences, the National Academy of Engineering, and the Institute of Medicine. The members of the committee responsible for the report were chosen for their special competences and with regard for appropriate balance.

This report has been reviewed by a group other than the authors according to procedures approved by a Report Review Committee consisting of members of the National Academy of Sciences, the National Academy of Engineering, and the Institute of Medicine.

The Institute of Medicine was chartered in 1970 by the National Academy of Sciences to enlist distinguished members of the appropriate professions in the examination of policy matters pertaining to the health of the public. In this, the Institute acts under the Academy's 1863 congressional charter responsibility to be an adviser to the federal government and its own initiative in identifying issues of medical care, research, and education. Dr. Kenneth I. Shine is president of the Institute of Medicine.

Support for this study was provided by the Office of the Assistant Secretary of Health, Department of Health and Human Services (contract no. 282-93-0045).

Library of Congress Cataloging-in-Publication Data

HIV and the blood supply : an analysis of crisis decisionmaking / Committee to Study HIV Transmission Through Blood and Blood Products, Division of Health Promotion and Disease Prevention, Institute of Medicine ; Lauren B. Leveton, Harold C. Sox, Michael A. Stoto, editors.

 p. cm.

Includes bibliographical references and index.

ISBN 0-309-05329-3

1. AIDS (Disease)—United States. 2. Blood banks—Risk management—United States. 3. Blood banks—Law and legislation—United States. 4. Medical Policy—United States. I. Leveton, Lauren B. II. Sox, Harold C. III. Stoto, Michael A. IV. Institute of Medicine (U.S.) Committee to Study HIV Transmission Through Blood and Blood Products.
RA644.A25H579 1995
362.1'969792—dc20 95-20469

 CIP

HIV and the Blood Supply: An Analysis of Crisis Decisionmaking is available for sale from the National Academy Press, 2101 Constitution Avenue, N.W., Box 285, Washington, D.C., 20055. Call 800-624-6242 or 202-334-3313 (in the Washington metropolitan area).

Printed in the United States of America.

The serpent has been a symbol of long life, healing, and knowledge among almost all cultures and religions since the beginning of recorded history. The image adopted as a logo-type by the Institute of Medicine is based on a relief carving from ancient Greece, now held by the Staatlichemusseen in Berlin.

COMMITTEE TO STUDY HIV TRANSMISSION THROUGH BLOOD AND BLOOD PRODUCTS

HAROLD C. SOX, Jr. (*Chair*), Dartmouth Medical School
SHULAMITH BAR-SHANY, Magen David Adom Blood Bank, TelAviv, Israel
DAVID BLUMENTHAL, Massachusetts General Hospital, Boston
ALLAN M. BRANDT, Harvard Medical School
BARBARA A. DEBUONO, State Health Commissioner, New York Health Department, Albany
MARTHA DERTHICK, University of Virginia
ROGER DETELS, University of California, Los Angeles
WILLIAM DULANY, Dulany & Leahy, Westminster, Maryland
MARK FEINBERG, University of California, San Francisco
JERRY MASHAW, Yale Law School
DOROTHY NELKIN, New York University
MADISON POWERS, Kennedy Institute of Ethics, Georgetown University
IRWIN M. WEINSTEIN, Hematologist, Los Angeles, California
CAROL O'BOYLE WILLIAMS, Minnesota Department of Health, Minneapolis

Project Staff

MICHAEL STOTO, Director, Division of Health Promotion and Disease Prevention
LAUREN LEVETON, Study Director
CYNTHIA ABEL, Program Officer
LAURA COLOSI, Research Assistant
KRISTINA BECKER, Project Assistant
DONNA THOMPSON, Division Assistant

Preface

The transmission of HIV through the blood supply in the early 1980s has led to considerable concern and controversy. Many individuals with hemophilia and many recipients of blood transfusions were infected with HIV through treatment with contaminated blood and blood products before there was an HIV antibody test for screening these products. These individuals—and their families, some of whom also became infected—face considerable suffering and emotional and financial hardship as a result. They believe they were betrayed by the very people and organizations with whom they had entrusted their safety. They ask if human error, or conflicting motivations, led to this tragic course of events. These questions become even more salient in so far as threats to the safety of the blood supply persist today (e.g., because of Creutzfeldt-Jakob disease, hepatitis C, and cytomegalovirus) (IOM 1992).

In April 1993, in response to concerns voiced by the hemophiliac community, Senators Edward Kennedy (D-MA), Robert Graham (D-FL), and Representative Porter J. Goss (R-FL) requested that Secretary of Health and Human Services Donna Shalala open an investigation into the events leading to the transmission of HIV to individuals with hemophilia from contaminated blood products. The Secretary agreed that it would be useful to gain a more complete understanding of the use of blood and blood products for the treatment of individuals with hemophilia and those receiving transfusions in the early years of the AIDS epidemic. Thus, with the intention of preparing for future threats to the blood supply, the Department of Health and Human Services requested that the Institute of Medicine (IOM) establish a committee to study the transmission of HIV through the blood supply. As a result, the Committee to Study HIV Transmission Through Blood and Blood Products was formed. Through this historical analysis, the Department of Health and Human Services expects to improve both decisionmaking and public health policy in meeting future challenges to the blood supply.

To carry out this year-long study, the IOM established a committee of 14 people. The creation of an IOM committee emphasizes the importance of providing an objective and impartial review of the decision-making processes and policies that surrounded the contamination of the blood supply with HIV. The Committee was asked to examine the decisions made from 1982 through 1986 to safeguard blood and blood products, and to evaluate the actions taken to contain the AIDS epidemic. The Committee held four meetings in which members formulated explanations and discussed information that had been collected to test their hypotheses. This report, the product of the Committee's efforts, attempts to provide both a comprehensive account of the events that led to the contamination of the U.S. blood supply and a critical assessment of the difficult decisions that were made in the context of the uncertainty of this period. This report does not seek to determine liability or affix blame for any individual or collective decisions regarding HIV transmission through blood or blood products during this time period. The Committee's conclusions and recommendations are intended to provide future leaders who will have responsibility for the blood supply with lessons gained from the experiences of those who tried to slow the tide of the AIDS epidemic among recipients of blood and blood products. The Committee undertook this assignment fully aware of the benefits and risks of hindsight. Hindsight offers an opportunity to do better the next time. The risk of hindsight is unfairly finding fault with decisions made by people who had to act long before scientific knowledge became available to dispel their uncertainty. To avoid this risk, the Committee has made every effort to conduct a thorough and objective review of what was known during 1982-1986 about the transmission of HIV through the blood supply. The Committee recognized the importance of conducting an organizational analysis of the major players involved in the blood supply system and attempted, in some instances, to understand and describe their various roles, responsibilities, and responses.

To understand the views of the many organizations involved in the blood supply, the Committee's first meeting included an opportunity to hear representatives of the Office of the Assistant Secretary for Health of the U.S. Public Health Service, the Food and Drug Administration (FDA), the Centers for Disease Control and Prevention (CDC), the National Institutes of Health (NIH), the American Association of Blood Banks, the Council of Community Blood Centers, the American Blood Resources Association, the American Red Cross, the National Hemophilia Foundation (NHF), the Committee on Ten Thousand, the HIV/Peer Association, and congressional staff of Senator Graham and Representative Goss. The Committee's second meeting included a public hearing in which the Committee heard presentations from interested parties. Fifty-nine speakers provided oral testimony to the Committee and an additional 50 provided written statements. A transcript of the public hearing is available through National Technical Information Services (Record Locator No. PB95142345). A list of all individuals who provided oral and written testimony appears in Appendix B. The Committee carefully considered all of this testimony as it formulated its conclusions and recommendations over the course of the following two meetings.

One of the advantages of conducting this study at this time is that many of the key participants in the 1982-1986 decisionmaking were available to speak to the Committee and staff. The Committee believed it was critical to hear firsthand accounts of the assumptions and beliefs that influenced critical decisions about the safety of the blood supply. Fact-finding interviews were held with 76 individuals knowledgeable about all aspects of the blood supply system. These interviews included representatives of FDA, CDC, NIH, NHF, the Office of the Assistant Secretary of Health, industry, and blood banks; physicians and scientists; and individuals with hemophilia. A list of all the people the Committee interviewed appears in Appendix A. The Committee also benefited from expert advice and background papers provided by consultants in plasma fractionation, blood supply systems, anthropology, risk assessment, virology, and organizational behavior. The Committee and staff also reviewed over 700 documents provided by each of the major organizations involved and other sources. Some of the key documents not readily available elsewhere are provided in Appendix D. Other documents reviewed by the Committee are available through the archives of the National Academy of Sciences.

A special acknowledgment is extended to those people who wrote background papers for the study—Jeffrey McCullough (whose paper provided much of the information contained in Chapter 2), Salman Kashevjee, Sheri Weiser, and Arthur Kleinman—and those who helped the Committee obtain important documentation—Val Bias, Wendy Donath, Corey Dubin, Bruce Evatt, Joseph Fratantoni, William Hammes, Dana Kuhn, Beth Leahy, Bruce Lesley, Jeanne Lusher, Clyde McAuley, Dick Merritt, Marla Persky, Andrea Posner, Dick Valdez, Jonathan Wadleigh, and many others. The Committee would also like to give special thanks to Lauren Leveton, Study Director, for her tireless efforts and guidance throughout the study. Thanks are also extended to the professional staff, Laura Colosi, Cynthia Abel, Kristina Becker and to summer law student intern Kathryn Astarita, for their commitment, assistance, and insight. Finally, the Committee thanks Michael Stoto, Director of the Institute of Medicine's Division of Health Promotion and Disease Prevention, for his contributions to this study.

REFERENCE

Institute of Medicine. *Emerging Infections*. Washington, D.C.: National Academy Press, 1992.

Contents

EXECUTIVE SUMMARY — 1

1 INTRODUCTION — 19
   HIV Infection via Blood Transfusion — 21
   The Committee's Charge — 22
   Organization of the Report — 24

2 THE U.S. BLOOD SUPPLY SYSTEM — 25
   Introduction — 25
   Blood and Blood Products — 25
   Blood Collection Organizations — 34
   Professional Associations — 36
   Hemophilia Organizations — 38
   Role of the U.S. Public Health Service — 41
   Blood and Blood Product Regulation — 47
   Regulatory Authority of the FDA — 51
   Summary — 53

3 HISTORY OF THE CONTROVERSY — 57
   Introduction — 57
   The Risk of AIDS — 60
   Immediate Responses to Evidence of Blood-Borne AIDS Transmission — 70
   Reconsidering the Evidence: Further Attempts to Formulate Policies — 74
   Research Activities — 76

4   PRODUCT TREATMENT   81
     Introduction   81
     Critical Time Period: 1970-1983   83
     Analysis and Conclusions   92
     Summary   95
     Afterword   96

5   DONOR SCREENING AND DEFERRAL   101
     Introduction   101
     Donor Screening Practices   103
     Analysis and Findings   105
     Conclusions   122
     Afterword   128

6   REGULATIONS AND RECALL   135
     Introduction   135
     Framework of Analysis   136
     Findings and Conclusions   142
     Influence and Responsibilities of Other Organization   160
     The Advantages of Marginal Thinking   163
     Summary   166

7   RISK COMMUNICATION TO PHYSICIANS AND PATIENTS   169
     Introduction   169
     Framework for Analysis   170
     Risk Reduction Options   175
     Case Studies   181
     Obstacles to Communication   192
     Conclusions   201

8   CONCLUSIONS AND RECOMMENDATIONS   207
     General Conclusions   207
     Recommendations   217

     APPENDIXES
A   Individuals Interviewed by the Committee   239
B   Individuals Providing Oral and Written Testimony   243
C   Chronological Summary of Critical Events, National   247
        Hemophilia Foundation (NHF) Communications, Knowl-
        edge Base, Risk Assessment, Clinical Options, and NHF
        Actions
D   Key Documents Provided to the Committee   263
E   Glossary of Acronyms and Terms   303
F   Committee and Staff Biographies   315

INDEX   323

TABLES AND FIGURES

Tables

2.1   Major Organizations Comprising the Blood Supply System and   26
      Their Functions

2.2   Components Produced by Blood Banks and the Medical Use of   29
      the These Components

2.3   Plasma Derivative Products and Their Uses   32

3.1   Chronology of Critical Events   58

3.2   Reported Cases of Opportunistic Infections and AIDS, Risk   61
      Groups Identified, and Evolving Knowledge Base: June
      1981 Through May 1985

4.1   Chronology of Fractionator License Applications and   92
      Approvals for Heat-Treated Factor VIII Concentrate

7.1   Summary of Clinical Options, Status and Sources of Recom-   176
      mendations, and Data Recommended

8.1   Triggers for Taking Actions in Response to Uncertain Risks   215

Figures

2.1   Organization of the plasma and plasma products industry   28
8.1   Blood Safety Council relationship   220

HIV AND THE BLOOD SUPPLY

Executive Summary

A nation's blood supply is a unique, life-giving resource and an expression of its sense of community. In 1993, voluntary donors gave over 14 million units of blood in the United States (Wallace, et al. 1993). However, the characteristic that makes donated blood an expression of the highest motives also makes it a threat to health. Derived from human tissue, blood and blood products can effectively transmit infections such as hepatitis, cytomegalovirus, syphilis, and malaria from person to person (IOM 1992). In the early 1980s blood became a vector for HIV infection and transmitted a fatal illness to more than half of the 16,000 hemophiliacs in the United States and over 12,000 blood transfusion recipients (CDC, MMWR; July 1993).

Each year, approximately four million patients in the United States receive transfusions of approximately 20 million units of whole blood and blood components. The blood for these products is collected from voluntary donors through a network of nonprofit community and hospital blood banks. Individuals with hemophilia depend upon blood coagulation products, called antihemophilic factor (AHF) concentrate, to alleviate the effect of an inherited deficiency in a protein that is necessary for normal blood clotting. The AHF concentrate is manufactured from blood plasma derived from 1,000 to 20,000 or more donors, exposing individuals with hemophilia to a high risk of infection by blood-borne viruses.

The safety of the blood supply is a shared responsibility of many organizations including the plasma fractionation industry, community blood banks, the federal government, and others. The Food and Drug Administration (FDA) has regulatory authority over plasma collection establishments, blood banks, and all blood products. Since 1973, the FDA has established standards for plasma collection and plasma product manufacture and a system for licensing those who met standards. The Centers for Disease Control and Prevention (CDC) has responsibility for surveillance, detection, and warning of potential public health risks within the blood supply. The National Institutes of Health (NIH) supports these efforts through fundamental research. During the 1950s and 1960s, blood shield laws were adopted by 47 states. These laws exempt blood and blood products from strict liability or implied warranty claims on the grounds that they are a service rather than a product. The laws were developed on the premise that given the inherently risky nature of blood and blood products, those providing them required protection if the blood system was to be a reliable resource.

As a whole, this system works effectively to supply the nation with necessary blood and blood products, and its quality control mechanisms check most human safety threats. The events of the early 1980s, however, revealed an important weakness in the system—in its ability to deal with a new threat that was characterized by substantial uncertainty. With intent to prepare the guardians of the blood supply for future threats concerning blood safety, the Department of Health and Human Services commissioned the Institute of Medicine to study the transmission of HIV through the blood supply. The Committee to Study HIV Transmission Through Blood and Blood Products undertook this assignment fully aware of the advantages and dangers of hindsight. Hindsight offers an opportunity to gain the understanding needed to confront the next threat to the blood supply. The danger of hindsight is unfairly finding fault with decisions that were made in the context of great uncertainty.

HISTORY

The Risk of AIDS

Starting with the identification of 26 homosexual men with opportunistic diseases in June 1981, the CDC's *Morbidity and Mortality Weekly Report* became the source for reports of the epidemic. By July 1982, enough cases had occurred with common symptomatology to name the new disease "acquired immune deficiency syndrome" (AIDS). By January 1983, epidemiological evidence from CDC's investigations strongly suggested that blood and blood products transmitted the agent causing AIDS and that the disease could also be transmitted through intimate heterosexual contact. The conclusion that the AIDS agent was blood-borne was based on two findings. First, AIDS was occurring in transfusion recipients and individuals with hemophilia who had received AHF concentrate; these patients did not belong to any previously defined group at risk for contracting AIDS. Second, the epidemiologic pattern of AIDS was similar to hepatitis B, another blood-borne disease.

Immediate Responses to Evidence of Blood-Borne AIDS Transmission

In the first months of 1983, the epidemiological evidence that the AIDS agent was blood-borne led to meetings and public and private decisions that set the pattern of the blood industry's response to AIDS, starting with a public meeting convened by the CDC in Atlanta on January 4, 1983. Later that month, the leading blood bank organizations, and, separately, the National Hemophilia Foundation (NHF) and the blood products industry, issued statements about preventing exposure to AIDS. In March 1983, the Assistant Secretary for Health promulgated the first official Public Health Services (PHS) recommendations for preventing AIDS, and the FDA codified safe practices for blood and plasma collection.

The government and private agencies quickly identified, considered, and in some cases adopted strategies for dealing with the risk of transmitting AIDS through blood and blood products. The recommended safety measures, however, were limited in scope. Examples include: questions to eliminate high-risk groups such as intravenous drug users, recent immigrants from Haiti, and those with early symptoms of AIDS or exposure to patients with AIDS; direct questions about high-risk sexual practices were generally not used. These questions reflected a lack of consensus about the magnitude of the threat, especially among physicians and public health officials who had trouble interpreting the unique epidemiological pattern of AIDS. The recommendations also reflected uncertainty about the benefits of identifying and deferring potentially infected blood and plasma donors, treatment of blood products to inactivate viruses, recall of products derived from donors known to have or suspected of having AIDS, and changes in transfusion practice and blood product usage. The costs, risks, and benefits of these and other potential control strategies were uncertain.

Opportunities to Reformulate Policy

In the interval between the decisions of early 1983 and the availability of a blood test for HIV in 1985, public health and blood industry officials became more certain that AIDS was a blood-borne disease as the number of reported cases of AIDS among hemophiliacs and transfused patients grew. As their knowledge grew, these officials had to decide about recall of contaminated blood products and possible implementation of a surrogate test for HIV. Meetings of the FDA's Blood Products Advisory Committee in January, February, July and December 1983 offered major opportunities to discuss, consider, and reconsider the limited tenor of the policies.

Despite these and other opportunities to review new evidence and to reconsider earlier decisions, blood safety policies changed very little during 1983. Many officials of the blood banks, the plasma fractionation industry, and the FDA accepted with little question estimates that the risk of AIDS was low ("one in a million transfusions"), and they accepted advice that control strategies (such as automatic withdrawal of AHF concentrate lots containing blood from donors suspected of having AIDS, or a switch from AHF concentrate to cryoprecipitate in mild or moderate hemophiliacs) would be ineffective, too costly, or too risky. During this period, there were missed opportunities to learn from local attempts to screen potentially infected donors or implement other control strategies that had been rejected as national policy.

Research Activities

From 1983 through 1985, research on AIDS included epidemiological analysis to understand patterns of spread and etiology, the search for methods to control or eliminate the disease, and evaluation of the efficacy of potential safety measures such as surrogate tests for the infection. Related research on methods to inactivate hepatitis B virus in AHF concentrate had begun in the 1970s and came to fruition in the early 1980s.

Scientists at the Pasteur Institute in Paris first isolated the retrovirus now known as HIV-1 in 1983. Investigators at the National Institutes of Health (NIH) provided convincing evidence that HIV-1 was the causative infectious agent of AIDS in 1984, and were also able to propagate HIV-1 in the laboratory, thus providing the basis for a blood test to identify individuals infected by the virus. Scientists at NIH isolated and characterized HIV in 1984. Viral inactivation methods for AHF concentrate were developed in laboratories of the plasma fractionators, and the FDA licensed the new processes quickly. Although the pace of viral inactivation research had been slow, it accelerated in the 1980s, largely in response to hepatitis, and had identified effective strategies by 1984. However, research into other potential ways to safeguard the blood supply such as the use of surrogate tests was not pursued vigorously, and there was relatively little research on blood safety issues per se.

FINDINGS

The Committee framed its approach by examining four topics that are essential components of a focused strategy for ensuring the safety of the blood supply: blood product treatment, donor screening and deferral, regulation of removal of contaminated products from the market, and communication to physicians and patients.

Product Treatment

Plasma products can be treated by a variety of physical and chemical processes to inactivate viruses and thus to produce a product free from contamination and relatively safe for transfusion. Shortly after the development of the technology to manufacture AHF concentrate, it was recognized that these products carried a substantial risk of transmitting hepatitis B. Although some blood derivative products had been treated with heat to destroy live viruses since the late 1940s, Factor VIII and IX concentrates in the United States were not subject to viral inactivation procedures until 1983 and 1984. If this technology had been developed and introduced before 1980 to inactivate hepatitis B virus and non-A, non-B hepatitis virus, fewer individuals with hemophilia might have been infected with HIV.

Overall, the record of the plasma fractionators and the FDA with respect to the development and implementation of heat treatment is mixed. The Committee's analysis focused on whether the basic knowledge and technology for inactivating viruses in AHF concentrate had been available before 1980 and whether industry had appropriate incentives (from FDA, NIH, NHF, or others) to develop viral inactivation procedures. In the Committee's judgment, heat treatment processes to prevent the transmission of hepatitis, an advance that would have prevented many cases of AIDS in individuals with hemophilia, might have been developed before 1980. For a variety of reasons (e.g., concern about possible development of inhibitors and higher costs), however, neither physicians caring for individuals with hemophilia nor the Public Health Service agencies actively encouraged the plasma fractionation companies to develop heat treatment measures earlier. The absence of incentives, as well as the lack of a countervailing force to advocate blood product safety, contributed to the plasma fractionation industry's slow rate of progress toward the development of heat-treated products. Once plasma fractionators developed inactivation methods, however, the FDA moved expeditiously to license them.

Donor Screening and Deferral Policies

The purpose of donor screening and deferral procedures is to minimize the possibility of transmitting an infectious agent from a unit of donated blood to the recipient of that unit, as well as to ensure the welfare of the donor. Donor screening includes the identification of suitable donors; the recruitment of donors; and the exclusion of high-risk individuals through methods and procedures used at the time of donation, such as questionnaires, interviews, medical exams, blood tests, and providing donors with the opportunity to self defer. Donor deferral is the temporary or permanent rejection of a donor based on the results of the screening measures.

By January 1983, in addition to suggesting that the agent causing AIDS was transmitted through blood and blood products and could be sexually transmitted, the epidemiological evidence also demonstrated that there were several groups who had an increased risk of developing AIDS. The highest incidence of the disease was in male homosexuals, who donated blood frequently in some geographic regions. The Committee found that organizations implemented donor screening measures in different ways at different times. Plasma collection agencies had begun screening potential donors and excluding those in any of the known risk groups as early as December 1982, and CDC scientists suggested in January 1983 that blood banks do likewise. Also in January, the blood-banking organizations (the American Association of Blood Banks, the American Red Cross, and the Council of Community Blood Centers) issued a joint statement that recommended the use of donor screening questions to detect early symptoms of AIDS or exposure to AIDS patients. The statement, however, did not advocate directly questioning donors about their sexual preferences. Blood banks did institute some screening measures in early 1983, but only a few asked potential donors questions about homosexual activities. At the same time, CDC scientists also suggested that all blood and plasma collection agencies employ an available surrogate test for hepatitis B core antigen (anti-HBc). Most blood and plasma collection agencies rejected this recommendation. Although the precise impact of these two actions is not known, earlier implementation of either probably would have reduced the number of individuals infected with HIV through blood and blood products. In March 1983 the PHS issued recommendations that identified high-risk individuals for AIDS and stated that these individuals should not donate plasma or blood.

Based on its review of the evidence, the Committee found that decisionmakers involved with donor screening and deferral acted with good intent in some instances. In other instances, however, preference for the status quo under the prevailing conditions of uncertainty and danger led decisionmakers to underestimate the threat of AIDS for blood recipients. The Committee concluded that when confronted with a range of options for using donor screening and deferral to reduce the probability of spreading HIV through the blood supply, blood bank officials and federal authorities consistently chose the least aggressive option that was justifiable. In adopting this limited approach, policymakers often passed over options that might have initially slowed the spread of HIV to individuals with hemophilia and other recipients of blood and blood products, for example, by screening male donors for a history of sexual activity with other males and screening donated blood for the anti-HBc antibody. The Committee believes that it was reasonable to require blood banks to implement these two screening procedures in January 1983. The FDA's failure to require this is evidence that the agency did not adequately use its regulatory authority and therefore missed opportunities to protect the public health.

Regulations and Recall

The FDA is the principal regulatory agency with authority for blood and blood products, but it exercises its authority largely through informal action. Recall—the removal of a product from the market—exemplifies the relationship between the FDA's potent formal powers and its informal modus operandi. Recall is a voluntary act undertaken by the manufacturer but overseen by the FDA, which has the authority to seize or revoke the license of a product. Regulation of blood and blood products has been generally based on establishing a scientific consensus. Because the FDA's resources are limited, it relies upon the blood industry and others for cooperation. The FDA's Blood Products Advisory Committee is a venue for consensus-building about blood regulatory policy. In an industry in which firm and product reputation is critical to market success, the FDA's collegial approach is usually effective.

The Committee analyzed the FDA's exercise of its regulatory powers by examining how it acted during four critical events: (1) letters issued by the FDA in March 1983 requiring particular practices related to donor screening and the segregation of high-risk plasma supplies; (2) a July 1983 decision not to recall plasma products "automatically" whenever they could be linked to individual donors who had been identified as having or as suspected of having AIDS; (3) a decision not to recall nontreated AHF concentrate when heat-treated AHF concentrate became available in 1983; and (4) a delay of years in the FDA's formal decision to recommend tracing recipients of transfusions from a donor who was later found to have HIV. For each of these, the Committee posed a series of hypotheses to explain the FDA's actions. These focused on the reach of the agency's legal powers, the information available at the time in relation to relevant public health considerations, the agency's resources, the FDA's institutional culture, the economic costs of particular actions, and the prevailing political climate.

The analysis of these four events led the Committee to identify several weaknesses in the FDA's regulatory approach to blood safety issues. The agency's March 1983 letters may have been unclear concerning whether all of their recommendations were required to be implemented by the addressed. Handling of the case-by-case recall decision suggested that the agency lacked both the capacity to structure its advisory process adequately and to analyze independently the recommendations that were made to it. In the Committee's judgment, these and other events indicate the need for a more systematic approach to blood safety regulation when there is uncertainty and danger to the public.

Communication to Physicians and Patients

As evidence accrued on the possibility that the blood supply was a vector for AIDS consumers of blood and blood products and their physicians found themselves in a complex dilemma about how to reduce the risk of infection. Restricting or abandoning the use of blood and blood products could lead to increased mortality and morbidity. On the other hand, continued use of these products apparently increased the risk of AIDS. The Committee investigated the processes by which physicians and patients obtained information about the epidemic and the costs, risks, and benefits of their clinical options.

A wide range of clinical options were available by late 1982 and might, in some instances, have reduced or eliminated dependence on AHF concentrate and thereby reduced the risk of HIV transmission. As often happens in times of intense scientific and medical uncertainty such as in the early 1980s, individuals with hemophilia and transfusion recipients had little information about risks, benefits, and clinical options for their use of blood and blood products.

The dramatic successes of treatment with AHF concentrate in the 1970s provided a context in which thresholds for abandoning or radically restricting the use of these products for individuals with severe hemophilia were high. Both physicians and individuals with hemophilia expressed reluctance about returning to the era of clinical treatment before the introduction of AHF concentrate. The National Hemophilia Foundation (NHF) and physicians, in their effort to find the right balance between the risks and benefits of continued use of AHF concentrate, tended to overweight the well-established benefits of AHF concentrate and underestimate the risks of AIDS, which were still uncertain.

In addition, the Committee found that prevailing assumptions about medically acceptable risks, especially regarding hepatitis, led to complacency and a failure to act with sufficient concern upon reports of a new infections risk. Ultimately, assumptions about medical decisionmaking practices in which patients played a relatively passive role led to failures to disclose completely the risks of using AHF concentrate and thereby did not enable individuals to make informed decisions for themselves. As the potential dimensions of the epidemic among individuals with hemophilia became clear, communication between physicians and patients was further compromised by physicians' reticence to discuss the dire implications of widespread infection with their patients and families.

Institutional barriers to patient-physician communications and relationships between relevant organizations also impeded the flow of information. If the NHF had received input from a wider group of scientific and medical experts, more explicit and systematic dissemination of a range of clinical options might well have been possible. In addition, the financial and other relationships between the NHF and the plasma fractionation industry created a conflict of interest that seriously compromised the perceived independence of NHF's recommendations.

No organization stepped forward to communicate widely the risks of blood transfusions to potential recipients. Many blood bank officials during this period publicly denied that AIDS posed any significant risk to blood recipients. In this context, and because many transfusions occurred on an emergency basis, patients were typically not appraised of the growing concerns about the contamination of the blood supply. For both individuals with hemophilia and recipients of blood transfusions, physician concern that their patients might refuse care deemed a "medical necessity" further contributed to failures to inform them of the risks.

CONCLUSIONS

Decisionmaking Under Uncertainty

The events and decisions that the Committee has analyzed underscore the difficulty of personal and institutional decisionmaking when the stakes are high, when knowledge is imprecise and incomplete, and when decisonmakers may have personal or institutional biases. The Committee attempted to understand the complexities of the decisionmaking process during this uncertain period and to develop lessons to protect the blood supply in the future. In retrospect, the system did not deal well with contemporaneous blood safety issues such as hepatitis, and was not prepared to deal with the far greater challenge of AIDS.

Although enough epidemiological evidence had emerged by January 1983 to strongly suggest that the agent causing AIDS was transmitted through blood and blood products and could be sexually transmitted to sexual partners, the magnitude of the risk for transfusion and blood product recipients was not known at this time. Policymakers quickly developed several clinical and public health options to reduce the risk of AIDS transmission. There was, however, substantial scientific uncertainty about the costs and benefits of the available options. The result was a pattern of responses which, while not in conflict with the available scientific information, were very cautious and exposed the decisionmakers and their organizations to a minimum of criticism.

Blood safety is a shared responsibility of many diverse organizations. They include U.S. Public Health Service agencies such as the CDC, the FDA, and the NIH, and private-sector organizations such as community blood banks and the American Red Cross, blood and plasma collection agencies, blood product manufacturers, groups like the National Hemophilia Foundation, and others. The problems the Committee found indicated a failure of leadership and inadequate institutional decisionmaking processes in 1983 and 1984. No person or agency was able to coordinate all of the organizations sharing the public health responsibility for achieving a safe blood supply.

Bureaucratic Management of Potential Crises

Federal agencies had the primary responsibility for dealing with the national emergency posed by the AIDS epidemic. The Committee scrutinized bureaucratic function closely and came to the following conclusions about the management of potential crises.

First, unless someone from the top exerts strong leadership, legal and competitive concerns may inhibit effective action by agencies of the federal government. Similarly, when policymaking occurs against a backdrop of a great deal of scientific uncertainty, bureaucratic standard operating procedures designed for routine circumstances seem to take over unless there is a clear-cut decision-making hierarchy. An effective leader will insist upon coordinated planning and execution. Focusing efforts and responsibilities, setting timetables and agendas, and assuming accountability for expeditious action cannot be left to ordinary standard operating procedures. These actions are the responsibilities of the highest levels of the public health establishment.

Second, the FDA and other agencies in the early 1980s lacked a systematic approach to conducting advisory committee processes. These agencies should tell their advisory committees what it expects from them, keep attention focused on high-priority topics, and independently evaluate their advice. Because mistakes will always be made and opportunities missed, regulatory structures must organize and manage their advisory boards to assure both the reality and the continuous appearance of propriety.

Third, agencies should not rely upon the entities they regulate for analysis of data and modeling of decision problems.

Fourth, agencies need to think far ahead. They must monitor more systematically the long-term outcomes of blood transfusion and blood product infusion to anticipate both new technologies and new threats to the safety of the blood supply. The Committee believes that the Public Health Service should plan what it will do if there is a threat to the blood supply. It should specify actions that will occur once the level of concern passes a specified threshold. The Committee favors a series of criteria or triggers for taking regulatory or other public health actions in which the response is proportional to the magnitude of the risk and the quality of the information on which the risk estimate is based. Taking on small steps allows for careful reconsideration of options, particularly as information about uncertain risks unfolds. Not all triggering events need lead to drastic action; some may merely require careful reconsideration of the options or obtaining new information.

RECOMMENDATIONS

The Committee's charge was to learn from the events of the early 1980s to help the nation prepare for future threats to the blood supply. From the record assembled for this study, the Committee identified potential problems with the system in place at that time and has identified some changes that might have moderated some of the effects of the AIDS epidemic on recipients of blood and blood products. The federal and private organizations responsible for blood safety and the public health more generally will have to evaluate their current policies and procedures to see if they fully address the issues raised by these recommendations.

The Public Health Service

Several agencies necessarily play important, often differentiated, roles in managing a public health crisis such as the contamination of blood and blood products by the AIDS virus. The National Blood Policy of 1973 charged the PHS (including the CDC, the FDA, and the NIH) with responsibility for protecting the nation's blood supply.

The Committee has come to believe that a failure of leadership may have delayed effective action during the period from 1982 to 1984. This failure led to less than effective donor screening, weak regulatory actions, and insufficient communication to patients about the risks of AIDS. In the event of a threat to the blood supply, the Public Health Service must, as in any public health crisis, insist upon coordinated action. The Secretary of Health and Human Services is responsible for all the agencies of the Public Health Service,[1] and therefore the Committee makes

Recommendation 1: The Secretary of Health and Human Services should designate a Blood Safety Director, at the level of a deputy assistant secretary or higher, to be responsible for the federal

---

[1] In the 1980s and now, the PHS agencies report to the Assistant Secretary of Health. As this report was beingwritten, the Department of Health and Human Services has proposed to eliminate the office of the Assistant Secretary, so that the PHS agencies would report directly to the Secretary.

government's efforts to maintain the safety of the nation's blood supply.

To be effective in coordinating the various agencies of the PHS, the Blood Safety Director should be at the level of a deputy assistant secretary or higher, and should not be a representative of any single PHS agency.

In considering the history of the contamination of the blood supply with HIV and the current surveillance, regulatory, and administrative structures for ensuring the safety of our nation's blood resources, the Committee became convinced that the nation needs a far more responsive and integrated process to ensure blood safety. To this end, the Committee makes

Recommendation 2: The PHS should establish a Blood Safety Council to assess current and potential future threats to the blood supply, to propose strategies for overcoming these threats, to evaluate the response of the PHS to these proposals, and to monitor the implementation of these strategies. The Council should report to the Blood Safety Director (see Recommendation 1). The Council should also serve to alert scientists about the needs and opportunities for research to maximize the safety of blood and blood products. The Blood Safety Council should take the lead to ensure the education of public health officials, clinicians, and the public about the nature of threats to our nation's blood supply and the public health strategies for dealing with these threats.

The proposed Blood Safety Council would facilitate the timely transmission of information, assessment of risk, and initiation of appropriate action both during times of stability and during a crisis. The Council should report to the Blood Safety Director (see Recommendation 1). The Council would not replace the PHS agencies responsible for blood safety but would complement them by providing a forum for them to work together and with private organizations. The PHS agencies would be represented on the Council.

The Blood Safety Council should consider the following activities and issues: to deliberate the need for a system of active surveillance for adverse reactions in blood recipients; to establish a panel of experts to provide information about risks and benefits, alternative options for treatment, and recommended best practices (see Recommendation 13); and to investigate methods to make blood products safer, such as double inactivation processes and reduction of plasma pool size.

When a product or service provided for the public good has inherent risks, the common law tort system fails to protect the rightful interests of patients who suffer harms resulting from the use of those products and services. To address this deficiency, the Committee makes

Recommendation 3: The federal government should consider establishing a no-fault compensation system for individuals who suffer adverse consequences from the use of blood or blood products.[2]

For such a no-fault system to be effective, standards and procedures would have to be determined prospectively to guide its operations. There needs to be an objective, science-based process to decide which kinds of adverse outcomes are caused by blood-borne pathogens and which individual cases of these adverse outcomes deserve compensation. As with vaccines, such a system could be financed by a tax or fee paid by all manufacturers or by the ultimate recipients of blood products. However, had there been a no-fault compensation system in the early 1980s, it could have relieved much financial hardship suffered by many who became infected with HIV through blood and blood products in the United States. The no-fault principles outlined in this recommendation might serve to guide policymakers as they consider whether to implement a compensation system for those infected in the 1980s.

The Centers for Disease Control and Prevention

The CDC has an indispensable role in protecting our nation's health: to detect potential public health risks and sound the alert. In order to improve CDC's efficacy in this critical role, the Committee makes

Recommendation 4: Other federal agencies must understand, support, and respond to the CDC's responsibility to serve as the nation's early warning system for threats to the health of the public.

One way to begin to implement this recommendation is for the Secretary of Health and Human Services to insist that an agency that wishes to disregard a CDC alert should support its position with evidence that meets the same standard as that used by the CDC in raising the alert.

In order to carry out its early warning responsibility effectively, the CDC needs good surveillance systems. The Committee, believing that the degree of surveillance should be proportional to the level of risk inherent in blood and blood products and should include both immediate and delayed effects, makes

---

[2] One Committee member (Martha Derthick) abstains from this recommendation because she believes that it fallsoutside of the Committee's charge.

Recommendation 5: The PHS should establish a surveillance system, lodged in the CDC, that will detect, monitor, and warn of adverse effects in the recipients of blood and blood products.

The Food and Drug Administration

The FDA has legal authority to protect the safety of the nation's blood supply, and it is the lead federal agency in regulating blood banking practice, the handling of source plasma, and the manufacture of blood products from plasma. The Committee's recommendations focus on decisionmaking and the role of advisory committees in formulating the FDA's response to crises.

In the Committee's judgment, a more systematic approach to blood safety regulation, one that is better suited to conditions of uncertainty, is needed. In particular, the Committee recommends (see Chapter 8) that the PHS develop a series of criteria or triggers for taking regulatory or other public health actions for which the response is proportional to the magnitude of the risk and the quality of the information on which the risk estimate is based. In order that the perfect not be the enemy of the good, the Committee makes

Recommendation 6: Where uncertainties or countervailing public health concerns preclude completely eliminating potential risks, the FDA should encourage, and where necessary require, the blood industry to implement partial solutions that have little risk of causing harm.

In all fields, decisionmaking under uncertainty requires an iterative process. As the knowledge base for a decision changes, the responsible agency should reexamine the facts and be prepared to change its decision. The agency should also assign specific responsibility for monitoring conditions and identifying opportunities for change. In order to implement these principles at the FDA, the Committee makes

Recommendation 7: The FDA should periodically review important decisions that it made when it was uncertain about the value of key decision variables.

Although the FDA has a great deal of regulatory power over the blood products industry, the agency appears to regulate by expressing its will in subtle, understated directives. Taking this into account, the Committee makes

Recommendation 8: Because regulators must rely heavily on the performance of the industry to accomplish blood safety goals, the

FDA must articulate its requests or requirements in forms that are understandable and implementable by regulated entities. In particular, when issuing instructions to regulated entities, the FDA should specify clearly whether it is demanding specific compliance with legal requirements or is merely providing advice for careful consideration.

In the early 1980s, the FDA appeared too reliant upon analyses provided by industry-based members of the Blood Products Advisory Committee (BPAC). Thus the Committee arrived at

Recommendation 9: The FDA should ensure that the composition of the Blood Products Advisory Committee reflects a proper balance between members who are connected with the blood and blood products industry and members who are independent of industry.

An agency that is well-practiced in orderly decisionmaking procedures will be able to respond to the much greater requirements of a crisis. This consideration leads to

Recommendation 10: The FDA should tell its advisory committees what it expects from them and should independently evaluate their agendas and their performance.

Advisory committees provide scientific advice to the FDA, but they do not make regulatory decisions for the agency. The FDA's lack of independent information and an analytic capability of its own meant that it had little choice but to incorporate the advice of BPAC into its policy recommendations. To ensure the proper degree of independence between the FDA and the BPAC, the Committee makes

Recommendation 11: The FDA should develop reliable sources of the information that it needs to make decisions about the blood supply. The FDA should have its own capacity to analyze this information and to predict the effects of regulatory decisions.

Communication to Physicians and Patients

One of the crucial elements of the system for collecting blood and distributing blood products to patients is the means to convey concern about the risks inherent in blood products. In today's practice of medicine, in contrast to that of the early 1980s, patients and physicians each accept a share of responsibility for making decisions.

In instances of great uncertainty, it is crucial for patients to be fully apprised of the full range of options available and to become active participants in the consideration and evaluation of the relative risks and benefits of alternative treatments. To encourage better communication, the Committee makes

> **Recommendation 12: When faced with a decision in which the options all carry risk, especially if the amount of risk is uncertain, physicians and patients should take extra care to discuss a wide range of options.**

Given the inherent risks and uncertainties in all blood products, the public and providers of care need expert, unbiased information about the blood supply. This information includes risks and benefits, alternatives to using blood products, and recommended best practices. In order to provide the public and providers of care with information they need, the Committee makes

> **Recommendation 13: The Department of Health and Human Services should convene a standing expert panel to inform the providers of care and the public about the risks associated with blood and blood products, about alternatives to using them, and about treatments that have the support of the scientific record.**

One lesson of the AIDS crisis is that a well-established, orderly decisionmaking process is important for successfully managing a crisis. This applies as much to clinical decisionmaking as to the public health decision process addressed by earlier recommendations. As the narrative indicates, there are both public health and clinical approaches to reducing the risk of blood-borne diseases. The Blood Safety Council called for in Recommendation 2 would deal primarily with risk assessment and actions in the public health domain that would reduce the chance that blood products could be vectors of infectious agents. The primary responsibility of the expert panel on best practices called for in Recommendation 13 would be to provide the clinical information that physicians and their patients need to guide their individual health care choices. To be most effective, this panel should be lodged in the Blood Safety Council (see Recommendation 2) so that both bodies can interact and coordinate their activities in order to share information about emerging risks and clinical options.

Recommendation 14: Voluntary organizations that make recommendations about using commercial products must avoid conflicts of interest, maintain independent judgment, and otherwise act so as to earn the confidence of the public and patients.

One of the difficulties with using experts to give advice is the interconnections that experts accumulate during their careers. As a result, an expert may have a history of relationships that raise concerns about whether he or she can be truly impartial when advising a course of action in a complex situation. One way to avoid these risks is to choose some panelists who are not expert in the subject of the panel's assignment but have a reputation for expertise in evaluating evidence, sound clinical judgment, and impartiality.

Financial conflicts of interest influence organizations as well as individuals. The standards for acknowledging, and in some cases avoiding, conflicts of interest are higher than they were 12 years ago. Public health officials, the medical professions, and private organizations must uphold this new, difficult standard. Failure to do so will threaten the fabric of trust that holds our society together.

REFERENCES

Centers for Disease Control. *Morbidity and Mortality Weekly Report* , July 23, 1993.
Institute of Medicine. *Emerging Infections*. Washington, D.C.: National Academy Press, 1992.
Wallace, E.L., et al. Collection and Transfusion of Blood and Blood Components in the United States. *Transfusion*, vol. 33, 1993.

1

Introduction

A nation's blood supply is a unique life-giving resource and an expression of its sense of community. In 1993, voluntary donors gave over 14 million units of blood in the United States (Wallace, et al. 1993). However, the characteristic that makes donated blood an expression of the highest motives also makes it a threat to health. Derived from human tissue, blood and blood products can effectively transmit infections such as hepatitis, cytomegalovirus, syphilis, and malaria from person to person (Institute of Medicine 1992). In the early 1980s, blood became a vector for HIV infection and transmitted a fatal illness to approximately half of the 16,000 hemophiliacs in the United States and to over 12,000 blood transfusion recipients (CDC, MMWR, July 1993).

Each year, approximately 4 million patients in the United States receive transfusions of over 20 million units of whole blood and blood components. The blood for the transfused products is collected from voluntary donors through a network of nonprofit community and hospital blood banks. Individuals with hemophilia depend upon blood coagulation products, called antihemophilic factor (AHF) concentrate to alleviate the effect of an inherited deficiency in a protein that is necessary for normal blood clotting. Bleeding due to this deficiency can cause serious damage to muscles, tissues, and joints, and can be fatal when there is bleeding into the brain. The AHF concentrate is manufactured from lots of "pooled" plasma derived from 1,000 to 20,000 or more donors, exposing individuals with hemophilia to the high risk of infection by blood-borne viruses.

The safety of the blood supply is a shared responsibility of many organizations—the plasma fractionation industry, community blood banks, the federal government, and others. Public concern about the inherent risks of blood and blood products has led the federal government, through the agencies of the Public Health Service, to take the lead in ensuring blood safety. The Food and

Drug Administration (FDA) has regulatory authority over plasma collection establishments, blood banks, and all blood products. The Centers for Disease Control and Prevention (CDC) has responsibility for surveillance, detection, and warning of potential public health risks within the blood supply. The National Institutes of Health (NIH) supports these efforts through fundamental research.

AIDS emerged as a threat to the safety of the blood supply in the early 1980s because of a unique confluence of events. Medical breakthroughs in cardiac surgery and other areas resulted in greater use of whole blood and its components. A new treatment for hemophilia, home infusion of AHF concentrate, grew rapidly and significantly improved the health and increased the life span of individuals with hemophilia. In addition, much of the medical community, as well as the country as a whole, believed that epidemics of infectious disease were a thing of the past. There were also many changes occurring in the government and society, such as a presidential mandate to lessen the regulatory role of government and increased public awareness that the homosexual population was enduring stigmatization and discrimination (Bayer 1983).

As evidence for blood-borne transmission of AIDS accumulated in 1982 and 1983, the Public Health Service had to deal with a very difficult problem. On the one hand, the U.S. blood supply was barely adequate to meet the urgent needs of day-to-day patient care. On the other hand, there was growing evidence that a blood transfusion posed a risk of causing a disease that was proving to be fatal for many. However, both the magnitude of the risk and the prognosis were still unknown. An examination of the efforts of the Public Health Service and others to cope with this problem provides a remarkable window into the making of public policy under duress and uncertainty.

The syndrome that came to be called AIDS was first noticed in homosexual men in 1981, but within a year epidemiologic evidence suggested that AIDS might also be a threat to recipients of blood and blood products. Several blood banks, blood collection agencies, and blood product manufacturers (i.e., plasma fractionators) took some actions to increase blood safety (e.g., donor education and screening to exclude known high-risk groups; terminating plasma collection from prisons; and encouraging autologous donations to reduce the risk of infection as early as January 1983), yet thousands of individuals and members of their families became infected before the implementation of a blood test for HIV in 1985.

Perhaps no other public health crisis has given rise to more lasting anger and concern than the contamination of the nation's blood supply with HIV. In response, blood recipients and individuals with hemophilia who were infected during this period, their families and their physicians, and public and private officials with responsibility for blood safety have asked a series of questions: Could this tragedy have been averted? What institutions, policies, or decision processes, had they been in place in the early 1980s, could have helped to reduce the number of people infected with HIV? What should be done now to thwart future blood-borne infections? Mindful of the risks of retrospective analysis, this report attempts to answer these questions.

HIV INFECTION VIA BLOOD TRANSFUSION

Transmission of HIV occurred via fresh blood (whole blood, packed cells) and fresh blood components (platelets, fresh frozen plasma, etc.) as well as AHF concentrate. Most of the individuals were tested when the HIV test became available in 1985 and thus, the number of those that became infected is well documented. In December 1987, the CDC reported that of the estimated 15,500 hemophiliacs in the United States, approximately 9,465 (63 percent) were infected with HIV (CDC, MMWR, 1987b). Estimates of HIV infection in other patients (medical and surgical) due to transfusion are more difficult to obtain. A study by the CDC summarized data up to June 1992, by which time 4,619 persons (excluding hemophilia patients) had been reported with transfusion-associated AIDS. This number is thought to be an under-reporting because patients die from their basic disease before developing AIDS (as 50 percent of patients receiving transfusions die within six months) (Barker and Dodd 1989). On the other hand, some patients that are infected may not have been tested up to this day.

In addition to the documented cases of transfusion-associated AIDS, the CDC routinely estimates the transmission of HIV to blood recipients, as there continue to be a few cases each year (even since the implementation of the ELISA test). According to the CDC,

> the number can be approximated using prevalence of infection in donors, the efficiency of transmission, and the number of units transfused per year. In 1985, 0.04 percent of donations were positive for HIV antibody by Western blot assay. If 0.04 percent had been the seroprevalence among donors the years prior to screening, if all seropositive units had transmitted infection, and if each unit had gone to a different recipient, then 7,200 of the approximately 18 million components transfused in 1984 might have transmitted infection. If 60 percent of these recipients have died from their underlying disease, then approximately 2,900 living recipients who acquired transfusion-associated HIV infection in 1984 would remain. Most of these would be asymptomatic. … Mathematical projections from reported transfusion-associated AIDS cases estimate that approximately 12,000 people now [1987] living in the United States acquired a transfusion-associated HIV infection between 1978 and 1984 [CDC, MMWR, 1987a].

THE COMMITTEE'S CHARGE

Individuals with hemophilia, transfusion recipients, and their families have raised serious concerns about why there were not better safeguards and warning systems to protect them from viruses transmitted by blood products. Could viral inactivation processes for blood products have been developed more rapidly? Were appropriate measures taken to eliminate high-risk donors from the blood supply? Were the necessary regulations to ensure the safety of blood and blood products enforced? Were consumers of blood and blood products appropriately informed of the possible risks associated with blood therapy and were alternatives clearly communicated?

In response to these concerns, the Secretary of the Department of Health and Human Services (DHHS) asked a Committee of the Institute of Medicine (IOM) to review the scientific evidence that was available to decisionmakers during the early 1980s when the AIDS epidemic emerged, to examine the decisionmaking processes, and to evaluate the actions taken to contain the epidemic. Of equal importance, the Secretary asked the Committee to recommend a framework for steps that could prepare the nation to deal effectively with future threats to the blood supply. The IOM established a committee whose charge was to review and evaluate the following areas: the history of efforts to assure blood and blood product safety, efficacy, and availability; the regulatory process for governing blood and blood products; the history of the transmission of the AIDS virus through the blood supply; the roles and responses of government and other agencies, health organizations, plasma fractionators, and medical care providers; research on blood and blood products; and the decisionmaking processes that followed the first suspicions that the blood supply was a vector for transmitting AIDS. The Committee's charge did not include the development of assertions about what should have been done at the time, nor did it include conducting a comprehensive organizational analysis.

Within the emotion-laden and potentially adversarial atmosphere of a public health tragedy, the Committee engaged in a systematic inquiry. The Committee framed its approach by examining four topics that are essential components of a focused strategy for ensuring the safety of the blood supply: blood product treatment; donor screening and deferral; regulation of removal of contaminated products from the market; and communication of risk to physicians and patients. The Committee then tested a range of hypotheses to explain why decisionmakers acted as they did. These hypotheses take account of the legal authority of relevant organizations; the information available to them; the countervailing public health considerations and scientific knowledge that influenced particular decisions; the resource limitations that constrained organizations; the institutional, social, and cultural obstacles; the public or private interest motivations of organizations; and the economic and political incentives that influenced decisions.

To understand how events unfolded over the course of the AIDS epidemic and to develop a chronology, the Committee sought to identify the critical events that would illuminate the decisionmaking process. The Committee asked each of the major organizations to list several events that they felt were the most important and to give the reasons for their choices. The Committee used this information to develop a chronology and focus its analysis on specific events.

Historical information was obtained from the key contacts at each of the organizations. The Office of the Assistant Secretary of DHHS identified sources of information within the federal service; and others representing nongovernment agencies made themselves known to the IOM Committee and staff. Among the topics for literature searches were: history of hemophilia; history of blood collection activities; scientific knowledge about HIV; viral inactivation processes; hepatitis; risk communication; social and ethical implications of AIDS; and regulations concerning blood products. The Committee obtained, largely through requests and voluntary contributions, court depositions, congressional hearings, internal office memoranda, minutes of meetings, and scientific articles.

The evaluation of policy decisions and actions taken over a decade ago is a problematic enterprise. On one hand, the historical record consists primarily of contemporaneous notes and explanations that make the decisions appear inevitable. On the other hand, the difficulties that beset decisionmakers at the time do not appear so compelling in light of our current knowledge— exemplifying the risk that hindsight knowledge can easily and anachronistically be transposed back to the period in question. Finally, the documentary record is often incomplete, ambiguous, or vague, and current testimony about past events may be filtered by years of subconscious reinterpretation in the light of new knowledge. Even when the record is reasonably complete and apparently "clear on its face," interpreting its meaning demands the reconstruction of an always elusive historical context, without which no individual actions or statements can properly be understood.

In addition to these difficulties, the events under discussion are highly charged emotionally, as pointed out above. The infection of individuals with HIV through the use of blood and blood products has created almost unimaginable suffering among those who were infected and their families (some of whom themselves became infected). Many, particularly in the hemophiliac community, believe that they were betrayed by the very scientific establishment, nonprofit organizations, physicians, and governmental agencies on whom they relied to assist them in managing their chronic conditions and acute episodes. Those in official positions, by contrast, almost uniformly believe that they did everything that could and should have been done given the scientific uncertainty and public health considerations that constrained the range of realistic options.

ORGANIZATION OF THE REPORT

Chapter 2 describes institutions and organizations that comprise the national blood supply system and presents an overview of how blood is collected and distributed. Chapter 3 presents the history of the unfolding AIDS epidemic and the evolving knowledge base about the risk of AIDS from blood and blood products.

The main analysis of this report appears in Chapters 4–7. Chapter 4 provides a review of the development of processes to inactivate viruses in blood products such as AHF concentrate, examining the efforts made by the FDA, NIH, and the plasma fractionators, going back to the 1970s when it first seemed possible to inactivate hepatitis B virus and thereby enhance the safety of blood products. Chapter 5 addresses strategies for protecting the safety of the blood supply by screening potential donors, examining closely the factors that influenced decisions regarding the implementation of donor screening measures. Chapter 6 examines the role of the FDA in regulating blood and blood product safety, highlighting several critical events, such as the FDA's guidance for implementing donor screening practices, recall of potentially contaminated products, and procedures to inform recipients of contaminated products. Chapter 7 describes how the risks of HIV and the options for risk reduction were communicated to individuals with hemophilia, to transfusion recipients, and to physicians. The chapter also addresses the institutional, social, and cultural obstacles to effective communication about risk. In Chapter 8, the Committee presents conclusions and makes several recommendations that draw upon the analysis in the preceding chapters.

REFERENCES

Barker, Lewellys F., and Dodd, Roger Y. Viral Hepatitis, Acquired Immunodeficiency Syndrome, and Other Infections Transmitted by Transfusion, from Petz, Lawrence D., and Swisher, Scott N. *Clinical Practice of Transfusion Medicine* (second edition). New York: Churchill Livingsone, Inc., 1989.

Bayer, Ronald. *Gays and the Stigma of Bad Blood.* Hastings Center Report; April 1983.

Centers for Disease Control. *Morbidity and Mortality Weekly Report,* July 23, 1993.

Centers for Disease Control. *Morbidity and Mortality Weekly Report,* March 20, 1987a.

Centers for Disease Control. *Morbidity and Mortality Weekly Report,* December 1987b.

Institute of Medicine. *Emerging Infections.* Washington, D.C.: National Academy Press, 1992.

Wallace, E.L., et al. Collection and Transfusion of Blood and Blood Components in the United States. *Transfusion,* vol. 33, 1993.

2

The U.S. Blood Supply System

INTRODUCTION

The U.S. blood supply system is comprised of many organizations with different management structures and philosophies. Table 2.1 lists each of the major organizations that function to meet the nation's blood needs. To provide the context for the Committee's analysis, this chapter provides information on blood and blood products, the organizations that collect, manufacture, and distribute them, and the professional and trade associations that represent these organizations. Because of the special role of hemophilia in the Committee's analysis, this chapter also provides background information on the National Hemophilia Foundation and related organizations. Finally, this chapter also presents information on the federal agencies responsible for blood safety, the history of blood and blood product regulations, and the regulatory authority of the FDA.

BLOOD AND BLOOD PRODUCTS

There are two different types of blood collection activities. One blood collection and supply system involves the cellular elements and plasma obtained from whole blood, and the other involves large-scale collection of the plasma portion of whole blood and the subsequent manufacture of derivatives produced from that plasma as a raw material. Before describing these two types of activities, a brief summary of the products produced from whole blood and plasma is helpful.

Table 2.1 Major Organizations Comprising the Blood Supply System and Their Functions

Organization	Function
Federal Agencies	
Department of Health and Human Services	Direction and oversight
Public Health Service	Direction and oversight
Food and Drug Administration	Regulation and review
Center for Biologics Evaluation and Review Blood Products Advisory Committee	Regulation, review, and research scientific advice
Centers for Disease Control and Prevention	Surveillance, investigation, and information dissemination
National Institutes of Health	Biomedical research
Blood Collection Organizations	
American Red Cross	Blood collection and supply, research
Community blood banks	Blood collection and supply, information exchange
Hospital blood banks	Blood collection and patient care
For-Profit	
Plasma fractionation industry	Plasma collection and supply, manufacturing, research
Professional and Trade Associations	
American Association of Blood Banks	Representing blood collection and transfusion services organizations, standard setting (inspection and accreditation program), and education
American Blood Resources Association	Advocacy for plasma fractionation industry, education

Organization	Function
Council of Community Blood Centers	Representing blood collection, information exchange
Nonprofit-Patient Advocacy	
National Hemophilia Foundation	
Medical and Scientific Advisory Council	Advocacy, education, and information dissemination Medical and scientific advice

Blood is composed of plasma and several cellular elements which include red cells (erythrocytes), five kinds of white cells (leukocytes, many with important subtypes), and platelets. Either whole blood can be collected or the plasma portion of the blood can be collected with the cellular portion returning to the donor. Whole blood is collected by blood banks, which prepare the cellular products and unprocessed plasma used directly for transfusion. Plasma is collected and used as raw material to commercially produce plasma "derivatives," which are concentrated forms of selected plasma proteins (Figure 2.1).

Whole Blood and Components

Whole blood is collected by venipuncture from healthy adults into plastic bags containing a liquid anticoagulant preservative solution. About 450 milliliters of blood can be collected as often as every 56 days without harm to the donor. The whole blood is separated into components within eight hours after collection. The components are red blood cells, platelet concentrate, and fresh frozen plasma. The fresh frozen plasma can be used in one of three ways: (1) for transfusion; (2) for further processing into cryoprecipitate (i.e., fresh or frozen plasma) to be used for transfusion, and cryoprecipitate poor plasma, which serves as a source of raw material for further manufacture of plasma derivatives; or (3) as a source of raw material for subsequent manufacture of plasma derivatives as described below.

As shown in Table 2.2, among the components prepared from whole blood are red blood cells, platelets, fresh frozen plasma, and cryoprecipitate. Blood banks make many modifications of these components to obtain blood products that will be effective for specific purposes. In addition, blood banks distribute

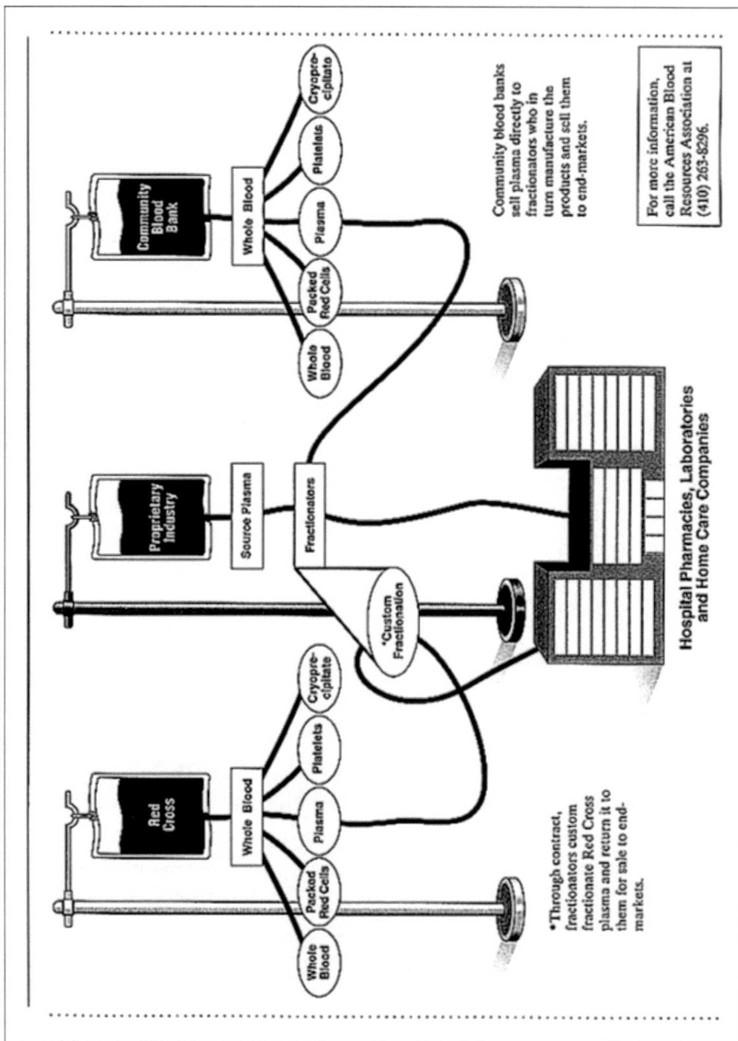

Figure 2.1 Organization of the plasma and plasma products industry. Reprinted with permission of the American Blood Resources Association.

many of the plasma derivative products as part of their total supply program for transfusion medicine therapy, but most of these other plasma products are actually manufactured commercially by plasma fractionation companies.

Table 2.2 Components Produced by Blood Banks and the Medical Use of the These Components

Component	Medical Use
Red blood cells	Oxygenate tissues
Platelets	Prevention or stopping of bleeding
Fresh frozen plasma	Stop bleeding
Cryoprecipitate	Stop bleeding
Cryoprecipitate poor plasma	Plasma exchange
Granulocytes	Treat infection
Frozen red blood cells	Store rare blood
Leukocyte-depleted red blood cells	Prevent reactions and certain diseases

Because the United States has a pluralistic system of blood collection, there is no central repository of data about the number of units of blood collected or the components produced or transfused. The American Red Cross (ARC) collects about 45 percent of the 14 million units of whole blood available for use annually in the United States. Other community blood banks collect about 42 percent, hospitals collect about 11 percent, and the remaining 2 percent is imported. In 1989, a total of 12,544,000 units of whole blood were collected by 190 blood centers and 1,685,000 units were collected by an estimated 621 hospitals (Wallace, et al. 1993).

Plasma and Derivatives

For the manufacture of derivatives, plasma can be obtained as the by-product from whole blood (plasma) or by plasmapheresis (source plasma). Plasma that is a by-product from whole blood collected by community blood banks or hospitals is sold to commercial companies in the plasma fractionation industry, who in turn manufacture the plasma derivatives and sell them in the pharmaceutical market. See Chapter 4 for a description of the role one such product—antihemophilic factor (AHF)—in the treatment of hemophiliacs. The blood banks' sale of their plasma to the commercial plasma fractionator may, but usually does not, involve an agreement to provide some of the manufactured derivatives back to the blood bank. For example, plasma from whole blood collected by the ARC is fractionated through a contract with Baxter Healthcare, which then returns all of the derivatives produced to the ARC for sale through their blood provision system.

The amount of plasma obtained from whole blood is not adequate to meet the needs for raw material to produce plasma derivatives. Therefore, much of the plasma that will be made into derivatives is obtained by plasmapheresis. This plasma is called source plasma, which is "the fluid portion of human blood collected by plasmapheresis and intended as the source material for further manufacturing use" [C.F.R., 1992]. Automated instruments are usually used to obtain 650–750 milliliters of plasma up to twice weekly from healthy adult donors (approximately 225 cc of plasma can be obtained from 450 ml of whole blood but most plasma is obtained directly through plasmapheresis). An individual can donate up to about 100 liters of plasma annually in the United States if the plasma protein levels and other laboratory tests and physical findings remain normal. The plasma is used as raw material for the manufacture of the derivatives shown in Table 2.3. The production of these plasma derivatives is a complex manufacturing process usually involving large batches of plasma (up to 10,000 liters) from as many 1,000–20,000, or more, donors.

The high demand for plasma products and the lengthy and often uncomfortable procedure of plasmapheresis led to the justification and legalization of compensation for plasma in the United States. Up to the early 1980s, plasma collection centers could be located in prisons and other areas where there was a high prevalence of hepatitis and other chronic infections. With the possible emergence of AIDS in the blood supply, plasma fractionators began closing their prison collection sites in December 1982, and in essence all were closed by January 1984.

Organizations and facilities need licenses for plasma collection (if shipped interstate) and the manufacture of AHF concentrate and other products from plasma.

Plasma Collection

Data regarding the plasma fractionation industry are proprietary and thus not readily available. The FDA does not routinely collect data on the nature of plasma donors, the amount of plasma each organization collects, or the number of derivative products produced. According to the American Blood Resources Association (ABRA), the U.S. plasma and plasma fractionation industry employs over 12,000 people nationwide (Scott 1990). U.S. plasma collection facilities perform approximately 13 million plasmapheresis donor collection procedures annually. Thus, if an average of 700 ml of plasma is obtained from each donation, it could be estimated that approximately 9 million liters of plasma would be collected annually in the United States by plasma centers. Individuals who donate plasma to support the plasma fractionation industry receive between $15 and $20 per donation. According to the ABRA, donors receive compensation of more than $244 million from plasma collection facilities annually (ABRA 1994). This is in contrast to whole blood donors, who donate voluntarily and do not receive compensation. Much of the plasma obtained from whole blood collected by blood banks is also used for production. Blakestone has estimated that in 1990 approximately 12 million liters of plasma were consumed in the manufacture of plasma derivatives (Blakestone 1994).

It is estimated that plasma fractionation worldwide sales exceed $4 billion annually, with U.S. firms providing more than 60 percent of the plasma products or $2.4 billion in domestic and export sales annually (ABRA 1994). Of the $2.4 billion in domestic and export sales, $645 million is the estimated export revenue from sales of U.S. plasma products in Europe.

Plasma Processing

The collected plasma is sent from the collection site to a fractionation laboratory, which in the United States, is either owned by a pharmaceutical company or by an outside company that sells the fractionated plasma to the pharmaceutical company. Fractionation involves further separation of the plasma into proteins such as albumin, immunoglobulin, and AHF concentrates. A pool size of at least 1,000 donors is required by the FDA for the production of immunoglobulin products used in the treatment of infectious disease, because increasing the pool size concentrates the therapeutic antibody portion of plasma. Pooling was more efficient for production in the manufacturing process of AHF concentrates because clotting factor proteins are found in extremely small quantities in plasma. Pooling plasma also has the negative effect of increasing chances for contracting infectious disease (see Chapter 4).

Table 2.3 Plasma Derivative Products and Their Uses

Plasma Derivative	Medical Use
Albumin	Restoration of plasma volume subsequent to shock, trauma, surgery, and burns
Alpha 1 proteinase inhibitor	Used in the treatment of emphysema caused by a genetic deficiency
Anti-inhibitor coagulant complex	Treatment of bleeding episodes in presence of Factor VIII inhibitor
Anti-thrombin III	Treatment of bleeding episodes associated with liver disease, antithrombin III deficiency, and thromboembolism
Cytomegalovirus immune globulin	Passive immunization subsequent to exposure to cytomegalovirus
Factor IX complex	Prophylaxis and treatment of hemophilia B bleeding episodes and other bleeding disorders
Fibrinogen	Treatment of hemorrhagic diathesis in hypo-, dys-, and afibrinogenemia
Fibrinolysin	Dissolution of intravascular clots
Haptoglobin	Supportive therapy in viral hepatitis and pernicious anemia
Hepatitis B immune globulin	Passive immunization subsequent to exposure to hepatitis B
IgM-enriched immune globulin	Treatment and prevention of septicemia and septic shock due to toxin liberation in the course of antibiotic treatment
Immune globulin (intravenous and intramuscular)	Treatment of agamma- and hypogamma-globulinemia; passive immunization for hepatitis A and measles

Plasma Derivative	Medical Use
Plasma protein fraction	Restoration of plasma volume subsequent to shock, trauma, surgery, and burns
Rabies immune globulin	Passive immunization subsequent to exposure to rabies
Rho(D) immune globulin	Treatment and prevention of hemolytic disease of fetus and newborn resulting from Rh incompatibility and incompatible blood transfusions
Rubella immune globulin	Passive immunization subsequent to exposure to German measles
Serum-cholinsterase	Treatment of prolonged apnea after administration of succinylcholine chloride
Tetanus immune globulin	Passive immunization subsequent to exposure to tetanus
Vaccinia immune globulin	Passive immunization subsequent to exposure to smallpox
Varicella-zoster immune globulin	Passive immunization subsequent to exposure to chicken pox

Blood and Blood Components Distribution

Traditionally, some areas of the United States have been able to collect more blood than needed locally and have provided these extra units to other communities. The misalignment of blood use and blood collection is a longstanding phenomenon. To deal with these blood shortages, blood is "exported" from areas of oversupply and "imported" into areas of shortage—a practice called "blood resource sharing." The lack of an adequate local blood supply and the need to import blood causes several difficulties including complex inventory management, technical disparities, emergency donor recruitment, higher costs, decreased independence, and higher risk-management costs (Scott 1990). Some blood centers import blood because they can obtain this blood for less than their own costs of production (Anderson 1990). For years, blood banks have participated in systems to exchange blood among themselves to alleviate shortages. Blood banks in metropolitan areas that serve large trauma, tertiary, and transplantation centers most frequently experience shortages of whole blood, components, and type-specific blood units. Although experience has demonstrated that the American public is ever-willing to donate blood in times of local disaster or national emergency, this same public has often not donated blood in sufficient supply to meet the daily needs of the local community. Less than 5 percent of the U.S. population donates blood and in certain communities the percentage is even lower. Without resource-sharing networks, many individuals would not receive the blood transfusions necessary to maintain or restore their health.

BLOOD COLLECTION ORGANIZATIONS

The United States blood collection system is heterogeneous owing to the "random development of blood centers without regard ... to patient referral patterns" (Scott 1990). The American Red Cross (ARC) collects approximately half the blood in the United States. In the non-ARC covered areas, blood is collected by one or more community or hospital blood banks. In most areas of the United States, there is only one local organization that collects blood. However, in some communities, including these where the ARC operates a blood program, blood may be collected by more than one organization. When this occurs, usually several hospitals and a community blood center (ARC or non-ARC) are involved.

The adequacy of the nation's blood supply varies at different times of the year and in different parts of the United States, but, in general, the United States is almost 100 percent self-sufficient in its blood supply. Approximately 2 percent of the U.S. blood supply is imported from western Europe (Wallace, et al. 1993). Sufficiency, however, varies among geographic areas of the United States on a continual basis. The extent to which the adequacy of the blood supply is related to the public image of blood banks and the association of blood with AIDS is not clear. Public opinion surveys indicate strong support for blood banks (Gallup 1991), and despite major public education efforts by blood banks, a high (35 percent) percentage of people believe they can contract AIDS or HIV by donating blood (CDC 1991).

Community Blood Banks

Blood is collected by blood centers and hospitals. Blood centers are freestanding organizations, virtually all of which are nonprofit. These centers are governed by a board of local volunteers and are organizations whose sole function is to provide the community's blood supply. Each blood center collects blood in a reasonably contiguous area and supplies the hospitals within the blood collection area. The blood center may or may not supply the total needs of the hospitals in its area or may supply hospitals in other areas as well. The area covered by each center is determined by historical factors and did not develop according to any overall plan. Rather, local interests dictated whether, how, and what kind of community blood program developed. Not every area of the United States is necessarily covered by a blood center. There are a total of approximately 180 blood centers in United States (Scott 1990). Approximately 45 of these (25 percent) are operated by the ARC and the remainder are community blood centers as described above.

The American Red Cross Service

The ARC is the organization that collects the largest number of units of blood in the United States. The ARC Blood Service is one of many humanitarian programs operated by the ARC. The ARC is a nonprofit, congressionally chartered (but not government sponsored or operated) organization that conducts programs supported by donated funds and through cost recovery. The mission of the ARC Blood Service is to "fulfill the needs of the American people for the safest, most reliable, most cost-effective blood, plasma … services through voluntary donations." In addition, the organization attempts to be the "provider of choice for blood, plasma … services … by commitment to quality, safety, and use of the best medical, scientific, manufacturing, and business practices" (ARC 1994).

Hospital Blood Banks

Some blood is collected by blood banks that are part of hospitals. These blood banks usually collect blood only for use in that hospital and do not supply other hospitals. Very few (possibly no) hospitals collect enough blood to meet all their needs. They purchase some blood from a local or distant community blood center. Most U.S. hospitals do not collect any blood but acquire all of the blood they use from a community center. Of those that do collect blood, there are no good data available to define the proportion of their needs that they collect. This can be presumed to be quite variable.

PROFESSIONAL ASSOCIATIONS

There are three major professional associations involved with blood banking. These are the American Association of Blood Banks (AABB), the Council of Community Blood Centers (CCBC), and the American Blood Resources Association (ABRA). Other organizations such as the American Medical Association, the College of American Pathologists, the American College of Surgeons, and the American Society of Anesthesiologists, may from time to time take positions on blood-bank-related issues and maintain blood bank or transfusion medicine committees. The AABB and CCBC are the only professional organizations devoted exclusively to blood banking and transfusion medicine. The ABRA is the trade association representing the plasma fractionation industry. Each organization is described briefly in the following section.

American Association of Blood Banks

Established in 1947, the American Association of Blood Banks (AABB) is a nonprofit scientific and educational association for individuals and institutions engaged in the many facets of blood and tissue banking and transfusion and transplantation medicine. It is the only organization devoted exclusively to blood banking and blood transfusion services. Institutional members of the AABB are classified either as a community blood center, a hospital blood bank, or a hospital transfusion service. The community blood center collects blood and distributes it to several hospitals but does not transfuse blood. A hospital blood bank both collects and transfuses blood, a hospital transfusion service transfuses but does not collect blood.

Member facilities of the AABB collect virtually all of the nation's blood supply and transfuse more than 80 percent. Approximately 2,400 institutions (community, regional, and ARC blood centers; hospital blood banks; and hospital transfusion services) and 9,500 individuals are members of the AABB. The services and programs of the AABB include inspection and accreditation, standard setting, certification of reference laboratories, operation of a rare donor file, accreditation of parentage testing laboratories, group purchasing programs, certification of specialists (technologists) in blood banking, educational programs, legislative and regulatory assistance to members, participation in the National Marrow Donor Program, participation in the National Blood Foundation, which provides funds for research in transfusion medicine and blood banking, and participation in the National Blood Exchange Program, which facilitates the movement of blood among centers with surplus and those with shortages.

AABB Inspection and Accreditation Program

The AABB operates a voluntary accreditation system in which most blood collection and transfusion organizations participate. The AABB accreditation program involves a biannual inspection by AABB volunteers. The AABB Inspection and Accreditation (I&A) program was initiated in 1958. The I&A program is designed to assist directors of blood banks and transfusion services in determining that knowledge, equipment, and physical plant meet established requirements. It is also a means for detecting deficiencies in practices and provides, when needed, consultation for their correction. The I&A program provides recognition through accreditation to those institutions functioning in accordance with existing published requirements of the AABB. While increased safety in obtaining and transfusing human blood and components is the major intent and benefit of the I&A program, certain ancillary benefits such as assistance in medico-legal problems may result. Inspection and accreditation by the AABB is a prerequisite for institutional membership in the association and for full participation in the AABB National Blood Exchange Program.

Council of Community Blood Centers

The Council of Community Blood Centers (CCBC) is an association of independent (non-ARC) not-for-profit community blood centers that serves the public by assisting its members in providing excellence in blood and related health services. The association was established in 1962 by the directors of six community blood centers who recognized the need for an organization that would represent the common interests of not-for-profit community blood programs and would provide a national forum to address the unique needs in the field of blood center operations. Its policies are determined by a board of trustees comprised of one voting representative from each institutional member.

Efforts to meet the goals of safety, quality, and efficiency in blood services are accomplished through a variety of activities and services that are developed and managed by volunteers. These efforts include group purchasing of supplies, services, and liability insurance; increasing volunteer blood donation; effective sharing of blood resources; strengthening of blood center management skills and the scope of services provided to the community; training programs to assure compliance with federal regulations; assuring fair and balanced resolution of disputes between blood centers and the public they serve; influencing federal and state regulations and policies; and promoting needed research and development in the blood services area.

The CCBC also promotes information exchange between members of operational practices, new programs, policies, and ideas through surveys, meetings of small working groups, and development of workable models. The weekly CCBC newsletter is a comprehensive chronicle of information about current government activities affecting blood centers as well as new developments in blood services and health care in general.

American Blood Resources Association

The American Blood Resources Association (ABRA) is a trade association founded in 1971 to represent the plasma collection and fractionation industry in both federal and state government relations. The ABRA's role is to educate the public at large about the commercial plasma and plasma products industry. The ABRA's mission is to promote and encourage research, to foster and monitor the promulgation of reasonable and just regulations, and to institute beneficial projects on behalf of the commercial plasma and plasma products industry. The ABRA provides facility and personnel certifications and develops industry manufacturing standards and guidelines. Its members operate under a strict code of ethics to ensure the high standards and quality. Its memberships operate over 80 percent of the U.S. commercial plasma collection facilities, and includes all of the commercial plasma product manufacturers in the United States and a majority of the manufacturers worldwide. Members manufacture and collect plasma in 42 states across the country.

HEMOPHILIA ORGANIZATIONS

The Nature of Hemophilia

Hemophilia is a rare, inherited, sex-linked disorder characterized by a deficiency in blood-clotting proteins. The estimated number of people with hemophilia in the U.S. population is approximately 15,000-16,000 (CDC, HRSA, MCHB, 1991, 1992, 1993). Hemophilia has been characterized by high mortality and a significantly lower mean age of death as compared to the general population (Chorba, et al. 1994).

There are two major types of hemophilia. The more common, hemophilia A, is characterized by a deficiency of antihemophilic Factor VIII clotting protein. The much less frequently occurring variety of hemophilia is hemophilia B, characterized by a deficiency of Factor IX clotting protein. About 85 percent of hemophilia cases are due to Factor VIII deficiency, about 14 percent to deficiencies of Factor IX. The remaining 1 percent involve the much more rare congenital clotting factors: V, VII, X, or XI (Hoffman, et al. 1994). The clinical severity of hemophilia is related to the degree to which the relevant factor is absent or deficient. The distinction of disease severity (i.e., mild, moderate, or severe) is critical in determining treatment of the disease. Mild or moderate hemophilia is rarely complicated by episodes of spontaneous bleeding (Hoyer interview). In severe cases, which are characterized by less than 1 percent of clotting factor activity, the disorder is accompanied by spontaneous bleeding into multiple joints of the body and muscles (Chorba, et al. 1984). This can be extremely painful, can lead to severe disabling musculoskeletal disease, and can be fatal. Most of the fatality associated with hemophilia results from central nervous system bleeding. Approximately 60 percent of hemophiliacs are classified as severe (Hoffman, et al. 1994).

Chapters 4 and 7 contain more detailed information on hemophilia treatment modalities available in the 1980s.

Hemophilia Treatment Centers

On July 29, 1975, Congress passed P.L. 94-63 authorizing federal funding to establish a network of comprehensive hemophilia treatment centers [Section 606 of P.L. 94-63 amended Title XI of the Public Health Service Act]. On October 1, 1976, a total of $3 million was appropriated to fund more than 20 regional hemophilia treatment centers [*Federal Register*, 1976, 1977] (Smith and Levine 1984). The Hemophilia Treatment Centers became a model program for the delivery of comprehensive care services for the diagnosis and treatment of hemophilia. The centers provided education, medical, psychosocial, orthopedic, dental, and genetic counseling expertise, and the means for early application of treatment. The comprehensive care provided was aimed at preventing or reducing the complications associated with hemophilia, as well as rehabilitation of those who already had severe musculoskeletal complications (Smith and Levine 1984).

National Hemophilia Foundation

The National Hemophilia Foundation (NHF) is a nonprofit health care organization founded in 1948. Its mission is to help meet the needs of all individuals with bleeding disorders. The NHF is organized into chapters, each of which has a locally elected board of directors and officers. Each chapter's president is the chief executive officer and serves without compensation. There are 46 chapters nationwide. Chapters are self-governed and determine their own priorities, programs, and uses of funds. They have the benefit and use of the NHF's advertising, public relations materials, publications, name, and affiliation. As an affiliated member, chapters pay a monthly participation fee to the NHF. There are several hemophilia societies not affiliated with the NHF.

The NHF provides financial support for particular programs and national legislative advocacy. The NHF board of directors serves as the policymaking body of the NHF, and the current board is comprised of 22 members. The board serves to elect NHF officers, grant and terminate chapter charters, determine territorial jurisdictions for chapters, and establish and enforce uniform rules. The decision-making process of the NHF involves the four vice presidents, the president, the chairman of the board, the Medical and Scientific Advisory Council (MASAC) chair, and the executive director. The board of directors also approves all MASAC recommendations before they become "official" NHF MASAC recommendations for dissemination.

Medical and Scientific Advisory Council

One important national activity of the NHF is MASAC. In 1982, the primary mission of MASAC was to advocate for continued development and expansion of an accessible comprehensive care network, to advocate for quality treatment and care for hemophilia, to support and be involved in hemophilia research, to discuss timely issues of relevance to the hemophilia community and make recommendations concerning them, and to continue to provide technical information, educational materials, and publications. The MASAC also provided advice to the NHF board of directors concerning medical and scientific issues of relevance, and reviewed research activities. The MASAC membership included representatives from six other individual committees of NHF: research and review, nursing, mental health, social work, education, and musculoskeletal.

Membership of MASAC is generally drawn from the regional treatment centers and represents both elected and appointed members (i.e., appointed members, regionally elected members, committee liaisons, and ex-officio members). The appointed members are generally elected for their expertise in a particular area (e.g., basic research in hemophilia, etc.). The chair of MASAC is appointed by the NHF president and has a three-year term, and MASAC members serve rotational twoand four-year terms.

In 1989, a committee of medical leadership was established by the NHF to facilitate more rapid communication about major issues in the hemophilia medical and scientific community. Members include the NHF vice president for medical and scientific affairs, the MASAC chair, the medical director, associate medical directors, the chair of the AIDS task force, the president of the NHF, the chairman of the NHF board and the executive director.

ROLE OF THE U.S. PUBLIC HEALTH SERVICE

National Blood Policy of 1973

The federal government regulates blood banking, monitors the safety and efficacy of blood products, and promotes research on blood diseases (OTA 1985). In late 1972, the U.S. Department of Health, Education and Welfare reported several problems within the blood supply system, including an inadequacy in the quantity of blood supplied, an unreliability in the quality of blood owing to the high rates of transfusion-related hepatitis, an inefficiency in the system itself owing to waste in some areas and shortages in others, and excessive costs of blood and blood services. On July 10, 1973, the Assistant Secretary for Health announced the National Blood Policy, which became "the focal point around which blood banking policy has evolved over the past decade" (OTA 1985). The National Blood Policy recognized that reliance on "commercial sources of blood and blood components for transfusion therapy has contributed to a significantly disproportionate incidence of hepatitis, since such blood is often collected from sectors of society in which transmissible hepatitis is more prevalent." For this reason, the National Blood Policy encouraged efforts to establish an all-volunteer blood donation system and to eliminate commercialism in the acquisition of whole blood and whole-blood components [*Federal Register* 1975] (Hutt and Merrill 1991).

The National Blood Policy listed four primary goals: to provide an adequate supply of blood; to ensure a higher quality of blood; to facilitate maximum accessibility to services; and to achieve total efficiency (U.S. Senate 1979). The first actions taken to meet these goals included the adoption of an all-volunteer blood collection system (for whole blood); coordination of all costs and charges; regionalization of blood collection and distribution; and an examination of the standards of care for hemophiliacs and other special groups. The policy did not address the commercial acquisition of plasma, the preparation and marketing of plasma derivatives, and the commercial acquisition of blood for diagnostic reagents (Hagen 1982).

In 1975, the American Blood Commission (ABC) was established and funded by the National Heart, Lung, and Blood Institute and was charged with implementing the "lion's share" of the objectives set forth in the National Blood Policy (OTA 1985). The progress of the ABC was hindered by lack of funds, disagreement between the two largest blood suppliers, resistance to regionalization of blood collection and distribution, problems in obtaining data from blood banks, and a lack of knowledge of blood banking by lay members of the commission (U.S. General Accounting Office 1978). In 1985 the ABC was formally disbanded.

Public Health Service

Public health management is the responsibility of the federal government through the Public Health Service (PHS). The Public Health Service Act of July 1, 1944 [42 U.S.C. § 201], consolidated and revised substantially all existing legislation relating to the PHS. The mission of the PHS is to promote the protection and advancement of the nation's physical and mental health. The Office of the Assistant Secretary for Health in the Department of Health and Human Services plans and directs the activities of the PHS. The federal system by which public health policy decisions are made comprises the Centers for Disease Control and Prevention, the agency that conducts surveillance and reporting of disease; the National Institutes of Health, the organization that conducts research; and the Food and Drug Administration, the regulatory arm of the PHS.

Centers for Disease Control and Prevention

The Centers for Disease Control and Prevention (CDC) was established as an agency of the PHS in 1973. The CDC is charged with protecting the public health of the nation by providing leadership and direction in the prevention and control of diseases and other preventable conditions, and responding to public health emergencies. The CDC also administers national programs for the prevention and control of communicable and vector-borne diseases which includes consulting with state and local public health departments. The CDC also collects, maintains, analyzes, and disseminates national data on health status and health services.

National Institutes of Health

The National Institutes of Health (NIH) is the federal government's principal biomedical research agency. Its mission is to pursue knowledge to improve human health. To accomplish this goal, the NIH seeks to expand fundamental knowledge about the nature and behavior of living systems, to apply that knowledge to enhance the health of human lives, and to reduce the burdens resulting from disease and disability. Two of the NIH institutes have a special role in protecting blood safety.

National Institute of Allergy and Infectious Diseases

The National Institute of Allergy and Infectious Diseases conducts and supports broad-based research and research training on the causes, characteristics, prevention, control, and treatment of a wide variety of diseases believed to be attributable to infectious agents (including bacteria, viruses, and parasites), to allergies, or to other deficiencies or disorders in the responses of the body's immune mechanisms.

National Heart, Lung, and Blood Institute

In 1948 the National Heart Institute was established, and in 1969 it was reorganized as the National Heart and Lung Institute. In the 1960s, epidemiological evidence demonstrated a correlation between high rates of post-transfusion hepatitis and blood from paid donors. This, coupled with the advances in surgical techniques (especially cardiac) that increased the need for whole blood for transfusion, created a demand to increase safety measures regarding the blood supply. In addition, an increase in the use of platelets and plasma derivatives also occurred, primarily because of advances in new technologies. As a result, the National Blood Resources Program was established in 1967. The primary objective in establishing the program was to develop safe and efficient blood collection and distribution (U.S. General Accounting Office 1978).

In 1970, Congress amended the Biologics Act, which, as discussed later in this chapter, was originally enacted in 1902 to provide the framework for federal regulation of biological products for human use, to include vaccines, blood, blood components or derivatives, and allergenic products. As a result, the Blood Resources Program became the Division of Blood Diseases and Resources at the National Heart, Lung, and Blood Institute.

Food and Drug Administration

The name "Food and Drug Administration" was established by the Agriculture Appropriation Act of 1931 [46 Stat. 392], although similar regulatory functions had been in existence under different organizational titles since January 1, 1907, when the Food and Drug Act of 1906 [21 U.S.C. §§ 1-15] became effective. The FDA's activities are directed toward protecting the health of the nation against impure and unsafe foods, drugs and cosmetics, biologics, and other potential hazards. One of the FDA's responsibilities is to administer regulation of biological products under the biological product control provision of the Public Health Service Act and applicable provisions of the federal Food, Drug, and Cosmetics Act. The FDA's legal authority is derived from the Food, Drug, and Cosmetics Act and related laws (Hutt and Merrill 1991).

Prior to 1972, regulation of the blood supply was carried out by the NIH (Hutt and Merrill 1991). Until 1947, the control of biological products had been under the supervision of the director of the Hygienic Laboratory of NIH. In 1948 it became part of the NIH National Microbiological Institute. In 1955, the NIH was reorganized and the Division of Biological Standards (DBS) for regulating biologics was created (Hutt and Merrill 1991).

In response to a 1972 General Accounting Office report that concluded that ineffective biologics were licensed under the Biologics Act because of the failure to apply the requirements for proof of effectiveness, the Secretary of Health, Education and Welfare delegated concurrently to the FDA and the DBS the authority to administer the drug provisions of the Food, Drug, and Cosmetics Act for all biological products. On July 1, 1972, the responsibility for implementing the Biologics Act was transferred from the DBS to the FDA [37 *Federal Register* 12,865, 1972]. Following its assumption of responsibility for administering the Biologics Act and the formation of the Bureau of Biologics, the FDA revoked NIH's announcement to review the effectiveness of all licensed biologics. The FDA then issued its own set of detailed procedures for the review of the safety, effectiveness, and labeling of all licensed biologics. The Bureau of Biologics was given lead responsibility for overseeing blood collection, processing, testing, and marketing. It was at this point that all blood banks became federally regulated and state licensed [37 *Federal Register* 17,419, 1972].

In 1982, through an FDA reorganization, the Center for Drugs and the Center for Biologics merged into one unit, and the Center for Drugs and Biologics (CDB) was established. The scientific director of the CDB was responsible for integrating the scientific and research activities for biologics between the NIH and FDA. The responsibilities of the Bureau of Biologics fell under this new center and the regulation for blood products and blood banking technologies was under the purview of the Office of Biologics Research and Review. The Office of Biologics in the Division of Blood and Blood Products was responsible for approval of license applications and amendments for new blood establishments and blood products, and for approval to market blood products and related technologies (OTA 1985).

In 1988, the CDB was reorganized again and the Office of Drugs and the Office of Biologics were separated into different centers. The Center for Biologics and Review assumed oversight for all activities that previously fell under the Office of Biologics and Review. In 1993, the Center for Biologics and

Review was renamed the Center for Biologics Evaluation and Research (Fratantoni 1994).

The Center for Biologics Evaluation and Research (CBER) administers regulation of biological products under the biological product control provisions of the Public Health Service Act and applicable provisions of the Food, Drug, and Cosmetics Act. CBER plans and conducts research related to the development, manufacture, testing, and use of both new and old biological products to develop a scientific base for establishing standards designed to ensure the continued safety, purity, potency, and efficacy of biological products. It also coordinates with the Center for Drug Evaluation and Research regarding activities for biological drug products, including research, compliance, and product review and approval. CBER also plans and conducts research on the preparation, preservation, and safety of blood and blood products; the methods of testing safety, purity, potency, and efficacy of such products for therapeutic use; and the immunological problems concerned with products, testing, and use of diagnostic reagents employed in grouping and typing blood.

The CBER is the dominant focus for coordination of the Acquired Immune Deficiency Syndrome (AIDS) program, works to develop an AIDS vaccine and AIDS diagnostic tests, and conducts other AIDS-related activities. It inspects manufacturers' facilities for compliance with standards, tests products submitted for release, establishes written and physical standards, and approves licensing of manufacturers to produce biological products. In carrying out these functions, the CBER cooperates with other Public Health Service organizations, governmental and international agencies, volunteer health organizations, universities, individual scientists, nongovernmental laboratories, and manufacturers of biological products.

Blood Products Advisory Committee

The FDA makes extensive use of technical advisory committees in the support if its evaluation and regulation of drugs, biologics, and medical devices for human use. Advisory committees are utilized by the FDA to obtain independent scientific and technical advice, opinions, or recommendations on a specific matter (FDA 1994). FDA advisory committees can be established in four ways: by order of the President of the United States; by congressional statute, by the Secretary of Health and Human Services, or by the FDA commissioner. The Secretary or the FDA commissioner must approve the establishment, renewal or rechartering, or amendment of all FDA public advisory committee charters (FDA 1994). Generally, the commissioner has direct authority to charter scientific and technical advisory committees, while the Secretary issues charters for committees advising on policy issues. All public advisory committees must be chartered, and their charters must be renewed biennially unless otherwise determined by law.

The CBER has four different standing advisory committees, one of which is the Blood Products Advisory Committee (BPAC), which provides evaluation of data related to safety, effectiveness, and labeling of blood and blood products and makes appropriate recommendations to the Secretary, the Assistant Secretary for Health, and the FDA commissioner (IOM 1992). Advisory committee nominations include candidates from relevant professional and scientific bodies, medical schools, academia, government agencies, industry and trade associations, and consumer and patient organizations. Committee members are appointed to terms not to exceed four years. Reappointment to a committee requires that one year elapse between appointments.

The general way in which an agenda is set for an FDA advisory committee involves two stages: (1) a meeting is formally scheduled and announced in the *Federal Register*; and (2) several days prior to the meeting, the FDA staff sends advisory committee members a detailed agenda and a list of specific questions on which their advice is sought. The FDA releases this list of questions to the public on the morning of the meeting (IOM 1992). An advisory committee meeting operates with the following separable portions: an open public hearing; an open committee discussion; a closed presentation of data; and closed committee deliberations. The BPAC's topics include investigational new drugs that meet the criteria of important diagnostic therapeutic, preventive, or other advances; novel and improved methods for product delivery; potential or apparently significant safety hazards; involvement of new biotechnology; and issues requiring additional expert review or clarification of study protocols. Product licensing agreements considered at BPAC meetings include those meeting the criteria of being a significantly new product; posing new uses for marketed products; having significant potential for risk compared to narrow therapeutic benefit; needing or being considered for postmarketing studies; presenting potential for withdrawal from market because of safety or questionable efficacy; and posing issues requiring additional expert review or clarification of study protocols.

The BPAC has 13 voting members and 2 nonvoting members. All voting members, consultants, and experts to advisory committees receive compensation for each day worked, travel, and per diem, unless waived. Industry and consumer representatives receive a salary if they have been cleared under the FDA's conflict of interest regulations as a special government employee. During the 1980s the BPAC was comprised of experts in relevant professional, scientific, and medical establishments, including academic blood banking, transfusion services, anesthesia and pharmacology, state public health departments, general medicine, biochemistry, pediatrics, laboratory medicine, infectious diseases, virology, hematology, and oncology.

BLOOD AND BLOOD PRODUCT REGULATION

Statutory Background

The history of blood and blood product regulation in the United States includes both congressional enactments (public laws) and rulemaking procedures of the FDA. The FDA regulates blood, blood components, and derivatives under two separate but overlapping statutes, one governing "biologics" and one governing "drugs." The biologics law requires that any "virus, therapeutic serum, toxin, anti-toxin, or analogous product" be prepared in a facility holding a federal license. A separate law, for food and drugs, includes drugs intended for the "cure, mitigation, or prevention of disease" and, thus, includes biologics such as blood and blood components or derivatives. Thus, blood banks and plasma product manufacturers are also subject to this drug regulatory process.

Biologics Act

In 1902, following several outbreaks of disease from contaminated vaccines, Congress enacted the Biologics Act [32 Stat. 728] which provided the framework for federal regulation of biological products for human use. The law required that biological drugs sold in interstate commerce must be licensed and produced in licensed establishments. The term *biologics* includes vaccines made from or with the aid of living organisms that are produced in animals or humans. Biologics also include antitoxins used to protect against diphtheria, tetanus, and whooping cough; serums for the treatment of disease; products for the treatment of allergies; and blood for transfusion and other medical purposes (Hutt and Merrill 1991).

In 1944, the Biologics Act was reenacted as part of the recodification of the Public Health Service Act [58 Stat. 682, 702, 1944], and is now codified at 42 U.S.C. § 262 (Hutt and Merrill 1991). The recodification hearings focused on the issue of possible duplicative regulatory authority of biological products under the Federal Drug and Cosmetics Act. Under the original act, the Public Health Service (PHS) licensed and controlled the manufacturing of virus serums, toxins, and other biologics. At the hearings, while PHS control of biologics was viewed as effective, the wording of the new act was seen to be suggestive of duplicative administrative control of the PHS and the FDA. In the event that some product dangerous to human life inadvertently entered the market, the FDA would have power of seizure [Section 351 of the PHS Act, referred to as the Biologics Act] (Hutt and Merrill 1991). Prior to 1970, the Biologics Act did not specifically include blood products. In 1970, Congress amended the Biologics Act "specifically to include vaccines, blood, blood components or derivatives, and allergenic products [84 Stat. 1297, 1308]" (Hutt and Merrill 1991).

Public Health Service Act

In 1974, the FDA promulgated regulations governing good manufacturing practices in the collection, processing, and storage of human blood components [39 *Federal Register* 18,614, 1974; 40 *Federal Register* 53,532, 1975]. By combining the jurisdictional and regulatory provisions of the Biologics Act and the Food, Drug, and Cosmetic Act, the FDA brought all blood and blood products produced and used in the United States under uniform federal requirements (Hutt and Merrill 1991).

Blood Shield Laws

During the 1950s and 1960s, blood shield laws were adopted by 47 different jurisdictions. The blood shield laws were developed to exempt blood and blood products from strict liability or implied warranty claims on the basis that blood and blood products provide a service, not a sale. Accordingly (as stated in the California Health and Safety Code 1606),

> the procurement, processing, distribution, or use of whole blood, plasma, blood products, and any blood derivatives for the purpose of infusing the same, or any of them, into the human body shall be construed to be, and is declared to be, for all purposes whatsoever, the rendition of a service by each and every person, firm, or corporation participating therein, and shall not be construed to be, and is declared not to be, a sale of such whole blood, plasma, blood products, or blood derivatives, for any purpose or purposes whatsoever (Westfall 1986).

Only four jurisdictions (New Jersey, District of Columbia, Rhode Island, and Vermont) did not adopt statutes protecting hospitals or blood donor services from strict liability or breach of implied warranty (Lipton 1986). Even in these jurisdictions, however, the likelihood that a court would hold a hospital or blood donor service liable under either breach or implied warranty or strict liability theories was considered remote (Lipton 1986).

In 1976 blood banks received exemption from liability under protection of blood shield law as providing a service and not a product. The court ruled that there was a rational basis for blood bank's exemption from liability, based on weighing the need for an available blood supply for surgery and other medical procedures against the "relatively minor risk of hepatitis which the blood recipient must take" (Westfall 1986). In addition, the court found that exemption of the blood bank from liability was constitutional because protection of blood banks was related to the state's purpose of encouraging the general blood supply.

In 1977, the courts extended this protection to blood product manufacturers on the same grounds: the distribution of blood products was a service and not a sale. In a wrongful death suit concerning a hemophiliac who had died from hepatitis after using a blood product [*Cutter v. Fogo* 1977], the court reasoned that because the blood product was unavoidably unsafe, and because the risk of hepatitis could not be eliminated despite every attempt to screen donors (i.e., through both biological tests and avoidance of high-risk donors), the blood product manufacturers were protected from strict product liability since the blood product had been instrumental in helping many hemophiliacs (Westfall 1986).

Federal Licensure of Blood Collection Organizations

Federal licensure is thought to ensure that the facility in which the biologic is produced will ensure its purity and quality. In addition to licensing the facility or establishment, this law requires that each biologic product itself be licensed by the government. Thus, to produce a licensed biologic, an organization must have an establishment license describing the facility in which the product is produced and a product license describing the specific product being produced. Over the years, this law has been specifically amended to include the terms *blood* and *blood component* or *derivative* to make it clear that blood and blood products are subject to the biologics regulation.

Establishment Licensure and Registration

Presently, there are 188 FDA-licensed organizations at 790 locations for collection and interstate shipment of blood and blood components. In addition, a total of 2,900 locations are registered to collect blood but not for interstate shipment. If an organization wishes to ship the components across state lines or engage in commerce by selling the products to other organizations, the organization must obtain an FDA license for this purpose. Even if an organization does not wish to produce blood components for interstate shipment, the FDA law requires that all organizations involved in "collection, preparation, processing, or compatibility testing ... of any blood product" register with the FDA (McCullough 1995). This registration allows the organization to collect blood and prepare blood components for its own use. Thus, for practical purposes, most hospitals that collect blood or prepare blood components for their own use are registered but not licensed since they do not ship blood in interstate commerce. Most blood centers are licensed since they supply multiple hospitals, some of which may be in other states. In addition, blood centers may wish to participate in blood resource sharing with blood centers in other states and thus need to be licensed for interstate shipment of blood.

Product Licensure

Along with the establishment license, the organization must file a product license application for each product it plans to produce in the facility.

For whole blood and components, the product application involves basic information about the manufacturer (organization), establishment, product, standard operating procedures, blood donor screening tests, frequency of donation, donor medical history, presence of a physician, phlebotomy supplies, venipuncture technique, collection technique, allowable storage period, storage conditions, disposal of contaminated units, supplies and reagents, label control processes, procedures for reissue of blood, and a brief summary of experience testing 500 samples.

For the manufacture of plasma derivatives, the product license application involves the manufacturer's (organization's) name; the establishment name; procedures for determining donor suitability including medical history, examination by physician, laboratory testing, methods of preparing the venipuncture site, and collecting the plasma; methods to prevent circulatory embolism and to assure return of red cells to the proper donor; minimum intervals between donation and maximum frequency of donation; techniques for immunizing donors; laboratory tests of collected plasma; techniques of preparing source plasma and storing it; methods to ensure proper storage conditions and identification of units; label control systems; and shipping conditions and procedures.

Blood banks and plasma derivative manufacturers must submit a report annually to the FDA indicating which products are collected, tested, prepared, and distributed.

Other Required Licensure

Blood banks are subject to several other requirements or licensure systems in addition to those of the FDA. Because blood banks carry out testing on human material that is in interstate commerce, and because they provide services to Medicare and Medicaid patients, they must comply with the Clinical Laboratories Improvement Act of 1988. Several states also require that blood banks have a license to operate or provide blood in that state. These licenses usually involve a specific application and inspection.

REGULATORY AUTHORITY OF THE FDA

Since 1972, the FDA has been the principal regulatory agency with respect to blood and blood products. Its statutory regulatory authority is extensive under the federal Food, Drug, and Cosmetics Act and the Public Health Service Act [codified as 42 U.S.C. § 262].

Compliance with Regulations

The FDA depends on the regulated industry for some amount of self-regulation. However, the FDA's enforcement cannot be by self-regulation, and the FDA's General Counsel determines if a violation of legislative mandates constitutes grounds for legal action (Hutt and Merrill 1991) (See Chapter 6, which focuses on FDA's regulation of blood and blood products during the period 1982–1986 when HIV contaminated the blood supply and before the development of a test to detect antibody to HIV, for more information).

A formal compliance program for the plasma fractionation industry was established in 1977. The responsibility for annual inspections was transferred from the Bureau of Biologics to the FDA field investigation office (OTA 1985). In addition, there was no ban on commercial collection of plasma at this time because the voluntary donor system could not meet the demand for plasma. To reduce the risks of transmission of hepatitis, source identification (as to whether the donor was paid or volunteer) was required as a federal regulation imposed by the FDA in 1978 for both whole blood and its components. This requirement, however, did not apply to source plasma or derivatives (OTA 1985).

In March 1980 a memorandum of understanding was established between FDA and the Health Care Financing Agency (HCFA) for coordination of the inspection of blood banks and transfusion services. The FDA exempted all transfusion services and clinical laboratories that are regulated by HCFA under Medicare [45 *Federal Register* 64,601; September 30, 1980]. HCFA adopted the FDA's blood regulation to assure uniform and efficient regulation of these facilities.

Recall Policy

The FDA's recall authority lies within the Public Health Service Act under the Biologics section [21 C.F.R. Part 7]. The FDA can issue a mandatory injunction to place the blood bank back into compliance with the regulations (Dubinsky, Falter, Foegel interviews). The FDA's *Regulatory Procedures Manual* requires CBER's technical staff to prepare a health hazard evaluation of a product before a recall action is initiated (FDA 1988). (A less formal discussion of recall appears in Chapter 6 and focuses on FDA's regulation of blood and blood products during the period 1982-1985 when HIV contaminated the blood supply and before the antiviral HIV test was developed.)

A recall is a method for removing or correcting marketed products that violate the laws administered by the FDA. The recall methods provide efficient and timely protection to the consumer, especially when a product has been widely marketed. Voluntary recalls may be undertaken at any time on the initiative of manufacturers to carry out their responsibility to protect the public health. The recall process is usually a voluntary action taken by a firm to remove a product from the market and may be taken as a result of FDA findings during inspections, reports from consumers, or scientific data indicating a risk (OTA 1985). If the firm decides against market withdrawal, the FDA can seize the product.

A market withdrawal is when a firm voluntarily removes a distributed product which involves a minor violation for which the FDA would not initiate legal action or which involves no violation. Requested recalls are initiated in response to a formal request from the FDA (FDA 1988). It is FDA policy that a recalling firm has the responsibility to determine whether the recall is progressing satisfactorily through the use of effectiveness checks. Because each recall is unique and requires its own strategy, the FDA reviews and/or recommends the firm's recall strategy and will develop its own strategy based on the agency's hazard evaluation and other factors, such as type or use of the product. The recall strategy is separate from, and not tied to, the class of recall selected (FDA 1988). Recall classification is a numerical designation assigned by the FDA to a product recall to indicate the relative degree of health hazard presented by the product being recalled. There are three classes of recall:

- Class I is defined as situations in which there is a strong likelihood that the use of, or exposure to, a violative product will cause serious, adverse health consequences, or death.
- Class II is defined as situations in which the use of, or exposure to, a violative product may cause temporary or medically reversible adverse health consequences or where the probability of serious adverse health consequences is remote.

- Class III is defined as situations in which the use of, or exposure to, a violative product is not likely to cause adverse health consequences.

Once the recall has been classified, FDA determines the depth of the recall, which depends upon the product's degree of hazard and the extent of distribution. The recall strategy will specify the level to which the recall should extend as follows [see 21 C.F.R. § 7.45]:

- consumer or user level, which may vary with the product, including any intermediate wholesale or retail level;
- retail level, including any intermediate wholesale level; or
- wholesale level.

The FDA issues a warning to alert the public that a product is being recalled and presents a serious hazard to health. This is usually reserved for urgent situations where other means for preventing the use of the recalled product may appear inadequate [21 C.F.R. § 7.45]. The FDA also surveys and monitors recall actions for all biologics by following up to make sure that the recall message (i.e., a letter to the manufacturer) was received and acted upon.

The FDA can implement stronger enforcement actions if the manufacturer is not acting in accordance with the recall. However, there must be scientific and medical evidence to justify stronger enforcement actions such as a court injunction or product seizure. FDA staff must present evidence to the FDA General Counsel and the Department of Justice on the necessity of such an action (Dubinsky, Falter, Foegel interviews).

SUMMARY

The nation's blood and plasma are collected by two distinct systems that are based on different donor sources and produce different products. The blood segment of the collection system is primarily not for profit, the plasma segment is primarily for profit. The federal government regulates blood banking, monitors the safety and efficacy of blood products, and promotes research on blood diseases. Both systems are regulated by the FDA in a similar manner, although the specific requirements differ because of differences between blood and plasma products.

Since the period 1982–1986, it appears that the number of units of whole blood collected in the United States has stabilized or slightly decreased. It also appears that the substantial increase in the collection of autologous blood that occurred during recent years is slowing. There is a slight decrease in the number of community blood centers and an increase in the average number of units collected, implying that the decrease in the number of centers may be due to mergers. Presently, members of the American Association of Blood Banks account for almost all blood collected in the United States. The number of AABB institutional members who collect blood has increased and those that transfuse blood has decreased. Because this could reflect the changing membership of the AABB, it is not proper to extrapolate these observations to changes in the blood collection or transfusion community. Membership in the Council of Community Blood Centers has increased substantially during the past decade.

It is not possible to provide accurate estimates of the amount of plasma or derivatives produced because this is proprietary information. There has been an increase in the kinds of plasma derivative products during the past decade. There has also been an increase in the number of plasma derivative manufacturers during the past decade. Although several companies that produced plasma derivatives in the early 1980s no longer do so, other companies have begun the production of plasma derivatives.

REFERENCES

American Blood Resources Association. Materials submitted to the Institute of Medicine; 1994.

Anderson, K. The Economics of Importing vs Collecting. In *Adequacy of the Blood Supply*, Council of Community Blood Centers conference proceedings; Clearwater, Florida. February 18, 1990.

Blakestone, M.S. Fractionation. *Plasmapheresis*, vol. 5, 1994.

Centers for Disease Control. *Morbidity and Mortality Weekly Report* , July 3, 1981.

Centers for Disease Control. *Morbidity and Mortality Weekly Report* , July 16, 1982.

Centers for Disease Control. *Morbidity and Mortality Weekly Report* , March 20, 1987.

Centers for Disease Control. *Morbidity and Mortality Weekly Report* , December 18, 1987.

Centers for Disease Control. HIV/AIDS Knowledge and Awareness of Testing and Treatment— Behavioral Risk Factor Surveillance . *Morbidity and Mortality Weekly Report*, vol. 40:704, 1991.

CDC, HRSA, and MCHB. *Minimal Data Set for Risk Reduction*; 1991, 1992, 1993.

Chorba, et al. Changes in Longevity and Causes of Death among Persons with Hemophilia A. *American Journal of Hematology*, vol. 45, 1994.

Food and Drug Administration. *Policy and Guidance Handbook for Advisory Committees*, 1994.

Food and Drug Administration. *Regulatory Procedures Manual*, May 16, 1988.

Fratantoni, J., Food and Drug Administration, Division of Hematology. Presentation to Committee, May 16, 1994.

Gallup Organization. *Attitudes of U.S. Adults Towards AIDS and the Safety of America's Blood Supply*. Princeton, New Jersey, 1991.

Hagen, Piet J. *Blood: Gift or Merchandise? New York:* Alan R. Liss, Inc., 1982.

Hoffman, et al. (editors). *Hematology: Basic Principles and Practice* (second edition). New York: Churchill Livingsone, 1994.

Hutt, Peter, and Merrill, Richard. *Food and Drug Law: Cases and Materials* . Westbury, New York: The Foundation Press, Inc., 1991.

Institute of Medicine, Committee to Study HIV Transmission Through Blood Products. Transcript of Public Meeting, September 12, 1994.

Institute of Medicine. *Food and Drug Administration Advisory Committees* . Washington, D.C.: National Academy Press, 1992.

Lipton, K. Blood Donor Services and Liability Issues Relating to Acquired Immune Deficiency Syndrome. *Journal of Legal Medicine*, vol. 7(2), 1986.

McCullough, Jeffrey. *The United States Blood Collection System*, 1995.

Office of Technology Assessment. *Blood Policy and Technology* Washington, D.C: U.S. GPO, OTA-H-260; January 1985.

Scott, E.P. Why My Blood Center Imports. In *Adequacy of the Blood Supply*, Council of Community Blood Centers conference proceedings, Clearwater, Florida, February 18, 1990.

Smith, Peter, and Levine, Peter. The Benefits of Comprehensive Care of Hemophilia: A Five-Year Study of Outcomes. *American Journal of Public Health*, vol. 74(June), 1984.

U.S. General Accounting Office [report to Congress]. Problems in Carrying Out the National Blood Policy. Washington D.C.: General Accounting Office, March 7, 1978.

U.S. Senate, Committee on Labor and Human Resources, Subcommittee on Health and Scientific Research . Hearing: Oversight on Implementation of National Blood Policy, June 7, 1979.

Wallace, E.L., et al. Collection and Transfusion of Blood and Blood Components in the United States. *Transfusion*, vol. 33, 1993.

Westfall, Pamela. Hepatitis, AIDS and the Blood Products Exemption from Strict Products Liability in California: A Reassessment. *Hastings Law Journal*, vol. 37(6), (1986).

3

History of the Controversy

INTRODUCTION

The events marking the emergence of HIV in the United States and its transmission through blood and blood products are best understood in four periods. (1) Through the end of 1982, people were struggling to understand an emerging disease and characterize the risk of infection. (2) In early 1983 official meetings took place and public and private decisions established the blood industry's early response to AIDS. (3) Meetings and other occasions for decisionmaking from mid-1983 through the end of 1983 provided many opportunities for blood banks, blood product manufacturers, regulatory organizations, and other agencies to reconsider the decisions of early 1983. (4) During 1982-1985, research on AIDS led to isolation of the virus and the development of a screening test. Concurrently, research efforts related to viral inactivation of the antihemophilic factor (AHF) concentrate, underway since the 1970s, were accelerated and completed. Table 3.1 provides a summary chronology of critical events.

The early 1980s were an unsettled time for the individuals and organizations responsible for blood safety in the United States. The public's confidence in government and public institutions generally was quickly eroding, and its hostility towards the involvement of government agencies in social matters was growing. The new Republican presidential administration had strong sentiments against government regulations, even those that addressed public health and safety.

In addition, the emergence of AIDS challenged every aspect of the country's public health infrastructure. It brought new focus to the importance of infectious diseases at a time when the attention and resources of both physicians and

Table 3.1 Chronology of Critical Events

Date	Event
July 16, 1982	CDC MMWR reports immune-suppressive disorder identified in three hemophiliac patients.
July 16, 1982	FDA's Bureau of Biologic meeting to discuss opportunistic infections in hemophiliacs.
July 16, 1982	Public Health Service Working Group on Opportunistic Infections in Hemophiliacs meeting to exchange information about the three cases of AIDS in hemophilia patients.
July 27, 1982	Working Group on Opportunistic Infections in Hemophiliacs second meeting to determine if other groups with acquired immunodeficiency showed similar etiology and if blood products were risk factors for AIDS.
December 10, 1982	CDC MMWR reports four additional cases in hemophiliacs, one suspect case in an infant who had received a blood transfusion.
January 4, 1983	CDC public meeting to identify opportunities to prevent AIDS.
March 4, 1983	Assistant Secretary for Health promulgates the first official PHS recommendations on the prevention of AIDS, including recommendations to avoid sexual contact with persons known or suspected of having AIDS and the increased probability of developing AIDS by having multiple sex partners.
March 24, 1983	FDA notification of all establishments collecting source plasma and human blood for transfusion and manufacturers of plasma derivatives of steps to be taken to decrease the risk of blood or plasma donation by persons who might be at increased risk of transmitting AIDS.
May 11, 1983	Baxter Healthcare recall of a lot of AHF concentrate when it discovers that the product was manufactured from pools containing plasma from an individual subsequently diagnosed as having AIDS.
July 19, 1983	FDA Blood Products Advisory Committee (BPAC) meeting to discuss the criteria for deciding to withdraw lots of AHF concentrate.

Date	Event
December 15, 1983	FDA's BPAC meeting to consider implementation of the hepatitis B core antibody test as a possible surrogate screening test for HIV.
April 1984	National Cancer Institute scientists report they have isolated a virus that causes AIDS.
October 26, 1984	CDC MMWR reports information on the viral inactivation of HIV through the use of heat treatment.
December 1984	First tests for detecting HIV developed and license application submitted to FDA.
March 1985	FDA grants two licenses for commercial use of the HIV tests, and notifies all blood facilities of the test's availability and schedules a workshop on its use.

public health officials was turning elsewhere. The AIDS epidemic called for emergency, focused, biomedical and behavioral research in a system based on investigator-initiated basic research. The exploding number of cases called for additional resources and new models of health care in a system increasingly concerned about costs. AIDS caused the nation to take note of homosexuality and drug use, which were easily avoided before these issues became such obvious matters of public health, and AIDS required clinicians and public health officials to address matters of personal behavior that had been heretofore taboo.

Personnel changes at the highest levels of the Public Health Service may have influenced the federal government's response to AIDS, and to concerns about the safety of the blood supply. Between 1982 and 1986, the position of director of the Centers for Disease Control (CDC) and NIH, administrator of the FDA, and Assistant Secretary for Health all changed hands, and there were substantial intervals during which these positions were filled on an acting basis.

Finally, the Committee was also struck by the way in which one historical event seems to have influenced individuals and organizational conduct and interpretations of the evidence about the HIV epidemic. This episode was the federal government's experience with the swine flu epidemic. In early 1976, at the urging of officials of the CDC, the federal government (with the visible participation of President Ford) engaged in a crash program to immunize every American against a disease that never materialized. Millions were vaccinated, however, and some died of complications that were attributed to the vaccine (Neustadt and Fineberg 1978). This episode seems simultaneously to have reduced the self-confidence of the CDC and increased the skepticism with which other public health service organizations regarded its warnings.

THE RISK OF AIDS

From the introduction of HIV into the United States through the end of 1982, most efforts were oriented to understanding an emerging disease and characterizing the risk of infection in a variety of settings. Following standard epidemiologic procedures, CDC epidemiologists and scientists, in collaboration with others, analyzed the characteristic manifestations of the new disease— opportunistic infections such as *Pneumocystis carinii* pneumonia (PCP) and Kaposi's sarcoma—and identified groups at high risk for the disease. Starting with the identification of 26 homosexual men with the opportunistic infections in June 1981 (see below), the CDC's MMWR became the source for reports of the epidemic. (Table 3.2 summarizes the information on the number of AIDS cases and the evolving knowledge base as reported in the CDC's *Morbidity and Mortality Weekly Report* [MMWR]).

Kaposi's Sarcoma and PCP in Homosexual Men

The first cases of the disease that would come to be known as AIDS came to light as early as October 1980, when Kaposi's sarcoma (KS) was diagnosed in several young homosexual men in Los Angeles. These and similar cases (21 in all) were reported in the following year (CDC, MMWR, June 5, 1981). Shortly thereafter, on July 3, 1981, the CDC reported five new cases of PCP in homosexual men in New York City, Los Angeles, and San Francisco (CDC, MMWR, July 3, 1981). Both KS and PCP are opportunistic infections that occur in individuals with severely weakened immune systems. In addition to reported cases of these diseases, there was an unusual increase in requests made to the CDC for a drug called pentamidine that is used for the treatment of PCP. At the time, this drug could only be dispensed through a physician's request to the CDC (Curran, Evatt interviews). With the possible outbreak of a new infectious disease in the United States coming to the attention of public health officials, the CDC established a task force in July 1981 to monitor the cases of opportunistic infections, to investigate additional cases, to formalize a definition of the disease, and to design a case/control study to examine the prevalence and epidemiology of the disease. The task force was headed by James Curran, chief of CDC's Venereal Disease Control Division (Curran, Foege interviews).

Table 3.2 Reported Cases of Opportunistic Infections and AIDS, Risk Groups Identified, and Evolving Knowledge Base: June 1981 Through May 1985

Date	No. of Cases (cumulative)	Risk Groups	Fatality Rate (%)	Knowledge of Disease and Modes of Transmission
June 5, 1981	5	5 Homosexual men	40	"The occurrence of pneumocystis in these 5 previously healthy individuals without a clinically apparent underlying immunodeficiency is unusual." (p. 1)
July 3, 1981	26	26 Homosexual men	31	"The occurrence of this number of KS cases during a 30-month period among young, homosexual men is considered highly unusual. No previous association between KS and sexual preference has been reported." (p. 3)
August 28, 1981	108	108 Homosexual men	40	"The apparent clustering of both *Pneuomocystis carinii* pneumonia and KS among homosexual men suggests a common underlying factor. Both diseases have been associated with host immunosuppression, and studies in progress are showing immunosuppression in some of these cases." (p. 5)
June 11, 1982	355	281 Homosexual and bisexual men 15 Heterosexual men 6 Heterosexual women 20 Men, unknown risk 33 IVDUs	43	"A laboratory and interview study of heterosexual patients with diagnosed KS, PCP or other OI is in progress to determine whether their cellular immune function, results of virologic studies, medical history, sexual practices, drug use, and life-style are similar to those of homosexual patients." (p. 9)
July 9, 1982		(34 Haitians)*	50	"The in vitro immunologic findings and the high mortality rate (nearly 50%) for these patients are similar to the pattern recently described among homosexual males and IV drug abusers." (p. 13)

Date	No. of Cases (cumulative)	Risk Groups	Fatality Rate (%)	Knowledge of Disease and Modes of Transmission
July 16, 1982		(3 Hemophiliacs)	67	"Although the cause of the severe immune dysfunction is unknown, the occurrence among the three hemophiliac cases suggests the possible transmission of an agent through blood products." (p. 15)
September 24, 1982	593	445 Homosexual men 77 IVDUs 36 Haitians 3 Hemophiliacs 32 Unknown risk	41	"CDC defines a case of AIDS as a disease, at least moderately predictive of a defect in cell-mediated immunity, occurring in a person with no known cause for diminished resistance to that disease….; The eventual case-mortality rate of AIDS, a few years after diagnosis, may be far greater than the 41% overall case-mortality rate noted…." (p. 18); "… The [case-mortality] rate exceeds 60% for cases diagnosed over a year ago." (p. 17)
December 10, 1982		(1 Infant)		"If the platelet transfusion contained an etiologic agent for AIDS, one must assume that the agent can be present in the blood of a donor before onset of a symptomatic illness and that the incubation period for such illness can be relatively long." (p. 27)
December 17, 1982		(4 Infants)		"Transmission of an 'AIDS agent' from mother to child, either in utero or shortly after birth, could account for the early onset of immunodeficiency in these infants." (p. 29)
January 7, 1983		(16 Prison inmates)		"Since male homosexuals and IV drug abusers are known to be at increased risk for AIDS, the occurrence of AID among imprisoned members of these groups might have been anticipated." (p. 32)

Date	Cumulative cases	Breakdown	Page	Quote
March 4, 1983	1,200	No breakdown given	Not stated	"Over 450 persons have died from AIDS, and the case-fatality rate exceeds 60% for cases first diagnosed over 1 year previously. …" (p. 32) "… The California cluster investigation and other epidemiologic findings suggest a 'latent period' of several months to 2 years between exposure and recognizable clinical illness and imply that transmissibility may precede recognizable illness." (p. 33)
June 24, 1983	1,641	1,165 Homosexual men 279 IVDUs 16 Hemophiliacs 82 Haitians 98 Unknown risk	39	"The cause of AIDS is unknown, but it seems most likely to be caused by an agent transmitted by intimate sexual contact, through contaminated needles, or, less commonly, by percutaneous inoculation of infectious blood or blood products. No evidence suggests transmission of AIDS by airborne spread." (p. 38)
August 5, 1983	1,972	No breakdown given	38	"… The ratio of male to female patients (14:1) has been almost constant over the last year." (p. 41)
September 9, 1983	2,259	1,604 Homosexual men 384 IVDUs 113 Haitians 26 Hemophiliacs 26 Heterosexual women 26 Transfusion 80 Unknown risk	41	"The occurrence of AIDS cases among homosexual men, IV drug abusers, persons with hemophilia, sexual partners of members of these groups, and recipients of blood transfusions is consistent with the hypothesis that AIDS is caused by an agent that is transmitted sexually, or, less commonly, through contaminated needles or blood." (p. 45)
January 6, 1984	3,000	2,130 Homosexual men 510 IVDUs 31 Transfusion 42 Pediatric 287 Unknown risk	43	"The 31 patients with 'transfusion-associated' AIDS include 18 men and 13 women who have no other known risk factor for AIDS and were transfused with blood or blood components within 5 years of their onsets of illness. These patients received transfusions between April 1978 and May 1983." (p. 50)

Date	No. of Cases (cumulative)	Risk Groups	Fatality Rate (%)	Knowledge of Disease and Modes of Transmission
June 22, 1984	4,918	3,541 Homosexual men 836 IVDUs 197 Haitians 49 Hemophiliacs 49 Heterosexual women 49 Transfusion 197 Unknown risk	45%	"… More than 76% of patients diagnosed before July 1982 are dead." (p. 60)
October 26, 1984		52 Hemophiliacs	58	"The possibility of blood or blood products being vehicles for AIDS transmission to hemophilia patients has been supported by the finding of risk of acquisition of AIDS for intravenous drug abusers and, subsequently, by reports of transfusion-associated AIDS cases. …" (p. 66) "Although the total number of hemophilia patients who have thus far developed clinical manifestations of AIDS is small relative to other AIDS risk groups, incidence rates for this group are high (3.6 cases/1,000 hemophilia A patients and 0.6 cases/1,000 hemophilia B patients)." (p. 67)
November 30, 1984	6,993	5,038 Homosexual men 1,190 IVDUs 249 Haitians 52 Hemophiliacs 54 Heterosexual women 93 Transfusion 263 Unknown/adult 54 Unknown/children	48	"Eighty-one adults and 12 children with transfusion-associated AIDS (TA-AIDS) have no other risk factors and were transfused with blood or blood components within 5 years of illness onset. TA-AIDS patients received blood from one to 75 donors (median 16 donors); interval from transfusion to diagnosis was 4 months to 62 months. …" (p. 72)

May 10, 1985	10,000	7,261 Homosexual men	49	"Since 1981, the proportion of AIDS cases in transfusion recipients has increased significantly. ..." (p. 91)
		1,685 IVDUs		
		71 Hemophiliacs		"Because the time from infection with HTLV-III/LAV to onset of AIDS may be several years, persons exposed to the virus through transfusion before institution of the self-deferral guidelines for blood donors in 1983 and screening of blood for HTLV-III/LAV antibody in 1985 may remain at risk of AIDS." (p. 93)
		81 Heterosexual women		
		149 Transfusion		
		672 Unknown risk		
		81 Unknown/children		

NOTE: CDC = Centers for Disease Control; HTLV-III = human T-cell lymphotropic virus, type III; IV = intravenous; IVDUs = intravenous drug users; KS = Kaposi's sarcoma; LAV = lymphadenopathy-associated virus; OI = opportunistic infection; and PCP = *Pneumocystis carinii* pneumonia.

* Cases in parentheses indicate the occurrence of the disease in a new risk group.

SOURCE: Centers for Disease Control. *Reports on AIDS Published in the* Morbidity and Mortality Weekly Report, *June 1981 Through May 1986*. Washington, D.C.: U.S. Government Printing Office, 1987.

Because the early cases appeared in the gay community, the new disease was first called "gay-related immunodeficiency disease" (GRID). Many scientists and public health officials initially hypothesized that behavioral elements of the homosexual lifestyle (multiple sex partners, for example) were the cause. Another early theory was that "poppers" (amyl nitrates), drugs frequently used by some gay men to enhance sexual pleasure, were the cause (CDC, MMWR, June 18, 1982).

Opportunistic Infections Among Heterosexual Intravenous (IV) Drug Users and Haitian Immigrants

In June 1982, the CDC reported 355 cases of opportunistic infections, with an increase in the number of heterosexual patients, particularly among IV drug users. According to the report, "a laboratory and interview study of the heterosexual patients [was] in progress to determine whether their cellular immune function, results of virologic studies, medical history, sexual practices, drug use, and lifestyle [were] similar to those of homosexual patients" (CDC, MMWR, June 11, 1982). One month later, the CDC reported 34 cases of opportunistic infections in Haitian patients. The pattern of infections was "similar to the pattern recently described among homosexual males and IV drug users" (CDC, MMWR, July 9, 1982).

On July 16, 1982, the CDC reported the first three cases of PCP among individuals with hemophilia. All three were reported to be heterosexual males. At this time, the CDC postulated that the immune dysfunction symptoms were transmitted through blood and blood products:

> The clinical and immunologic features these three patients share are strikingly similar to those recently observed among certain individuals from the following groups: homosexual males, heterosexual IV drug users, and Haitians. Although the cause of the severe immune dysfunction is unknown, the occurrence among the three hemophiliac cases suggests the possible transmission of an agent through blood products [CDC, MMWR, July 16, 1982].

On the same date, the FDA's Bureau of Biologics convened a meeting to discuss opportunistic infections in hemophiliacs. The meeting included representatives from the CDC, the National Hemophilia Foundation (NHF), the American Red Cross, the American Blood Resources Association (ABRA) (who represented the plasma fractionators), and the National Institutes of Health (NIH). The CDC presented an update of the epidemic of opportunistic infections, noting that the one common thread among all groups affected (i.e., homosexual men, IV drug users, Haitians, and individuals with hemophilia) was the presence of markers for hepatitis in more than 90 percent of each group (Hansen 1982).

In conjunction with the first cases among hemophiliacs, CDC Director William Foege asked public health officials to inform physicians caring for patients with hemophilia about the three cases of PCP among patients with hemophilia. He wrote to inform state and territorial health officers, industry representatives, the Assistant Secretary for Health, the FDA Commissioner, the Director of NIH, and all CDC regional offices that the CDC was conducting surveillance of the new disease and gathering additional information to determine the significance of the incidence reports. In addition, he asked physicians to immediately report cases of opportunistic infections or suspected acquired immune deficiency through state health departments to the CDC (Foege 1982a).

At the July 16, 1982, PHS meeting, a Committee on Opportunistic Infections in Patients with Hemophilia was established to exchange information about the cases, to characterize their similarity to other risk groups, and to conduct surveillance of both hemophilia cases and antihemophilic factor (AHF) concentrate (Public Health Service July 1982). The committee held its second meeting on July 27, 1982; representatives from the PHS, CDC, FDA, NHF, ABRA and NIH attended. The committee, chaired by Dr. Foege, adopted the term "acquired immunodeficiency syndrome" (AIDS), and decided to focus on two goals: to determine if the underlying immunodeficiency seen in hemophiliacs had the same etiology as in other groups with acquired immunodeficiency, and to determine if certain blood products were risk factors for AIDS (Foege 1982b) (see further discussion below).

By September 1982, 593 cases of AIDS had been reported to the CDC. Of these cases, 445 of the patients were homosexual men, 77 were IV drug users, 36 were Haitians, 3 were hemophiliacs, and 32 had no defined risk; 41 percent had died (CDC, MMWR, September, 24, 1982). In an editorial note, the CDC defined AIDS as:

> ... a disease, at least moderately predictive of a defect in cell-mediated immunity, occurring in persons with no known cause for diminished resistance to that disease. Such diseases include Kaposi's Sarcoma (KS), Pneumocystis Carinii Pneumonia (PCP), and other serious opportunistic infections. ... This case definition does not include the full spectrum of AIDS manifestations, which range[s] from absence of symptoms, to specific diseases that are insufficiently predictive of cellular immune deficiency to be included in incidence monitoring [CDC, MMWR, September 24, 1982].

The reference to an "absence of symptoms" suggests that as early as the autumn of 1982 researchers were beginning to establish that the new disease might have had an asymptomatic incubation period.

Increased Risk Among Individuals with Hemophilia and a
Similarity to Hepatitis B

In a December 10, 1982, update on AIDS among patients with severe hemophilia A, the CDC reported that all three of the cases reported in the July 16, 1982, MMWR had died and that, in the intervening four months, four additional confirmed cases and one suspected case of AIDS in heterosexual patients had been reported. Two of the patients were children under 10 years of age. In an accompanying editorial note, the CDC stated that the hemophilia patients had all received large amounts of a commercially manufactured anticoagulant known as AHF (antihemophilic factor). None of the patients had any prior opportunistic infections, all had been profoundly lymphopenic, and all had exhibited reversed ratios of CD4:CD8 lymphocytes. According to the CDC, these cases provided a new perspective on AIDS by showing that children with hemophilia were at risk for the disease. The report also stated that the number of cases was continuing to increase and that patients with hemophilia might be at significant risk for AIDS. The CDC also reported that a national survey of hemophilia treatment centers had determined that 30 percent or more of all hemophiliacs had abnormal immunological tests. The coincidence of symptoms of AIDS and serologic evidence of hepatitis in the individuals with hemophilia added weight to the theory that AIDS was a disease with a pattern of transmission that mimicked that of hepatitis B (CDC, MMWR, December 10, 1982).

By December 1982, a total of 788 AIDS cases had been reported. Of the 788 reported cases, 42 (5.3 percent) belonged to no known risk group (e.g., homosexuals, IV drug users, hemophiliacs, and Haitians). Two of the 42 cases with no known risk factors were patients who had received blood products (not related to the treatment of hemophilia) within two years of the onset of AIDS (CDC, MMWR, December 10, 1982).

Further Evidence of Sexual and Blood-Borne Transmission
of AIDS

The December 10, 1982 MMWR also reported a suspected case of transfusion-associated AIDS in a 20-month-old San Francisco infant who had none of the known risk factors for AIDS. One of the 19 donors of the blood components received by the infant during his first month of life was subsequently reported to have AIDS. The report suggested that blood transfusion was the means by which the infant had acquired AIDS. In an accompanying editorial note, CDC stated that

> ... if platelet transfusion contained an etiologic agent for AIDS, one must assume that the agent can be present in the blood of a donor before onset of

symptomatic illness and that the incubation period for such illness can be relatively long. This model for AIDS transmission is consistent with findings described in an investigation of a cluster of sexually related AIDS cases among homosexual men in southern California [CDC, MMWR, December 10, 1982].

One week later, the CDC reported four additional cases of AIDS in children (all less than two years old) (CDC, MMWR, December 17, 1982). None of the four infants were known to have received any blood or blood products. The mother of one was a prostitute and IV drug user; two were the children of Haitian immigrants; and one was the child of an IV drug user mother who had died of immune deficiency. According to the report, although the nature of the immune function described in the four cases was unclear, it was possible that these infants had AIDS and that the death of one of the mothers from PCP was probably secondary to AIDS. The CDC further stated that although the etiology of AIDS remained unknown, a series of epidemiological observations suggested it was caused by an infectious agent (CDC, MMWR, December 17, 1982).

The similar patterns of transmission of AIDS and hepatitis B and the latency period in both diseases led the medical and scientific community to discount the hypothesis that "poppers" were the cause of AIDS (CDC, MMWR, November 5, 1982; Panem 1988). A few months later, some physicians, scientists, and consumers of blood and blood products endorsed the theory that blood products may be transmitting the infectious agent. Others, however, were unconvinced and continued to hypothesize that the cases in hemophiliacs may have been due to immune suppression from using AHF concentrate (FDA, BPAC, 1983; Foege 1983; Aledort, Bove, Osborn interviews). They were skeptical because of the small number of known diagnosed cases among hemophilia patients compared to the number who were exposed to blood products.

Evidence for heterosexual transmission of AIDS appeared on January 7, 1983, when the CDC reported immunodeficiency in two female sexual partners of men with AIDS. The editorial note contained in this MMWR stated that

> ... epidemiological observations increasingly suggest that AIDS is caused by an infectious agent. The description of a cluster of sexually related AIDS patients among homosexual males in southern California suggest[s] that such an agent could be transmitted sexually or through other intimate contact. The present report supports the infectious-agent hypothesis and the possibility that transmission of the putative "AIDS agent" may occur among both heterosexual and male homosexual couples. At this time, CDC has received a total of 43 previously healthy females who have developed PCP or other opportunistic infections typical of AIDS [CDC, MMWR, January 7, 1983].

On the same date, the CDC also reported on the occurrence of AIDS in 16 prison inmates. All inmates were reported to have had a history of chronic IV drug use. The report added weight to the hypothesis that AIDS was caused by an infectious agent transmitted sexually or through exposure to blood or blood products (CDC, MMWR, January 7, 1983).

Summary

By January 1983, epidemiological evidence from CDC's investigations strongly suggested that blood and blood products transmitted AIDS and that the disease could be transmitted through intimate sexual contact. The evidence that the AIDS agent was blood-borne was the result of two findings. First, AIDS was occurring in transfusion recipients who did not belong to any known high-risk group and in individuals with hemophilia who had received AHF concentrate. Second, the epidemiological patterns of AIDS was similar to that of hepatitis B, another blood-borne disease.

IMMEDIATE RESPONSES TO EVIDENCE OF BLOOD-BORNE AIDS TRANSMISSION

In the first months of 1983, the epidemiologic evidence that the AIDS agent was blood-borne led to official meetings and public and private decisions that set the pattern of the blood industry's response to AIDS, starting with a public meeting convened by the CDC in Atlanta on January 4, 1983. Later that month, the leading blood bank organizations and, separately, the National Hemophilia Foundation (NHF) and the plasma fractionation industry issued statements. In March 1983, the Assistant Secretary for Health promulgated the first official PHS recommendations for preventing AIDS, and the FDA codified safe practices for plasma collection.

The CDC's Public Meeting

The purpose of the public meeting on January 4, 1983, was to identify opportunities to prevent AIDS. The CDC's objectives for the meeting were to tell the blood services community about the evidence they had gathered; to enlist the help of other PHS agencies, especially the FDA; and to formulate recommendations for the prevention of AIDS. According to data presented by the CDC, the manifestations of AIDS appeared 4–17 months after transmission of infection (Foege 1983).

The meeting produced a great deal of debate but no consensus on specific action (Bove, Curran, Evatt, Francis, Foege, McAuley, Sandler interviews). Donald Francis, assistant director for medical science of the Division of Virology at the CDC, recommended that the blood banks question donors directly about their sexual behavior and run blood donations through a series of surrogate tests (the use of nonspecific laboratory markers), including a test for the hepatitis B core antibody, which showed an 88 percent correlation with patients who had AIDS (Foege 1983; Evatt, Foege, Francis interviews). Some meeting participants opposed this recommendation because of the cost of the tests and other reasons (see Chapter 5). Gay activist groups objected to screening measures, claiming that they were discriminatory toward their members. Many meeting participants were not convinced by the evidence that AIDS was transmitted by blood or blood products (Bove, Curran, Evatt, Foege, Pindyck interviews).

Dennis Donohue, Director of the FDA's Division of Blood and Blood Products, stated that research on processes for inactivating viruses in blood products was under way. Oscar Ratnoff, a prominent hemophilia specialist, stated there was enough information about the danger of AHF concentrate to stop using it in favor of cryoprecipitate (Johnson 1983). Dr. Francis tried to establish a time frame for action or a minimum number of transfusion-related AIDS cases after which the FDA's Blood Products Advisory Committee would agree to take action to implement donor screening policies.

The Blood Bank Community's Statement

A week after the Atlanta meeting in January 1983, the American Association of Blood Banks, the Council of Community Blood Centers, and the American Red Cross issued a joint statement that "direct or indirect questions about a donor's sexual preference are inappropriate." The statement recommended questions to detect possible AIDS exposure (i.e., a donor health history), but did not recommend any laboratory screening tests. At this time, the PHS agencies had not completed their own recommendations (Donohue, Foege interviews), and the FDA did not issue any recommendations.

Position of the National Hemophilia Foundation

The next day, the Medical and Scientific Advisory Council (MASAC) of the NHF met and recommended that cryoprecipitate (a blood product produced from the serum of a small number of donors), rather than AHF concentrate, be used for newborn infants and children under four, newly diagnosed patients, and those with mild hemophilia. According to the report, there was insufficient evidence to develop specific recommendations about blood product use (i.e., AHF concentrate or cryoprecipitate) in the treatment of severe hemophilia. Additional recommendations included delaying all elective surgical procedures and the use of a synthetic substance, DDAVP (desmopressin acetate), to elevate

Factor VIII levels in patients with mild or moderate hemophilia A. MASAC also stated that it was important to screen and exclude all high-risk donors from the blood and plasma supply for the production of blood products used for treatment of hemophilia. The NHF directed their recommendations to treating physicians, regional and community blood collection centers, and plasma fractionators; in some instances, the NHF also told their chapters to distribute the information to the chapter members.

Position of the Plasma Fractionation Industry

On January 28, 1983, the American Blood Resources Association (ABRA), which represents the plasma industry, issued recommendations about donor screening and deferral to reduce the risk of AIDS. The recommendations focused on donor education, donor screening, and surrogate laboratory testing. The ABRA recommended issuing a brochure that would describe AIDS, tell how individuals in high-risk groups could reduce their risk of exposure, and discourage high-risk persons from donating. The ABRA also recommended that prospective donors, prior to donating, be required to read the information about AIDS and indicate that they were not members of a high-risk group. Individuals who identified themselves as members of high-risk groups or were unwilling to reply would be excluded from donating plasma (donor deferral). The ABRA recommended against large-scale surrogate testing of donated blood until ABRA had evaluated its feasibility.

On December 17, 1982, prior to ABRA's recommendations, Alpha Therapeutics, one of the four commercial manufacturers of AHF concentrate, had begun excluding all plasma donors who identified themselves as having been in Haiti, having used IV drugs, or if male, having had sexual contact with another man. Alpha had notified all its affiliates that this policy was effective immediately and that unscreened plasma should no longer be sent to Alpha. By the early part of 1983, each of the companies had in place donor education and screening programs requesting members of high-risk groups to identify themselves and refrain from donating plasma (FDA, BPAC, 1983b).

Federal Recommendations on the Prevention of AIDS

In a March 4, 1983 report, the PHS promulgated its first official recommendations on the prevention of AIDS. The recommendations stated that the evidence suggested the disease was a severe disorder of immune regulation caused by a transmissible agent (CDC, MMWR, March 4, 1983). As evidence, the report indicated that the transmission routes of AIDS paralleled that of hepatitis B and that blood or blood products appeared to be responsible for transmitting AIDS to hemophilia patients. Suspected cases of transfusion-associated AIDS had been reported, but none were yet proven. According to the report, the evidence suggested a latency period of two months to two years between exposure and onset of symptoms. Brandt noted that a significant proportion of individuals in high-risk groups had no symptoms of AIDS, suggesting that the pool of persons potentially capable of transmitting an AIDS agent may be considerably larger than the known number of AIDS cases.

The PHS made the following recommendations for preventing AIDS transmission:

- Sexual contact should be avoided with persons known to have or suspected of having AIDS.
- Avoid sex with multiple partners or those who may have multiple partners.
- Members of groups at increased risk for AIDS should not donate plasma and/or blood products.
- Studies be conducted to evaluate screening procedures for their effectiveness in identifying and excluding plasma and blood with a high probability of transmitting AIDS—including lab tests and physical exams.
- Physicians should adhere strictly to medical indications for transfusions.
- Work should continue toward development of safer blood products for use by hemophilia patients.

About three weeks later, on March 24, 1983, the FDA notified all establishments collecting source plasma and human blood for transfusion and all manufacturers of plasma derivatives of steps to be taken to decrease the risk of blood or plasma donation by persons who might be at increased risk of transmitting AIDS. These steps included implementing standard operating procedures to quarantine and dispose of any products collected from donors known or suspected of having AIDS. The FDA also advised the blood and plasma collection facilities to establish educational programs to inform persons at increased risk for AIDS that they should stop donating and to train personnel who screen donors to recognize the early signs of AIDS. The FDA also announced that it had approved a new heat treatment to inactivate viruses in AHF concentrate. The treatment was purported to help protect individuals with hemophilia from hepatitis B, and perhaps from AIDS (Petricciani 1984).

Summary and Comment

Government and private agencies identified, considered, and in some cases adopted strategies for dealing with the risk of transmitting AIDS through blood and blood products. The recommended safety measures were limited in scope, which reflected a lack of consensus about the nature and magnitude of the threat (especially among physicians and public health officials who were unprepared for the unique epidemiological pattern of AIDS), and uncertainty about the costs, risks, and benefits of the proposed control strategies.

RECONSIDERING THE EVIDENCE: FURTHER ATTEMPTS TO FORMULATE POLICIES

In the interval between the decisions of early 1983 and discovery of the virus that causes AIDS in early 1984, public health and blood industry officials became more certain that AIDS was a blood-borne disease as the number of reported cases of AIDS among hemophiliacs and transfused patients increased. As their knowledge grew, these officials had to decide about recall of contaminated blood products and possible implementation of a surrogate test for HIV. Major opportunities to reconsider the policies of early 1983 arose at meetings of the FDA's Blood Product Advisory Committee (BPAC) in July and December 1983.

On May 11, 1983, Hyland Therapeutics recalled a lot of AHF concentrate when it discovered that the product had been manufactured from pools containing plasma from an individual subsequently diagnosed as having AIDS. The NHF issued a medical bulletin and a chapter advisory in conjunction with the recall, stating:

> It is not the role of the NHF to judge the appropriateness of corporate decisions made by individual pharmaceutical companies. However, we urge that patients and treaters recognize the need for careful evaluation of blood products and note that such a recall action *should not cause anxiety or changes in treatment programs.* ... The NHF recommends that patients maintain the use of concentrates or cryoprecipitate as prescribed by their physicians. If you have any questions regarding this matter, they should be directed to your treating physician and/or the NHF [NHF, 1983].

On June 22, 1983, the American Association of Blood Banks, the Council of Community Blood Centers, and the American Red Cross issued a second joint statement, stating that "it appears at this time that the risk of possible transfusion-associated AIDS is on the order of one case per million patients transfused. There is a risk that widespread attempts to direct donations, while not increasing the safety of transfusions, will seriously disrupt the nation's blood donor system." Directed donation is the process by which the patient in need of blood or blood components identifies persons (usually friends and family) to provide the needed units rather than utilizing blood from the hospital blood supply. The directed donation programs were an administrative and logistical burden for blood banks, and blood bank officials were not convinced that these programs significantly increased the safety of the recipient (Bove, Perkins, Pindyck, Sandler interviews). The joint statement thus strongly recommended against conducting directed donation programs.

On July 19, 1983, the FDA's Blood Products Advisory Committee (BPAC) discussed the criteria for deciding to withdraw lots of AHF concentrate, and recommended product withdrawal only if there was good evidence that plasma from a donor with AIDS had been present in the pooled plasma from which the lot had been manufactured. The Pharmaceutical Manufacturers Association expressed concern about the impact of a recall on the supply of AHF concentrate. The NHF's Medical and Scientific Advisory Council (MASAC) had stated that recall of a product should be automatic if a donor was either suspected of having or diagnosed with AIDS. Dr. Louis Aledort, medical director of the NHF, stated his personal view that the NHF/MASAC recommendation would adversely impact the continued supply of AHF concentrate (Aledort, Hoyer interviews). Because of concern about maintaining an adequate supply of AHF concentrate, and skepticism that blood products were a vector for transmitting AIDS, the BPAC advised the FDA to recommend a case-by-case decision rather than automatic withdrawal for each lot that included plasma from an individual who had AIDS or was suspected of having AIDS (see Chapter 6 for further discussion).

On December 15–16, 1983, the BPAC met to consider all possible options of surrogate marker tests. The discussion focused on the implementation of the hepatitis B core antibody (anti-HBc) test as a possible surrogate screening test for HIV. Arguments against using the test in blood banks included (a) it would eliminate too many noninfected donors and would therefore threaten the adequacy of the blood supply; (b) the test was not useful in differentiating high-risk homosexuals (e.g., those with multiple partners) from other male homosexual donors; and (c) the prevalence of anti-HBc antibodies was high among certain ethnic groups (e.g., Asians) and would cause deferral of these donors. The BPAC did not recommend surrogate testing, but agreed with a suggestion to create an industry task force to consider the logistics of testing plasma for anti-HBc as a surrogate for AIDS.

Summary and Comment

Blood safety policies changed very little during 1983. Many officials of the blood banks, the plasma fractionation industry, and the FDA accepted with little question estimates that the risk of AIDS was low ("one in a million transfusions"), and they accepted advice that control strategies (such as automatic withdrawal of AHF concentrate lots containing blood from donors suspected of having AIDS, or a switch from AHF concentrate to cryoprecipitate in less severe hemophiliacs) would be ineffective, too costly, or too risky. During this period, there were missed opportunities to learn from pilot tests to screen potentially infected donors or implement other control strategies that had been rejected as national policy. (These local attempts to screen are discussed briefly below, and in more detail in Chapter 5.)

RESEARCH ACTIVITIES

During 1983 through 1985, research on AIDS included epidemiological analysis to understand patterns of spread and etiology, methods to control or eliminate the disease, and evaluation of the efficacy of potential safety measures such as surrogate tests for the infection. Related research on methods to inactivate the hepatitis B virus in blood products that had begun in the 1970s came to fruition in the early 1980s (see Chapter 4 for a detailed discussion).

The Public Health Service Effort

As discussed earlier, the PHS Committee on Opportunistic Infections in Patients with Hemophilia held its second meeting on July 27, 1982. On the same date, the committee distributed two recommendations to the assistant secretary for health, the FDA commissioner, the NIH director, CDC regional offices, and state and territorial health officers. The first recommendation was to establish an active surveillance system at once to identify new suspected cases of AIDS occurring in individuals with hemophilia. In November, the CDC, the NHF, and the regionally based network of hemophilia treatment centers agreed to cooperate in this effort. The second recommendation called for (a) laboratory studies of the immunologic competence of individuals with hemophilia who had no symptoms of opportunistic infections, and (b) applied research to determine practical techniques for eliminating the risk of infection from AHF concentrate (Foege 1982b). The meeting summary also noted concerns about the adequacy of funding to support these activities, stating that existing federal grants and contract mechanisms were not "responsive to rapid funding of urgent problems" (Foege 1982b).

The PHS committee also recommended studies to evaluate the effectiveness of screening procedures for identifying and excluding high-risk donors but did not propose a source of funding for the studies. Several blood banks did initiate pilot studies on safety measures such as anti-HBc as a surrogate for HIV (Irwin Memorial Blood Bank), the use of a reversed T-cell ratio test (a test indicating immune dysfunction) to exclude high-risk donors (Stanford University Blood Bank), and confidential unit exclusion to allow donors to self-defer (New York

Blood Center). The results of the studies did not provide strong enough evidence to convince those who attended the December 15–16, 1983, BPAC meeting (discussed above) to recommend surrogate testing or other measures to reduce AIDS transmission.

In March 1983 Assistant Secretary of Health Edward Brandt announced the formation of a PHS Executive Committee on AIDS. The purpose of the committee was to coordinate the activities of PHS agencies and share information on upcoming meetings, grant awards, and new developments. In addition, Assistant Secretary Brandt directed the NIH, in collaboration with the CDC and FDA, to support studies to evaluate screening procedures, including laboratory tests, for their effectiveness in identifying and excluding blood and plasma donors at increased risk for AIDS (Brandt 1983). In response to this request, the NIH director, Dr. James Wyngaarden, designated the National Heart, Lung, and Blood Institute (NHLBI) to lead NIH's effort in determining if any test "would merit experimental validation and possible preparation for an Request for Application (RFA)" (Wyngaarden 1983). In the following year, the NHLBI sponsored several conferences on AIDS.

Early in 1983, NIH redirected some of its research budget ($165,000 in supplemental funding) to scientists working on studies of Kaposi's sarcoma (Thomas 1983; Panem 1988). In addition, the NHLBI established an interagency agreement with the CDC to evaluate immunologic changes in hemophiliacs and patients receiving blood and blood products (Sloand 1994). A total of $61,500,000 was allocated to the PHS budget in fiscal year 1984 for AIDS-related research; this represents a 114 percent increase from the $28,700,000 allocated in fiscal year 1983 (Stoto, et al. 1988).

Isolation of the Virus and Development of a Screening Test

Investigators at the Pasteur Institute in Paris reported the isolation of novel virus that they termed LAV from an individual with lymphadenopathy syndrome in 1983. These investigators suspected that LAV might be involved in the causation of AIDS, but due to difficulties they experienced in propagating the virus in large quantities and the lack of an effective serologic test to identify LAV-infected persons, this hypothesis could not be proved at the time. In April 1984, researchers at the National Cancer Institute of the NIH reported the isolation of a virus they called HTLV-III from a number of persons suffering from AIDS and from asymptomatic or moderately symptomatic persons from groups of persons at risk of AIDS (Popovic, et al., 1984). The NIH investigators described for the first time a method to prepare large quantities of HTLV-III in the laboratory and provided convincing evidence that this virus was the etiologic agent of AIDS.

The discovery that a virus caused AIDS shifted some research efforts toward a focus on the biological aspects of transmission of the disease and its interactions within the human body. The public's reaction to the discovery of HTLV-III (later renamed HIV) included an increased fear of casual transmission and of infection through the act of donating blood (Fee and Fox 1988; Brandt 1987). As a result of the isolation of HTLV-III, blood and plasma collection organizations, anticipating the quick development of a direct test for the virus, did not implement any additional donor screening procedures until such a test was developed. Meanwhile, during 1982–1984, U.S. manufacturers were completing the development of a process for inactivating the hepatitis B viruses by heating AHF concentrate (see Chapter 4). In October 1984, the CDC announced that laboratory experiments showed that the heat treatment process also inactivated HIV.

During 1984, however, researchers remained focused on developing a screening test for HIV. Once the virus was identified, several companies began developing tests to screen blood by detecting antibodies that would indicate exposure to the virus. In April 1984, NIH developed and patented a prototype screening test for antibodies to HIV, and by May it had solicited applications from companies interested in commercial use of the tests. Five companies were selected in June. The first tests used an enzyme-linked immunosorbent assay (ELISA), and the FDA received an application for licensure from a company in December 1984. By March 1985, the FDA had granted two licenses for commercial use of the tests; it also notified all blood facilities that the test was available, and it scheduled a workshop on its use [50 *Federal Register* 28477]. Subsequently, all blood banks and plasma collection centers implemented the ELISA.

The first ELISA tests detected 96–98 percent of HIV-infected blood samples. However, despite a high degree of specificity, false seropositive results occurred. For this reason, a second, more costly, less sensitive, but more specific screening test called the Western Blot was used to confirm or refute the positive results of the ELISA test. Neither test could detect HIV antibodies during the six-to-eight-week window period (i.e., the time between HIV infection and the evidence of antibodies in a donor's blood). Since the implementation of the initial ELISA test, several more sensitive tests have replaced it because they reduce the length of the window period. Through the widespread use of this test, the current risk of HIV transmission through screened blood is estimated to be less than 1 in 420,000 units (Lackritz, et al. 1995; Busch, et al. 1995).

Summary and Comment

In the early 1980s, the CDC's surveillance program identified AIDS patients and characterized the disease swiftly and thoroughly. Dr. Gallo at the NIH isolated and characterized HIV in less than two years. Meanwhile, laboratories of the plasma fractionation industry were developing viral inactivation methods for AHF concentrate. The pace of virus inactivation research in the 1970s had been slow, but accelerated in the 1980s in response to hepatitis and was complete by 1984. Most of the PHS research effort was concentrated on identifying and characterizing the virus. Research into other potential ways to safeguard the blood supply, such as surrogate tests, was not pursued vigorously, and there was relatively little research on blood safety issues perse.

REFERENCES

Brandt, Allan. *No Magic Bullet*. Oxford University Press, New York, New York; 1987.

Brandt, Edward, Assistant Secretary for Health. Memorandum to Agency Heads; March 2, 1983.

Busch, et al. Presentation at the National Institutes of Health consensus conference; January 1995.

Centers for Disease Control, *Morbidity and Mortality Weekly Report* , June 5, 1981.

Centers for Disease Control, *Morbidity and Mortality Weekly Report* , July 3, 1981.

Centers for Disease Control, *Morbidity and Mortality Weekly Report* , June 11, 1982.

Centers for Disease Control, *Morbidity and Mortality Weekly Report* , June 18, 1982.

Centers for Disease Control, *Morbidity and Mortality Weekly Report* , July 9, 1982.

Centers for Disease Control, *Morbidity and Mortality Weekly Report* , July 16, 1982.

Centers for Disease Control, *Morbidity and Mortality Weekly Report* , September 24, 1982.

Centers for Disease Control, *Morbidity and Mortality Weekly Report* , December 10, 1982.

Centers for Disease Control, *Morbidity and Mortality Weekly Report* , December 17, 1982.

Centers for Disease Control, *Morbidity and Mortality Weekly Report* , November 5, 1982.

Centers for Disease Control, *Morbidity and Mortality Weekly Report* , January 7, 1983.

Centers for Disease Control, *Morbidity and Mortality Weekly Report* , March 4, 1983.

Fee, Elizabeth and Fox, Daniel, eds. *AIDS: The Burdens of History*. University of California Press, Berkeley, California; 1988.

Foege, William H., M.D., Director, Centers for Disease Control. Letter to State and Territorial Health Officers; July 9, 1982a.

Foege, William H., M.D. *Summary Report on Open Meeting of Public Health Service Committee on Opportunistic Infections in Patients with Hemophilia*; August 6, 1982b.

Foege, William H., M.D. *Summary Report on Workgroup to Identify Opportunities for Prevention of Acquired Immune Deficiency Syndrome*; January 4, 1983a.

Food and Drug Administration. Blood Products Advisory Committee; February 7, 1983b.

Food and Drug Administration. Blood Products Advisory Committee; July 19, 1983.

Hansen, K.B. Armour Pharmaceuticals. Interoffice Correspondence to Bessler, et al.; July 19, 1982.

Johnson, Robert. Letter to list [Armour Pharmaceutical interoffice correspondence]; January 12, 1983.

Lackritz, et al., Presentation at the National Institutes of Health consensus conference; January 1995.

Neustadt, R. and Fineberg, H. *The Swine Flu Affair: Decisionmaking on a Slippery Disease.* U.S. Department of Health, Education, and Welfare; 1978.

National Hemophilia Foundation. *Chapter Advisory #8*; May 11, 1983.

Panem, Sandra. *The AIDS Bureaucracy.* Harvard University Press, Cambridge, Massachusetts; 1988.

Petricciani, John C. M.D., Food and Drug Administration, Director Division of Blood and Blood Products, Center for Drugs and Biologics. Letter issued August 8, 1984.

Popovic, M., et al. Detection, Isolation, and Continuous Production of Cytopathic Retroviruses (HTLV-III) from Patients with AIDS and pre-AIDS. *Science*; 1984.

Sloand, Elaine. Submission to the Institute of Medicine, "Chronology of Major NHLBI Intramural Activities on AIDS"; April 8, 1994.

Stoto, et al. Federal Funding for AIDS Research: Decision Process and Results in Fiscal Year 1986. *Reviews of Infectious Diseases*, Vol. 10; March-April 1988.

Thomas, R. Anne, Director, Division of Public Information, National Institutes of Health. Memorandum issued May 17, 1983.

Wyngaarden, Director, National Institutes of Health, Memorandum to NHLBI Director; March 14, 1983.

4

Product Treatment

INTRODUCTION

Plasma products can be treated by a variety of physical and chemical processes to reduce the risk of contamination from viruses and other infectious agents, thus increasing the safety of their use. Currently available product treatment procedures use physical heat or chemical detergents to virally inactivate plasma products that will be used in medical treatment of clotting disorder diseases such as hemophilia. Owing to a variety of technical obstacles that remain today, there are no effective methods to inactivate viruses present in whole blood or in nonplasma blood components such as cellular blood products (e.g., red blood cells and platelets) used for transfusion purposes.

Shortly after the development of the technology to manufacture antihemophilic factor (AHF) concentrate, it was recognized that blood products carried a substantial risk of hepatitis to their recipients. Although some blood derivative products (e.g., albumin) have been treated with heat to destroy live viruses since the late 1940s, Factor VIII and IX AHF concentrates in the United States were not subjected to procedures of viral inactivation until 1983–1984. In fact, the methods used to manufacture AHF concentrate can also inadvertently concentrate certain viruses, present in the original plasma donation, within the final product preparation. The fact that AHF concentrate is prepared from pooled plasma from thousands of donors greatly increases its risks for transmitting disease.

This chapter describes the development and implementation of treatment methods used to inactivate viruses in AHF concentrate. The events leading to the development and implementation of these methods unfolded over the period from 1970 to March 1983, during which time AHF concentrate became widespread as the standard medical treatment for individuals with hemophilia. Although inactivation of hepatitis viruses was the goal of the first product treatment methods developed to increase the safety of AHF concentrate, review of the history of their development is important to consider for several reasons. First, because the product treatment methods used to inactivate hepatitis viruses also inactivate HIV, their availability prior to 1981 would have minimized, if not prevented, the widespread HIV infection of persons with hemophilia. Second, consideration of the development of viral inactivation methods helped shed light on important aspects of the prevailing scientific, medical, and regulatory environments of the early 1980s. The Committee framed its analysis of the development and implementation of viral inactivation methods of four questions:

- When did the information that facilitated the development of viral inactivation methods become available?
- Could the technology to accomplish viral inactivation of AHF concentrate have been developed earlier to decrease the transmission of hepatitis and AIDS?
- What were the internal and external pressures that influenced the rate at which viral inactivation methods for AHF concentrate were developed and implemented?
- What was the role of the Food and Drug Administration and the National Institutes of Health in encouraging or supporting research on viral inactivation methods to improve the safety of AHF concentrate?

The Committee developed two hypotheses to explain the actions that were taken during the period from 1970 to 1983:

- Plasma fractionators and other organizations responsible for the safety of blood products did not begin research on viral inactivation of AHF concentrates until the onset of the AIDS epidemic.
- Hepatitis was viewed as an acceptable risk by the government regulatory agencies responsible for the safety of blood and blood products, the plasma fractionation industry, the physicians who treated the individuals with hemophilia, and the individuals with hemophilia. As a result, little incentive was available to improve AHF product safety through the expeditious development and implementation of viral inactivation technologies.

Testing these hypotheses against the evidence gathered through documents and fact-finding interviews, the Committee concluded they were able to reject the first hypothesis but unable to reject the second.

CRITICAL TIME PERIOD: 1970-1983

Two important elements frame the period from 1970 to 1983: (1) the discovery of hepatitis as an infectious agent associated with the use of blood and blood products, and (2) the development of viral inactivation procedures for increasing the safety of AHF concentrate. With respect to both elements, it is important to establish when certain scientific information was available in relation to decisions about blood and blood product safety.

Hepatitis

The transfer of blood and blood derivatives between humans is considered one of the greatest and most successful therapeutic practices in modern medicine. However, accompanying the development and increased use of blood transfusion practices, there has been a growth in rates of blood-borne diseases.

Iatrogenic transmission of hepatitis has a long history dating back to at least the 1880s when vaccination against smallpox, using glycerinated lymph of human origin was occasionally practiced. So-called serum hepatitis (now known to result from hepatitis B infection) was also seen in many individuals who received preparations of yellow fever vaccine that had been stabilized by the addition of human serum.

By 1943, hepatitis had been recognized as a complication following transfusion of whole blood and plasma. Supporting evidence accrued during World War II as the constant demand for blood and plasma administration during battle led to the recognition that a serious transmissible illness was affecting large numbers of soldiers following transfusion. Studies conducted in the United States and England following World War II identified two viruses, one with a short incubation period that could be transmitted both orally and parenterally, and the other with a long incubation period and transmissible only parenterally.

The identification of two viruses, made in the late 1940s, was confirmed two decades later with the availability of sera to distinguish between the two types of viruses responsible for the distinct clinical presentations (Seeff 1988). The virus causing hepatitis B (serum hepatitis) was discovered in 1965, and the virus causing hepatitis A in 1973. By 1968, a direct test for the presence of an antigenic component of hepatitis B, or HBsAg (hepatitis B surface antigen) was developed and used to detect individuals suffering from active chronic or acute hepatitis infections. Ultimately, a highly effective vaccine to prevent hepatitis B infection became available in 1982; a second generation recombinant vaccine has been available since 1986. An effective vaccine to prevent hepatitis A has recently been developed.

Despite the widespread use of diagnostic tests for hepatitis A and B, a significantly large number of cases of post-transfusion hepatitis continued to be observed. It was then realized, between 1976 and 1978, that other undiscovered agents were responsible for what became known as non-A, non-B (NANB) hepatitis.

Hepatitis A was found to be responsible for a transient infection that causes a self-limited disease of mild to moderate severity. A mortality rate of 0.2 percent or less is seen following hepatitis A infection and the infection never becomes chronic. Hepatitis A is commonly transmitted by a fecal-oral route, either the result of person-to-person transmission or ingestion of contaminated food or water. The virus usually appears in the bloodstream during the incubation period and the early acute phase of hepatitis A infection. Transmission by blood transfusion or by contaminated AHF concentrate has also been reported, however, such instances of blood-borne transmission are rare.

Hepatitis B (HBV) infection frequently causes a transient infection that in most cases is cleared by the host immune response and leaves the individual immune from reinfection by hepatitis B upon subsequent exposure (i.e., through development of immunity thought to be mediated primarily by antiviral antibodies). However, acute HBV infection can be severe and sometimes fatal (i.e., there is a 0.2–2 percent mortality rate), and a minority of infected persons experience a persistent infection that is associated with progressive liver disease and a type of liver cancer known as hepatocellular carcinoma. Though HBV infection is less likely to be severe, it is more likely to become chronic in young persons, with 90 percent of infected newborns developing chronic infection while only 2–7 percent of infected adults do so. Transmission of HBV principally results from exposure to blood or blood products, although sexual transmission is also common. During the 1960s, up to 10 percent of persons who received massive transfusions acquired HBV infection and more than 80 percent of individuals with hemophilia were infected through their use of contaminated pooled AHF concentrate.

In 1977 another virus, the delta hepatitis virus (HDV) was discovered; HDV is an incomplete RNA virus that can be transmitted only in the company of HBV. Infection with HDV can occur either as a co-infection with HBV or as a "superinfection" in individuals with pre-existing chronic HBV infection. HDV infection is usually severe with complications of fulminant hepatitis and progressive chronic hepatitis. An overall mortality rate of 2–20 percent has been reported. Chronic HDV infections are seen in 1–3 percent of HBV infections and 70–80 percent of superinfections. The transmissible nature of HDV was established in 1980 by transmission of the virus to HBV-infected chimpanzees.

The identification of the viruses responsible for the hepatitis syndromes permitted the development of serologic tests to screen blood donors for potential infection and resulted in a substantial reduction of post-transfusion hepatitis B.

During the years 1970-1972, the HBsAg test was required and implemented in all blood and plasma collection organizations. In July 1975, the use of a third-generation test for HBsAg with a greater degree of sensitivity, utilizing radioimmunoassay or reversed passive hemagglutination, was required by the FDA. In 1977, the World Health Organization Committee on Viral Hepatitis adopted the terms *hepatitis A* for the hepatitis virus transmitted orally, and *hepatitis B* (HBV) for the virus transmitted sexually and through transfusion of blood or blood products.

As a result of the implementation of HBsAg testing during the period from 1972–1975, AHF concentrate testing positive for HBsAg decreased from 25 percent to 3 percent of Factor VIII lots tested by the FDA, and from 67 percent to 2 percent of Factor IX lots tested by the FDA. After 1975, according to Dr. Robert Gerety, chief of the Hepatitis Branch, Division of Blood and Blood Products in the Bureau of Biologics at the FDA at the time, no lots of either Factor VIII or Factor IX submitted to the bureau contained detectable HBsAg; but despite this, the problem of HBV infection following administration of the AHF concentrate would remain serious (Gerety and Barker 1976).

By 1975, even though third-generation testing was in practice, some donations of blood or plasma had levels of HBsAg that were below the level of assay detection and HBV-infected donations continued to enter the pools used in the plasma lots. Even though these lots contained undetectable levels of HBsAg, owing to the extraordinary infectivity of HBV, they were still able to transmit the infection to susceptible recipients of the affected blood products. However, in 1976, although 80 percent of individuals with hemophilia were identified as positive for the antibody to hepatitis B (evidence of previous infection with the virus), the majority did not develop clinically apparent hepatitis. The percentage of individuals with hemophilia with chronic HBV infection ranged from 2.5 to 7.8 percent and the percentage of those who had clinically recognizable hepatitis ranged from 6 to 26 percent. Gradually, it was believed by the medical community treating individuals with hemophilia that many adults with hemophilia had developed an immunity to HBV as a result of prior exposure to the virus (Aledort, Dietrich, Levine interviews). Administration of the AHF concentrate to children and adolescents with hemophilia, however, often resulted in clinical and chronic HBV infections (Gerety and Barker 1976). Once screening for HBV markers resulted in the exclusion of HBV carriers in the donor pool, NANB virus was responsible for 80–90 percent of the hepatitis cases. Prospective studies performed in the late 1970s and early 1980s indicated that the incidence of post-transfusion hepatitis (HBV and hepatitis C [HCV]) was 7–21 percent in recipients of blood from volunteer donors (Barker and Dodd 1989). The infectious nature of NANB hepatitis was first established in 1978 by experimental transmission to chimpanzees. The virus itself was not identified until 1989, and is now referred to as HCV.

Following the identification of the etiologic agent of the majority of cases of NANB hepatitis in 1988, the natural history and severity of this infection became better known. In prospective studies, 50–70 percent of persons with acute hepatitis C infection were shown to become carriers of chronic HCV. It is known now that chronic hepatitis C infection is often silent, is one of the major causes of cirrhosis, hepatocellular carcinoma, or both, in the United States, and is a common precipitant of liver failure necessitating liver transplantation.

Viral Inactivation of AHF Concentrate

Early Methods

According to a Department of Health, Education and Welfare Conference on Hemophilia in 1976, research at that time had already begun to develop alternate means, other than testing for HBsAg, of removing HBV from final products while maintaining the therapeutic activity of the clotting treatment. Pilot studies had been undertaken to evaluate two methods of viral removal: solidphase immunoabsorption and polyethylene glycol precipitation. However, results of inoculating chimpanzees with the treated products were equivocal (Barker and Dodd 1989). In 1978, hepatitis continued to present a major risk in the use of pooled plasma products, including fibrinogen, AHF concentrates (i.e., Factors VIII and IX), and Factors II, VII, and X (Trepo, et al. 1978).

Two other methods of viral inactivation were also being developed during the 1970s. These methods provided the foundation for most of the subsequent development in this area. First, Dr. Edward Shanbrom, the codeveloper of Factor VIII concentrates, who by this time had left Hyland Laboratories (Baxter Healthcare) and was self-employed, developed a nonionic detergent method for treating plasma before it was fractionated into Factor VIII and the other plasma derivatives (Shanbrom interview). Second, a German pharmaceutical company, Behringwerke, A.G., initiated studies in 1977 on heat inactivation methods for AHF concentrate (Weidmann and Hoechst 1993).

Dr. Shanbrom's method required adding a detergent to the fractionation column, and this method was chosen for experimentation because it was known that viruses containing lipid membranes are readily inactivated by detergentinduced disruption of membrane integrity (Shanbrom pers. com. 1995). The application of the inactivation process before the plasma was fractionated, however, would have required relicensure of all the products of fractionation (Bacich, Shanbrom interviews). Although Dr. Shanbrom tried to interest the various plasma fractionation companies in his detergent process, for several reasons none responded favorably (Shanbrom interview). According to one of the plasma fractionators, they were already involved with heat-treated viral inactivation research, and interrupting these research efforts to begin experimentation on the effectiveness of the detergent method would delay licensing (Bacich interview). There was also a question whether there were sufficient data to support the effectiveness of the detergent process against HBV (Mozen interview). Further, Dr. Shanbrom approached both Armour Pharmaceutical and the federal Centers for Disease Control to test the procedure in chimpanzees to confirm its ability to inactivate hepatitis viruses, but was told that there were too few chimpanzees and that confirming the efficacy of this process was not a priority (Favero 1992).

The process used by Behringwerke was (and still is) a pasteurization procedure that requires the heating of AHF concentrate at 60°C for 10 hours, using sucrose and glycine as stabilizers, before lyophilization. Behringwerke's "heat sterilized" Factor VIII was licensed in Germany in May 1981 (Weidmann and Hoechst 1993). Behringwerke claimed (at that time) that the loss of potency or yield (i.e., factor protein) of the treated Factor VIII was approximately 50 percent, but U.S. manufacturers claimed the loss was 90 percent or more according to their internal studies (Feldman pers. com. 1994).

The reasons for the discrepancies in the results obtained by different companies in testing this method are not clear. However, owing to the loss of activity resulting from this process, the cost of the Behringwerke product was approximately 10 times that of non-heat-treated concentrate (Feldman pers. com. 1994). Although Behringwerke's pasteurized Factor VIII was used in Germany upon its licensure, the company was simultaneously producing non-heat-treated material; also, Germany continued to import Factor VIII from the United States. The loss of yield due to the application of heat resulted in the need to obtain larger plasma volumes according to testimony from a Behringwerke representative. This led to significant supply problems, as larger plasma volumes were difficult to obtain at the time (Weidmann and Hoechst 1993). In 1981, there was only enough pasteurized product to treat about 50 patients, and in 1982 only 100. In addition, while the Behringwerke pasteurized product was shown to be effective against HBV, it remained unknown whether it was effective against non-A, non-B hepatitis.

The heat-treated Behringwerke product was not universally accepted for use among the German hemophilia population for several reasons, including the limited supply. One reason was the belief by some physicians that the stabilizer added to the product during the heating process would also stabilize the virus, hindering full viral inactivation (Feldman interview). There was also a concern about the risk of heat-induced alterations in the structure of the treated Factor VIII preparation (neoantigenicity). Neoantigenicity can lead to the formation of inhibitors, or antibodies, to the altered product after infusion into the patient.

The medical community feared that the formation of such inhibitors to the product would render the patient more difficult to treat effectively (Aledort, Dietrich, Levine interviews). Behringwerke's heat-treated product was also considerably more expensive, and German insurance companies covered its cost only for special circumstances (Weidmann and Hoechst 1993; Federal Minister of Health 1992). Behringwerke initiated testing the pasteurized product for inactivation of NANB hepatitis in 1985, and a successful clinical trial was completed during 1986–1987 (Weidmann and Hoechst 1993).

Studies by U.S. Plasma Fractionation Companies

There were basically three methods utilizing heat for viral inactivation used by U.S. manufacturers in the early 1980s: (1) In 1979, the Baxter Healthcare company initiated studies on heat inactivation of AHF concentrate using a "dry heat" process. The dry heat process involved the application of heat at a specified temperature and time to the concentrate in the lyophilized (freezedried) state (Persky pers. com. 1995); (2) the "wet heat" process, a term coined by Alpha Therapeutics, involved suspending powder of lyophilized concentrate in heptane solvent and heating at 60°C for 20 hours. Following the heating process, the solvent was removed and the concentrate revialed (McAuley pers. com. 1995); and (3) in liquid pasteurization, Factor VIII, albumin, or other proteins in the completely soluble liquid state were heated with the addition of various stabilizers.

By the early 1980s, all of the plasma fractionators had initiated studies on inactivation by application of various amounts of heat for different durations of time (McAuley pers. com. 1995; Persky pers. com. 1995; Leahy pers. com. 1995; Hammes pers. com. 1995). They also began experimenting with the addition of different stabilizers and organic solvents to protect the protein and enhance the heat effect. There was, however, little if any communication between the different manufacturers regarding the results of the ongoing experiments, because of antitrust laws, regulations, and the normal business consideration of competitive advantage (Bacich pers. com. 1994; Feldman pers. com. 1994; Hammes pers. com. 1995).

Problems of Viral Inactivation Development

As the Behringwerke experience illustrates, to some extent the possibility of using heat to inactivate viruses in AHF concentrate, as used in other plasma derivatives (e.g., albumin), would be accompanied by three major concerns that impeded progress. The first concern was that heat would denature the labile factor protein to varying degrees depending on the amount and duration of the heat. Denaturing of the factor protein could cause the development of new antigens that would stimulate blocking antibodies (inhibitors) and reduce the amount of active factor protein in the recipients. Subsequently, this would further increase the amount of factor protein required to obtain a normal clotting response. The second concern was the potential additional cost of implementing the process. In addition to the heating process itself, a lower yield of active concentrate would increase the need for plasma, resulting in added cost. Finally, there was a concern about the adverse effects on the patient of a possibly unstable heat-treated product with varying degrees of purity. Higher-purity products, those in which extraneous proteins such as fibrinogen were removed (e.g., the Behringwerke product), were found to be less stable at room temperature after reconstitution, according to the analysis conducted by one manufacturer (Feldman pers. com. 1994).

Impact of the First Reported Cases of AIDS in Individuals with Hemophilia

One of the purposes of the July 27, 1982, meeting of the PHS Committee on Opportunistic Infections in Patients with Hemophilia was the need to determine if certain blood products, particularly AHF, were risk factors for AIDS (see Chapter 3). The group issued a recommendation to urgently determine practical techniques for decreasing or eliminating the infectious risks from AHF concentrate. Meeting participants discussed several viral inactivation methods that were under study and that a meeting of the FDA's Blood Products Advisory Committee (BPAC) later in the year would discuss and evaluate the various approaches (Foege 1982). During a December 3–4, 1982, meeting of the BPAC there was discussion of a minimal criterion for virus inactivation in high-risk products such as AHF concentrate. Dr. Aronson, the director of FDA's Coagulation Branch in the Division of Blood and Blood Products, described several experimental methodologies, including heat inactivation, inactivation with propiolactone and ultraviolet irradiation, removal by affinity chromatography, antibody inactivation, immunoabsorbence by immobilized antibody, and polyethylene glycol precipitation. Hepatitis B was selected as a marker to determine the degree of inactivation per method because materials and methods were not yet available for NANB.

The CDC convened a meeting, held in Atlanta in early January 1983, to which those concerned with blood and blood products were invited (see also Chapter 3 and Chapter 5). The recommendations that stemmed from the meeting, however, made no mention of changing the current usage of AHF concentrate. On the other hand, it was mentioned that viral inactivation procedures for Factor VIII were on the horizon (Foege 1982).

Federal Research Support for Viral Inactivation

The National Institutes of Health is the major federal source of funding to support research in areas relevant to health. Within the NIH, the institute with primary responsibility for blood research is the National Heart, Lung, and Blood Institute (NHLBI), and in particular its Division of Blood Diseases and Resources (DBDR) (see Chapter 2). A charge of the DBDR is to support research to improve the quality, safety, and availability of blood and blood products for therapeutic use. Consistent with this charge, the five-year plan published by the DBDR in 1982 identified as a research priority, the development of methods to decrease the transmission of infectious pathogens, particularly the hepatitis viruses, via AHF concentrate and other blood products. However, the Committee did not find any evidence that the NHLBI actually provided any support for intramural or extramural research between 1982 and 1983 to develop viral inactivation methodologies to limit hepatitis transmission by AHF concentrate.

Beginning in 1982, NHLBI did support several studies aimed at evaluating the potential transmission of the etiologic agent of AIDS through blood and blood products. These efforts included an interagency agreement with the CDC to evaluate immunologic abnormalities in recipients of blood and blood products, initiated in November 1982, and investigation of the possible transmission of the etiologic agent of AIDS to chimpanzees in May 1983. In July 1983, a request for applications was released by the NHLBI for the development of tests (so-called surrogate markers) to identify individuals who might act as carriers of the AIDS agent. Seven grants, totaling $1.5 million, were awarded for the purpose in April 1984; their utility was eclipsed, however, by the discovery of HIV at about the same time, and the money was devoted to studies of more specific test methods. In October 1984, the NHLBI issued a request for proposals for the development of HIV inactivation methods for plasma derivatives. Although the NIH and NHLBI might have been expected to take similar action with respect to viral inactivation methods focused on hepatitis, there is no evidence that the agency devoted any substantial effort to this end.

Specific Viral Inactivation Methods

By February 1983, all the major plasma fractionators had results from their research on the development of a heat-treated AHF concentrate. The major, if not exclusive, goal of these inactivation methods was the elimination of hepatitis viruses in AHF concentrate. Each plasma fractionation company subjected the AHF concentrate to varying temperatures and conditions for different durations.

Each company used stabilizers to protect the Factor VIII against the heat, but there was uncertainty whether the stabilizers also provided protection for pathogens as well. Using stabilizers such as sucrose resulted in a less than 20 percent loss of potency (Hwang 1982). Each of the manufacturers also initiated chimpanzee studies to determine if the hepatitis virus had been inactivated. Alpha Therapeutics reported that they had also looked for evidence of neoantigenicity but found none after heat treatment (McAuley 1994).

Testing for the Effectiveness of the Inactivation Process

As stated above, the major rationale for developing a viral inactivation procedure for AHF concentrate was to eliminate the hepatitis viruses. Proof that hepatitis had been inactivated, however, required inoculating the treated AHF concentrate into chimpanzees, a time-consuming, expensive, and resource-intensive effort. From 1981 through 1984 each of the plasma fractionators initiated chimpanzee studies to determine whether their viral inactivation processes inactivated HBV and NANB hepatitis virus. The results of initial studies conducted by Armour Pharmaceutical indicated that HBV was not completely inactivated by their heat treatment process, but that NANB was (Feldman pers. com. 1994). Armour Pharmaceutical was licensed for a process in January 1984 that was proven to inactivate NANB hepatitis in chimpanzee studies; but the company was unable to successfully inactivate HBV with their initial heat treatment process (Leahy pers. com. 1995; Rodell interview).

FDA Approval and Licensing of Treated Factor VIII

Table 4.1 summarizes the dates of license application and the FDA's approval of each plasma fractionator's heat-treated Factor VIII concentrate. Baxter's licensing was accomplished in only 8 months and licensing for the other fractionators took about 12 months from initial application. All plasma fractionators were licensed for sale of Factor VIII concentrate by February 1984. Upon licensure of the change in processing of the AHF concentrate products, the plasma fractionators immediately began producing a proportion of their production output using the added heat treatment step (Hammes pers. com. 1995; Leahy pers. com. 1995; McAuley pers. com. 1995; Persky pers. com. 1995). The four relevant plasma fractionators claim to have begun processing and distributing heat-treated AHF concentrate immediately after obtaining FDA licensure. However, none of the companies had entirely converted their manufacturing processes to produce only heat-treated products at the time they were licensed by the FDA to produce heat-treated AHF concentrate.

Table 4.1 Chronology of Fractionator License Applications and Approvals

Plasma Fractionator and Method for Heat-Treated Factor VIII Concentrate	Date Applied for FDA Licensing	Date License Granted by FDA
Baxter Healthcare (dry heat, 60°C for 72-74 hours)	June 1982	March 1983
Miles, Inc. (formerly Cutter Biological) (liquid pasteurization, 60°C for 10 hours)	August 1983	January 1984
(dry heat, 68°C for 72 hours)	November 1983	February 1984
Alpha Therapeutics (wet heat, 60°C for 20 hours)	December 1982	February 1984
Armour Pharmaceutical (dry heat, 60°C for 30 hours)	December 1982	January 1984

SOURCE: Persky 1995; Rodell 1982; Petricciani 1983; Hammes 1995; Mozen 1995; McAuley 1995; and Feldman 1994.

ANALYSIS AND CONCLUSIONS

As with other areas of scientific investigation, technical advances to improve the safety of blood and blood products relies on the imagination and abilities of individual researchers, the availability of sufficient financial resources to encourage and support new research directions, and the encouragement or pressure applied by regulatory agencies or consumer advocates. Progress in improving the safety of AHF concentrate could have potentially been encouraged by a variety of sources including the plasma fractionation industry, the NIH, the FDA, and the National Hemophilia Foundation. In evaluating the adequacy of the response of each of these groups, the Committee reviewed the sources of technical innovation and research funding for viral inactivation technologies for the hepatitis viruses and HIV. Furthermore, as scientific progress can be greatly facilitated by the open exchange of research findings, the Committee attempted to analyze the communication that took place among these different groups about their efforts to develop effective viral inactivation methods. After reviewing the data on the development of viral inactivation, the Committee concluded that although viral inactivation methods had begun in the late 1970s to eliminate hepatitis, they were not given a high priority for several reasons.

First, most individuals with hemophilia had already been exposed to HBV, which led to the perception that these individuals did not need to be protected through viral inactivation of the AHF concentrate (see Chapter 7) and that initial exposure to the hepatitis virus caused the development of protective antibodies in the majority of individuals with hemophilia (Aledort interview). Also, the anticipated availability of a vaccine against HBV led to the expectation that uninfected individuals and infants would be protected against it. This protection, provided by the vaccine, would be accomplished without resorting to methods to improve the safety of AHF concentrate (Pindyck interview). It was not known until sometime between 1976 and 1978, after introduction of the third-generation screening test for hepatitis B in 1976 and continued observation of transfusion-associated hepatitis, that the majority of these transfusion-associated hepatitis cases were due to other agents, especially the virus subsequently identified as HCV. This fact, together with the lack of knowledge of the virulence of NANB hepatitis at that time, further contributed to the limited impetus for and the slow pace of the development of viral inactivation technology. In addition, plasma fractionators, government, the medical community, and society as a whole did not seem to realize that new serious pathogens, or latent agents (e.g. Creutzfeldt-Jakob disease), might also be present in the untreated concentrate. Hepatitis was viewed to be an acceptable risk for individuals with hemophilia because it was considered a medically manageable complication of a very effective treatment for hemophilia (see Chapter 7).

According to the record, all of the product treatment methods that were ultimately proven to be effective in inactivating the hepatitis B and C viruses, and HIV, were developed within the laboratories of the plasma fractionators or by individuals closely associated with these industries. With the exception of Behringwerke, A.G., in Germany, each of the major plasma fractionators developed their inactivation methods at approximately the same time and entirely independently of each other. Dr. Edward Shanbrom, once employed by Hyland Laboratories (Baxter Healthcare), advocated a detergent method for viral inactivation after leaving the company. Without adequate support for the development or testing of this method, however, it did not gain widespread attention or acceptance. The record thus clearly indicates that, regardless of potential input or support from other sources, the impelling motive and decision to develop viral inactivation methods depended almost entirely on the plasma fractionation industry.

Given the FDA's role in licensing and ensuring the safety and efficacy of AHF and other plasma-derived materials, it would be natural to expect the agency to have had an interest in fostering, supporting, and possibly even conducting research on ways of inactivating hepatitis viruses and other infectious agents present in these preparations. However, review of the FDA's activities in this area uncovered only limited evidence of proactive effort to encourage industry to develop viral inactivation methods to limit hepatitis transmission by AHF. The FDA had essentially no significant internal research activities in this area. The FDA did convene a BPAC meeting in December 1982 to review the approval process for viral inactivation methods, with a particular focus on the details of the requisite chimpanzee challenge experiments. Several BPAC sessions in 1983 were devoted to viral inactivation and marker viruses (Franantoni 1995); however, this type of activity primarily served to facilitate, rather than actively encourage, the implementation of viral inactivation technologies.

The Committee identified several apparent reasons for the limited level of activity by the FDA, but their relative importance is difficult to determine. In discussions with FDA officials, certain useful perspectives emerged (Aronson, Donohue interviews). First, like most other persons with knowledge of this area, officials at the FDA appear to have been complacent about the risk of hepatitis transmission from AHF concentrate. Thus, although viral inactivation was considered a laudable goal, there seems to have been no sense of urgency in encouraging its development. Second, FDA officials believed that the appropriate expertise for developing viral inactivation methods resided in industry and that innovations would eventually emerge. Only a very limited number of personnel were available for the regulatory oversight of coagulation products in the early 1980s, and much of their time and effort was devoted to the emerging methods for thrombolytic therapy for myocardial infarctions. In addition, the FDA had only very modest internal facilities and support for research on viral inactivation technologies.

Given these factors, it is perhaps not surprising that the FDA looked to industry to provide the specific direction for progress in viral inactivation. However, the factors that influenced the pace of viral inactivation technologies developed by industry included interest in gaining competitive advantage and concerns over yield and cost. While these concerns are understandable from the perspective of a manufacturer, in the absence of active encouragement by the FDA these concerns probably inhibited expeditious progress in inactivation technologies. Further, with the primary responsibility for the development of viral inactivation methods left to industry, inherent limitations were placed on the free exchange of scientific and technical information that might expedite product development efforts. Operating in a competitive market, manufacturers are not inclined to share the details of their research efforts; and the FDA is legally barred from sharing a company's research findings among competitors. Companies interacting among each other could be in violation of antitrust laws and face potential criminal charges, fines, and sanctions. Furthermore, the very nature of the competitive world of business is one that normally would cause a company to preserve manufacturing processes and research results for its own benefit, to enable the marketing of products at a competitive advantage.

The Committee found that the plasma fractionators did not seriously consider alternative inactivation processes (e.g., the detergent process) because they placed a low priority on developing inactivation procedures for AHF concentrate and because heat inactivation had been successful for other blood products. Further, inactivation of pooled source plasma before fractionation would have required individual relicensure of all plasma products (Bacich, Hammes, Shanbrom interviews). In addition, inactivation methods used on plasma products could cause neoantigenicity, a problem that would negate the clinical effectiveness of AHF concentrate and possibly render the patient untreatable with these concentrates. The difficulty of testing the efficacy of inactivation procedures was due to the lack of correlation between antigen testing and infectiousness, and the absolute need for (and scarcity of) chimpanzees, which slowed progress in developing inactivation methods (Shanbrom pers. com. 1995; Epstein and Fricke 1990).

Once the initial inactivation methods were developed and shown to be effective in limiting the transmission of hepatitis B and NANB infection in experimentally inoculated chimpanzees, there was a relatively short interval between the product licensing application submission to the FDA and the licensure of the heat-inactivated products. The fact that the plasma fractionation industry was able to produce an inactivated product for license consideration concurrent with, and shortly after, the first reports of AIDS in individuals with hemophilia suggests that hepatitis infection (rather than AIDS) provided the major motivation for the ultimate development of viral inactivation methods.

SUMMARY

Overall, the record of the plasma fractionators and the FDA with respect to the development and implementation of heat treatment is mixed. The Committee's analysis focused on whether scientific information and technology was available earlier for the development of viral inactivation methods for AHF concentrate, and whether industry had appropriate incentives (from the FDA, the NIH, the National Hemophilia Foundation, or others) to develop these processes. In the Committee's judgment, heat treatment processes to prevent the transmission of hepatitis could have been developed before 1980, an advance that would have prevented many cases of AIDS in individuals with hemophilia.

Treaters of hemophilia and Public Health Service agencies did not, for a variety of reasons, encourage the companies to develop heat treatment measures earlier. Strong incentives to maintain the status quo and a weak countervailing force concerned with blood product safety, combined to inhibit rapid development of heat-treated products by plasma fractionation companies.

Once inactivation methods were developed, the plasma fractionators and the FDA moved expeditiously to license them. Following licensure of the first heat-treated AHF concentrate, however, many treating physicians and the National Hemophilia Foundation were slow to encourage their patients to use the new product (see Chapter 6).

AFTERWARD

Subsequent Events

In 1988, the CDC reported the results of a study of 75 HIV infected recipients of Factor VIII. Among this group of 75, they identified 18 sole recipients of a batch of Factor VIII from a single manufacturer that had been heat treated at 60°C for 30 hours. Subsequently, the manufacturer withdrew the product from the market and the lyophilized Factor VIII treated for 30 hours or less was no longer produced by any of the manufacturers. Armour Pharmaceutical modified their heating process by heating at 68°C for 72 hours (Feldman pers. com. 1994).

In 1992, investigators in France and Holland reported the development of a high incidence of inhibitor formation in hemophilia patients treated with a specific European manufacturer's preparation of AHF concentrate (Rosendaal, et al. 1983). This event alerted the medical community worldwide to the possibility of inhibitor formation following treatment with virally inactivated products, which had been extensively discussed previously but had not been reported. Although the development of inhibitors to AHF concentrate (heat-treated and non-heat-treated) had been seen in the first few years of treatment of a hemophilia patient, it was rarely observed in multitransfused patients (Rosendaal, et al. 1983).

Current Procedures and Challenges

Since the mid-1980s, each of the plasma fractionators has revised their manufacturing and viral inactivation procedures for Factor VIII and IX. Current procedures used in the United States for viral inactivation include (a) heating in solution (pasteurization), and (b) use of an organic solvent such as N-Butyl phosphate with a detergent such as Triton X-100 or polysorbate 80. Current techniques for purifying the Factor VIII proteins to reduce the amount of virus in the product, include monoclonal antibody affinity chromatography and processes of intensified ultrafiltration. In addition, individual units of plasma are currently screened with the following tests before pooling: HBsAg, anti-HIV 1 and 2, ALT, anti-HCV 2.0, and syphilis (Leahy pers. com. 1995; McAuley pers. com. 1995; Mozen pers. com. 1995; Persky pers. com. 1995).

The production of AHF using genetic engineering techniques is a major advance in blood product safety. Recombinant Factor VIII has been available since 1993 and recombinant Factor IX is currently in clinical trial (Mozen pers. com. 1995). Recombinant factor is produced by synthesizing a glycoprotein from a genetically engineered Chinese hamster ovary cell line, which secretes recombinant antihemophilic factor (rAHF) into a cell culture medium. The rAHF is extracted from the culture medium by immobilizing the monoclonal antibody in a series of chromatography columns to selectively isolate the rAHF in the medium (Persky pers. com. 1995). DNA research in factor proteins had begun at the start of the 1980s and Miles, Inc., cloned the factor VIII gene in 1984 (Mozen pers. com. 1995).

In March 1995, two pharmaceutical companies initiated precautionary voluntary withdrawals of immune globulin products manufactured before December 1994 for possible hepatitis C transmission. The FDA's Center for Biologics Evaluation and Research acknowledged that "there is no epidemiologic evidence of hepatitis C transmission by intramuscular immune globulins" but evidence exists for transmission of HCV by nonvirally inactivated intravenous immune globulin manufactured after the institution of the anti-HCV testing (Council of Community Blood Centers 1995). According to the Council of Community Blood Centers (1995), the FDA began testing samples of immune globulins lots not subjected to a viral inactivation step in December 1994. This testing program follows a May 1993 recommendation to immune globulin manufacturers to develop viral inactivation procedures for all their products. The FDA recommends positive or untested lots be used only if lots known to be negative are not available (Council of Community Blood Centers 1995).

Finally, the Committee examined recent modifications instituted by several European countries to improve blood supply safety. It was found that blood supply safety measures adopted internationally included implementation of two-stage viral inactivation processes. Other measures included: decreased reliance on blood products imported from other countries; increased centralized oversight, control authorities and processes; regulation of epidemiological surveillance systems; expert advisory panels for research, testing, and quality control; and establishment of a computerized tracking system for monitoring treatment.

REFERENCES

Bacich, John, Baxter Healthcare. Personal communication to the Institute of Medicine; November 16, 1994.

Barker, Lewellys F., Dodd, Roger Y. "Viral Hepatitis, Acquired Immunodeficiency Syndrome, and Other Infections Transmitted by Transfusion," from Petz, Lawrence D., Swisher, Scott N. *Clinical Practice of Transfusion Medicine* (second edition) Churchill Livingsone, Inc., New York, NY; 1989.

Council of Community Blood Centers. Newsletter; March 10, 1995.

Epstein, Jay S., M.D., Fricke, William A., M.D., "Current Safety of Clotting Factor Concentrates," *Archives of Pathology and Laboratory Medicine*, Vol. 114; March 1990.

Favero, Martin S., Assistant Director for Laboratory Science Centers for Disease Control. Letter to Dr. Edward Shanbrom; September 8, 1982.

Federal Minister of Health. *Report by the Federal Minister of Health to the Committee on Health of the German Parliament;* 1992.

Feldman, Frederick, Armour Pharmaceutical. Personal communication to the Institute of Medicine; November 18, 1994.

Foege, William H., M.D., Assistant Surgeon General and Director Centers for Disease Control. Memorandum to Assistant Secretary for Health; August 6, 1982.

Frantantoni, Joseph C., M.D. Letter to the Institute of Medicine; 1995.

Gerety, Robert J., Barker, Lewellys F. "Viral Antigens and Antibodies in Hemophiliacs" proceedings from *Unsolved Therapeutic Problems in Hemophilia Conference* sponsored by the Bureau of Biologics, FDA Division of Blood Diseases and Resources, NHLBI, and the National Hemophilia Foundation; 1976.

Hammes, William J., Associate Counsel, Miles, Inc. Letter to Institute of Medicine; February 13, 1995.

Hwang, D. "Hepatitis-Free AHF," Alpha Therapeutics, interoffice memorandum to Dr. C. Heldebrant; September 17, 1982.

Leahy, Beth, Director Public Affairs, Armour Pharmaceutical. Letter to IOM ; March 17, 1995.

McAuley, Clyde, M.D., Medical Director, Alpha Therapeutic. Letter to Institute of Medicine; February 8, 1995.

McAuley, Clyde, M.D. Medical Director, Alpha Therapeutic. "Alpha Information Re: AIDS," submission to the Institute of Medicine; September 8, 1994.

Mozen, Milton, Ph.D., Scientific Affairs, Miles, Inc. Personal communication to the Institute of Medicine; January 20, 1995.

Persky, Marla, Associate General Counsel, Biotech Group Baxter Healthcare. Letter to the Institute of Medicine; February 24, 1995.

Petricciani, John C. Letter to Michael B. Rodell, Travenol Laboratories; March 21, 1983.

Rodell, Michael B. Letter to Harry M. Meyer, Jr., Food and Drug Administration; June 14, 1982.

Rosendaal, et al."A Sudden Increase in Factor VIII Inhibitor Development in Multitransfused Hemophilia A Patients in the Netherlands." Blood; April 15, 1983.

Seeff, Leonard B. Transfusion Associated Hepatitis: Past and Present. *Transfusion Medicine Reviews,* Vol 2.; December, 1988.

Shanbrom, Edward. Personal communication to the Institute of Medicine; January 19, 1995.

Trepo, C., et al. "Different Fates of Hepatitis B Virus Markers during Plasma Fractionation," *Vox Sang*, vol. 35; 1978.

Weidmann, Ernst, M.D. and Hoechst AG. U.S. District Court Northern District of Illinois Eastern Division, *Gruca v. Alpha Therapeutic, Co.*; November 8, 1993.

5

Donor Screening and Deferral

INTRODUCTION

The purpose of donor screening and deferral procedures is to minimize the possibility of transmitting an infectious agent from a unit of donated blood to the recipient of that unit, as well as ensuring the welfare of the donor himself. Donor screening and deferral includes measures taken prior to and during the collection of blood or plasma. Specifically, donor screening includes the identification of suitable donors; the exclusion of high-risk groups (e.g., prisoners); use of questionnaires, interviews, and medical exams at the time of donation; and providing donors with the opportunity to self-defer by privately coding the unit label as "do not transfuse" or "not for transfusion" (self-deferral is discussed in detail at the end of this chapter). Donor screening also includes laboratory tests performed on the unit of blood collected for the presence of markers of infectious disease. Two types of tests can be used to detect an infectious agent; a surrogate test (e.g., antibody to hepatitis B core) or a direct test for the virus (anti-HIV using the ELISA test as of March 1985; see Chapter 3). These tests are performed because donors may be unaware that they are asymptomatic carriers of an infectious agent or may be unwilling to identify themselves as a member of a high-risk group. Donor deferral is the temporary or permanent rejection of a donor, based on the results of the screening measures listed above.

By January 1983, the CDC had accumulated enough epidemiological evidence to suggest that the agent causing AIDS was being transmitted through blood and blood products, and also through sexual contact. The evidence also demonstrated that there were several groups in the United States with an increased risk for developing AIDS. The highest incidence of the disease was reported in male homosexuals, who were donating blood frequently in some geographic regions. In the early 1980s, the increased evidence of infections in IV drug users suggested that AIDS was an infectious disease similar to hepatitis B in modes of transmission. As a result, debates began regarding the possibility of increasing the safety of the blood supply through the exclusion of high-risk groups as blood and plasma donors. This chapter describes donor screening and deferral measures before the test for HIV (ELISA) became available in 1985 and addresses whether the actions taken were reasonable given the information available at the time.

Critical Events

Donor screening issues arose in mid to late 1982, when the first cases of AIDS in hemophiliacs were reported and the first possible case of transfusion-associated AIDS was reported in an infant (CDC, MMWR, July 16, 1982; CDC, MMWR, December 10, 1982). As a result, the blood bank community began discussing the costs and benefits of several types of donor screening measures in late 1982 and early 1983. Between December 1982 and December 1983, there were two critical events that presented opportunities for the blood services community to enact new donor screening and deferral policies to reduce the threat of HIV transmission through blood and blood products.

Critical Event 1

On January 4, 1983, the Public Health Service (PHASE) held a meeting convened by the CDC in Atlanta on opportunistic infections in hemophiliacs. At the meeting, the blood services community first heard preliminary data on the possibility of a transmissible agent within the blood supply. Scientists from the CDC recommended that blood banks implement specific donor screening measures such as questioning donors about their risk behaviors and running blood donations through a series of tests, among which the most important was for the hepatitis B core antibody insofar as it occurred in most individuals who had AIDS (Curran, Evatt, Foege, McAuley, Pindyck, Rodell interviews; Foege, 1983). There was broad resistance to the implementation of specific donor screening measures, and the meeting ended with no consensus on the validity of such measures for the exclusion of high-risk donors.

Critical Event 2

On December 15-16, 1983, the Blood Products Advisory Committee (BPAC) of the FDA met to discuss, in detail, all possible options of surrogate marker tests for HIV (see also Chapter 3). This meeting is notable for being a second attempt to address the need to implement surrogate tests as a means to increase the safety of the blood supply and a second occasion when testing was proposed but not recommended.

Explanatory Hypotheses

The Committee identified three hypotheses to guide its analysis of the issues of donor screening and deferral:

1. There was a lack of consensus about the costs and benefits of implementing various donor screening procedures as a means to reduce the risk of transmission of HIV through the blood supply, which resulted in limited responses among organizations to the issues of donor safety.
2. Information available at the time might have been sufficient to convince blood and plasma collectors of the need to directly question donors about their risk behaviors (e.g., sexual preference, drug use) or to use anti-HBc testing as a means to exclude high-risk donors, but other constraints in the environment in which they operated prevented the collectors from implementing a specific policy in the early 1980s.
3. Inappropriate incentives inhibited reasonable decisionmaking by the responsible parties.

Testing these hypotheses against the documentary and personal evidence, the Committee concluded that they were able to support the first and second hypotheses, but unable to support the third. Before turning to a detailed examination of these conclusions, we present a brief history of donor screening practices.

DONOR SCREENING PRACTICES

Hepatitis

Cases of post-transfusion hepatitis were described as early as 1943 (Bensen 1943) and syphilis screening tests were introduced in 1946. In 1965, identification of the virus causing "serum hepatitis" led to a direct test for the presence of an antigenic component of the virus. Prior to 1970, the incidence of post-transfusion hepatitis was 8-17 percent among transfusion recipients (Seeff 1988). During the period from 1970-1972, all blood and plasma collection agencies implemented the test for the presence of hepatitis B virus. Subsequently, hepatitis cases continued to appear in approximately 5-18 percent of transfusion recipients (OTA 1985), strong evidence that viruses in the blood supply other than hepatitis B caused hepatitis (non-A, non-B hepatitis).

Donor Pools

In the late 1970s and early 1980s, blood donor pools included many groups at high risk for AIDS. The homosexual population volunteered to donate blood frequently during this time frame in efforts to help develop a hepatitis B vaccine and to gain a social acceptance (Evatt, Curran, McAuley, Perkins interviews). In addition to homosexuals, other populations who were at a high risk for infectious diseases, such as prison inmates and persons in other institutional settings (e.g., mental hospitals), served as blood or plasma donors (McAuley, Perkins, Rodell, Shanbrom interviews). People in these groups constituted a large proportion of the paid donors in the United States. Thus, both the paid and volunteer donor pool included many individuals from the high-risk populations.

Early Donor Screening Practices

Efforts to have "safe" donors started in the early 1950s. The aim was to eliminate persons who carried the two known blood-borne infectious agents, those causing syphilis and hepatitis. Blood bank personnel obtained every donor's medical history and deferred any donors who had a history of hepatitis. Blood from volunteer donors was known to be safer than blood from paid commercial donors (Allen, et al. 1959; Eckert 1986). In July 1973, the Secretary of Health, Education and Welfare called for a transition to an all-volunteer blood donation system (for whole blood) as part of a national blood policy. In November 1975, the FDA required that all blood units collected be labeled as from either a paid or a volunteer donor (U.S. Comptroller General 1975). At this time (and currently), paid donors were the principal source of plasma for fractionation into blood products such as AHF concentrates.

In 1982 the American Association of Blood Banks (AABB) standards required that each donor meet the following criteria: the donor had to appear in good health, the skin at the venipuncture site had to be lesion-free, the donor should not have received blood or blood components (known to be a possible source of hepatitis) in the preceding six months, and the donor's arms had to pass inspection for repeated sites of venipuncture prior to donation. In addition, the standards required permanent deferral of a donor if the donor had a history of viral hepatitis, a history of reactive tests for hepatitis B surface antigen, or had donated the only unit of blood or blood components transfused to a patient who developed post-transfusion hepatitis within the six months following transfusion. Recent travel to areas considered endemic to malaria led to deferral for six months after return, and donors with clinically active hepatitis were unacceptable (AABB 1982). These standards applied to American Red Cross collection centers and to all other community blood banks that were members of the AABB.

In 1982 the AABB required that all its member blood collection sites perform the following tests on each unit collected: determination of ABO type, determination of Rh type, tests for "unexpected antibodies" prior to cross-match, tests for hepatitis B surface antigen, and a confirmatory test on blood type and Rh type after labeling the unit to discover any labeling errors (AABB 1982).

ANALYSIS AND FINDINGS

January 4, 1983, CDC Meeting

As a follow-up to meetings in July 1982 (see Chapter 3), the meeting in Atlanta on January 4, 1983, was convened to consider opportunities to prevent AIDS transmission, both person-to-person, and through blood and blood products. This meeting was widely publicized, and over 200 people attended, including representatives of the CDC, the FDA, NIH, the National Hemophilia Foundation, the National Gay Task Force, blood banks, and the plasma fractionation industry. While there was a consensus among most plasma and blood collection organizations and PHS agencies that steps should be taken to reduce the risk of AIDS transmission through the blood supply, members of the scientific and medical community disagreed on measures for detecting high-risk donors.

William Foege, director of the CDC, opened the meeting, which was chaired by Jeffrey Koplan, assistant director for public health practice at the CDC. James Curran and Bruce Evatt of the CDC presented data they had collected on AIDS in hemophiliacs and transfused patients. They concluded that AIDS was transmitted by sexual contact and through blood (Curran, Evatt, Foege interviews). They also stated that this infectious agent might have entered the blood supply through donations from infected people, particularly male homosexuals. By January 1983 more than 700 cases of AIDS had been reported, of which approximately 70 percent were in homosexual men. The CDC officials suggested changing the donor screening process to identify homosexual donors with multiple sexual partners by asking male donors whether they had ever had sex with a man (Foege 1983).

At the meeting, CDC scientists also recommended performing a surrogate test for AIDS (to detect antibodies against hepatitis B core antigen) on all blood units. Surrogate testing is "the use of nonspecific laboratory markers" to detected infectious agents that show a correlation with HIV infection. The CDC predicted that implementing the anti-core test for hepatitis B would detect 90 percent of donors with AIDS. There was no agreement that the test would be effective, and there was no consensus to use it.

Outcomes of the Meeting

A series of responses followed the meeting. On January 6, 1983, Donald Francis, assistant director for medical science of the Virology Division at the CDC, wrote a memo to Dr. Koplan, stating that the CDC should proceed to promulgate its recommendations in the hope that the FDA would agree. One of the CDC recommendations was deferral of all blood and plasma donors who

- are IV drug users (already in place);
- are sexually (heterosexually or homosexually) promiscuous (more than an average of two different people per month for the previous two years);
- have had sexual (heterosexual or homosexual) contact with someone who is sexually promiscuous or an IV drug user in the past two years;
- have lived in Haiti in the past five years; and
- have a serologic test positive for anti-HBc.

Francis estimated that this deferral process would eliminate over 75 percent of AIDS-infected donors (Francis 1983).

The blood banks (American Association of Blood Banks, American Red Cross, and Council of Community Blood Centers) issued a joint statement entitled "Acquired Immune Deficiency Syndrome Related to Transfusion" on January 13, 1983. They recommended that donor screening include specific questions to detect early symptoms of AIDS or exposure to patients with AIDS, but they did not recommend asking about high-risk sexual practices. The joint statement addressed the question of whether it was appropriate to limit voluntary blood donation from groups at high-risk for AIDS, and pointed out that this question involved many medical, ethical, and legal issues that were not easily resolved. The recommendations held that despite pressure on the blood banks to restrict blood donation by gay male donors, "direct or indirect questions about a donor's sexual preference are inappropriate." The joint statement also encouraged the use of autologous donations, especially in elective surgery, and called upon blood banks to prepare to handle increased requests for cryoprecipitate (AABB, et al. 1983).

During the early months of 1983, prior to any PHS recommendations, many blood banks added to their donor questionnaires inquiries about symptoms associated with AIDS, such as presence of enlarged lymph nodes, night sweats, and weight loss. On January 14, 1983, the Medical and Scientific Advisory Council (MASAC) of the National Hemophilia Foundation (NHF) recommended that the plasma product industry take steps to eliminate high-risk donors (e.g., IV drug users, homosexuals) from plasma donation. The plasma fractionators began questioning donors and excluding high-risk donors in the first months of 1983, but did not implement surrogate testing (NHF 1983).

The American Blood Resources Association (ABRA), a trade organization for the manufacturers of blood products, issued its recommendations on donor deferral on January 28, 1983. One of the three focal areas of ABRA's recommendations was surrogate laboratory testing. At the time, ABRA recommended against large scale surrogate testing pending an assessment of the issues underlying the implementation of surrogate testing, specifically determining "the adequate availability of testing reagents and equipment of any of the several possible tests under consideration, their economic and logistical impact upon the plasma supply network, the efficacy of the test to exclude high-risk individuals, and other potential consequences to plasma products resulting from the imposition of additional testing requirements" (ABRA 1983).

The PHS promulgated its first official recommendations on the prevention of HIV on March 4, 1983. Individuals at high risk for AIDS were required to refrain from donating plasma and/or blood. Persons at increased risk of AIDS included the following:

- persons with symptoms and signs suggestive of AIDS,
- sexual partners of AIDS patients,
- sexually active homosexual or bisexual men with multiple partners,
- Haitian entrants to the United States,
- present or past abusers of IV drugs,
- patients with hemophilia, and
- sexual partners of individuals at increased risk for AIDS.

Prior to the issuance of these recommendations, donor selection policies (AABB 1982 Standards for Transfusion Services) for both the collection of whole blood and plasma already sought to identify people in the following high-risk groups as being at increased risk of infectious diseases: drug abusers, persons with residence in or recent travel to Haiti, and those with a history of recent treatment with blood products. The PHS made the following new recommendations for preventing transmission of AIDS through blood and blood products:

- Sexual contact should be avoided with persons known to have or suspected of having AIDS.
- Members of groups at increased risk for AIDS should not donate blood and/or plasma; centers collecting plasma or blood should notify donors of this recommendation.
- Studies should be conducted to evaluate screening procedures, including lab tests and physical examinations, for their effectiveness in identifying and excluding plasma and blood with a high probability of transmitting AIDS.
- Physicians should adhere strictly to medical indications for transfusions and encourage autologous donations.
- Work should continue toward development of safer blood products for use by hemophilia patients.

The PHS did not recommend directly questioning donors about high-risk sexual behavior nor did it recommend surrogate testing of donated blood (CDC, MMWR, March 4, 1983).

Later in March 1983, the FDA notified all establishments collecting source plasma and whole blood for transfusion, and manufacturers of plasma derivatives, of the steps needed to decrease the risk of blood or plasma donation by persons who might be at increased risk of transmitting AIDS. The FDA advised the blood and plasma facilities to train personnel who screen donors to recognize the early signs of AIDS and to establish educational programs to inform persons at increased risk for AIDS that they should stop donating. The FDA issued three letters on the reduction of the risk of transmission of HIV through blood and blood products (see Appendix D for the text of these letters, and Chapter 6 for further discussion). The letters recommended the following steps for whole blood and plasma collection centers:

(a) educational programs should be instituted to inform persons at risk of AIDS that until the AIDS problem was resolved or a definitive test for AIDS became available, they should refrain from donating blood;

(b) personnel responsible for donor screening should be retrained to recognize signs and symptoms of AIDS; and

(c) the standard operating procedure should include the quarantine and disposal of any products collected from a donor that was known to have AIDS or was suspected of having AIDS (Petricciani 1983a,b).

The following additional steps applied only to plasma collection centers:

(d) if plasma was collected from a donor belonging to a high-risk group, label each unit to identify it for restricted use only;

(e) examine donors for lymphadenopathy; and

> (f) keep an accurate record of each donor's weight and monitor for significant weight loss (Petricciani 1983c).

These advisories constituted an interim measure to protect recipients of blood and blood products until specific laboratory tests became available.

The FDA recommendations for plasma fractionators stated that "extensive discussions among licensed manufacturers, the Office of Biologics and concerned groups such as the NHF, have led to a consensus concerning an appropriate approach to decreasing the potential risk of transmitting AIDS by certain plasma derivatives." The recommendations included (a) do not fractionate plasma collected from donors at increased risk of AIDS into derivatives already known to have a high risk of disease transmission; (b) use plasma from donors in high-risk groups only for the manufacture of albumin, plasma protein fraction, globulin, or in vitro diagnostic products; and (c) all establishments must label products containing plasma proteins from high-risk donors with "caution, for use in ..." (Petricciani 1983c). The memo made the restrictions effective immediately. Although the FDA did not call the recommendations in these letters regulations, blood and plasma collection organizations promptly implemented them (Bove, Perkins, Petricciani, Sandler interviews).

Donor Questioning and Opposition to It

A representative from Alpha Therapeutics, a commercial manufacturer of AHF concentrate, announced at the January 4, 1983, meeting that the company had instituted direct donor questioning designed to exclude high-risk individuals from plasma donation. On December 17, 1982, Alpha Therapeutics had required the exclusion of all donors who had been in Haiti, used IV drugs, or, if male, had had sexual contact with another man. The announcement of this action met with a great deal of opposition from many groups, including the volunteer blood banks and the gay community. These groups took the position that donor sexual preference was a private matter and that the questionnaire was an invasion of privacy. Additionally, Alpha Therapeutics took the position at the January 4, 1983, meeting that AIDS should be a reportable disease, in order to assist in donor screening (Alpha Therapeutics 1994).

Representatives from other plasma fractionation companies also present at the January 4, 1983, meeting discussed the potential threat to the safety of plasma and their manufactured products. One representative from the Pharmaceutical Manufacturers Association stated: "The fractionation industry voluntarily led the way several months ago in designing and implementing donor-processing programs that were aimed at minimizing participation in plasma collection by members of AIDS high-risk groups. By the early part of

1983, each of the companies ... had in place donor education and questioning programs specifically requesting members of high-risk groups to identify themselves and refrain from donating plasma" (FDA, BPAC 1983a). One explanation for the plasma fractionators' aggressive approach to donor screening may have been the profit motive that drives one company to distinguish itself from its competitors. Executives at Alpha Therapeutics and other companies may have acted upon their belief, or strong suspicion, that AIDS was caused by a blood-borne infectious agent, and as a result implemented screening policies to protect both their company from product liability and the recipients of their products from harm. In addition, Alpha's insistence on the exclusion of high-risk donors in late 1982 may have led other companies, which did not want their products to appear less safe than Alpha's, to implement donor screening policies in 1983.

Some nonprofit blood centers initiated projects directed towards excluding donors or removing infected blood from the available supply. For example, by February 1983, the Greater New York Blood Program was providing donors with information about AIDS, high-risk groups, and the possibility of transmitting AIDS through blood. They asked donors either not to give blood or to give it for research purposes if they identified themselves as a member of a high-risk group (self-deferral). Medical screening resulted in the deferral of an additional 2 percent of donors, and a confidential questionnaire resulted in self-deferral by 1.4 percent of the donors (Pindyck, et al. 1985). The prevalence of anti-HBc in the group who indicated their blood was for research only was approximately 12 percent, compared to 6 percent among those donations marked for transfusion. These gains were weighted against the estimated cost of the anti-HBc test ($3.00 per test) and the cost of discarding a unit and replacing a donor (FDA, BPAC 1983c; Pindyck, et al. 1985). As a result, the New York program relied on "confidential unit exclusion" as a safety measure, rather than implementation of a routine anti-HBc surrogate test. (Confidential unit exclusion involves use of a bar code sticker to label a unit "do not transfuse" or "not for transfusion." See Afterward below.)

Although blood banks did not implement direct questioning of donors about their sexual preferences at the same time plasma collectors did, they did comply with the FDA's recommendations issued on March 4, 1983. These recommendations included the following steps: to expand medical screening of donors, to provide written educational materials to donors about those groups at increased risk of AIDS and the necessity of refraining from donation if identified as a member of the high-risk groups, as well as allowing for individual methods (e.g., confidential unit exclusion) for confidential self-deferral (OTA 1985).

Some people viewed direct questioning about sexual behavior and drug use as a violation of an individual's right to privacy. Public health officials countered by saying that the individuals' rights were less important than the collective public health. Many in the gay community objected to direct questioning and donor deferral procedures as discriminatory and persecutory. Many in the blood bank community questioned the appropriateness of asking direct or indirect questions about a donor's sexual preference (Bove, Curran, Evatt, Foege, Sandler interviews). Other individuals and organizations were concerned about providing the public with information about AIDS that might scare them away from donating blood (Curran, Evatt, Foege interviews). The National Hemophilia Foundation, physicians, and hemophilia treatment centers were concerned about AHF concentrate shortages and favored conveying a "let's not panic" attitude to the public (Curran interview).

The blood banks began with the view that a volunteer blood donor is an altruistic person who, despite the inconvenience, takes the time to donate blood. The idea of confronting such a donor with a prying and personal question about his sexual behavior seemed reprehensible and potentially very damaging to donor motivation (Bove, Sandler interviews). In addition, the blood banks perceived that the gay community might not cooperate if gay donors were rejected on the basis of sexual orientation, and furthermore, that they might donate on purpose or out of spite (Evatt, Silvergleid interviews). Because of their fear of blood shortages, the blood banks strongly opposed implementation of direct questioning. It appears that they decided that informal, "out of the spotlight," negotiations with the gay community were more likely to reduce the number of high-risk donors then implementing direct questioning of donors (Bove, Curran, Evatt, Sandler interviews). As one blood banker representative expressed it, "direct questioning will be counterproductive in most ARC regions, given the public nature of the blood donation process. How many men … are going to step forward, out of their closet, in front of their peers and admit they are 'queers'? Or even call in later to have their donation discarded" (Cumming 1983).

With respect to hepatitis, donor selection practices had changed in late 1982 and early 1983 to restrict donations by some populations with a prevalence of hepatitis B greater than the general population (e.g., prison inmates). Although there was recognition that the male homosexual population had a prevalence rate of infection with hepatitis B that exceeded the prevalence rate in the prison population, homosexual men were not included in the exclusionary criteria (Dodd 1982). No one articulated a convincing rationale for failing to exclude the donor group with the highest prevalence of hepatitis (i.e., male homosexuals) while acting swiftly to exclude other groups (Haitians) whose prevalence was lower.

Prior to the January 4 meeting, the CDC had worked with gay groups to enlist their support for deferring from blood donations (Curran, Evatt interviews). By early 1983, the male homosexual population had established groups that defended their interests in the political arena. Spokespersons for some of these groups were present at the Atlanta meeting and appeared to express concerns that any restriction on blood donations by male homosexuals would be a form of discrimination. Although some representatives of gay groups characterized male homosexuals as willing to undergo testing of donated blood (but not questioning of donors about sexual preference), some expressed doubts that homosexual males would answer direct questions about sexual activities truthfully, in light of the stigma attached to homosexuality (Foege 1983). Representatives of the National Gay Task Force opposed the suggestion to defer homosexual men. The CDC took the position that donor screening procedures were the only way to minimize the risks of infection at the time (Evatt interview).

In sum, the plasma fractionators favored donor questioning as a way to protect their products, and the users of their products from harm and, possibly, to protect themselves from product liability. The gay community saw donor questioning as an infringement of their rights. The CDC viewed it as the sole means of protecting the public health at the time. The blood banks saw donor questioning as damaging to donor motivation and possibly counterproductive to risk reduction. Generally, decisionmakers who did not insist upon direct questioning of donors had several reasons: they were unsure of the propriety of asking donors about sexual activities; they did not believe that direct questions would obtain reliable answers from donors about a sensitive issue such as sexual behavior; and they were concerned about the legal and political ramifications of direct questioning (see for example, American Red Cross memo from Dr. Cumming to Mr. de Beaufort, February 5, 1983, enclosed in Appendix D).

Surrogate Testing and Opposition to It

At the January 4, 1983, Atlanta meeting, CDC scientists also recommended testing all blood units with an anti-HBc test, predicting that the anti-core test for hepatitis B would detect 90 percent of donors with AIDS.

Published data on the accuracy of surrogate marker testing varied in the reported proportion of AIDS patients who had positive tests for anti-HBc. Unpublished data presented by the CDC showed a high prevalence of anti-HBc in AIDS patients, based on data from a cohort of homosexual men with AIDS who attended a sexually transmitted disease (STD) clinic (Foege 1983). Data from several studies based on different groups resulted in findings dissimilar from those reported by the CDC. These studies estimated that the implementation of anti-HBc would detect only between 25 percent and 40 percent of blood donors with AIDS (Foege 1983; Bove, Pindyck interviews). These studies suggest that there may have been variations between groups from different geographic areas. The Irwin Memorial Blood Bank conducted a pilot test on anti-HBc and found a higher correlation between ethnicity and prevalence of hepatitis B than between homosexuals and hepatitis B. The significance of such data did not clearly illustrate the benefit of using the test as a means to identify donors at high risk of transmitting AIDS (Perkins, Pindyck interviews; FDA, BPAC 1983c).

A careful reading of the evidence shows why people could not agree about the frequency of anti-HBc in people who could transmit AIDS. The CDC claimed that 90 percent of AIDS patients had anti-HBc. This statement appeared in public statements and letters, but the Committee was unable to find any 1982-1984 account that described the clinical characteristics and size of their AIDS study population, the methods for measuring anti-HBc, or a table of results. In other words, the standard basis for evaluating a scientific claim, a published report, was missing.

Because those that claimed a much lower impact on anti-HBc published their work, it is possible to evaluate its relevance to preventing the transmission of AIDS by excluding donors who had anti-HBc. These investigators described the frequency of anti-HBc in various high-risk groups (homosexuals, donors who designated their blood for research rather than transfusion, and residents of San Francisco census tracts that had a high proportion of homosexual men). Of course, only a fraction of these populations were infected with HIV. Therefore, the prevalence of anti-HBc in these high-risk populations would be much lower than in a population of people infected with HIV.

In early 1985, the CDC did publish a well-designed study that showed that 62 percent of donors to whom the CDC had traced a transfusion-related AIDS case had anti-HBc (McDougal, et al. 1985). The ELISA test and the Western Blot would be available within a few months (the 1985 article contained the results of using the ELISA and Western Blot to test their study subject's serum for HIV), and a surrogate test for HIV infection was no longer needed. When it was important to know the effect of surrogate testing on AIDS transmission, however, the evidence was inadequate or unpublished. Apparently, no one examined the evidence from all these studies and did what is commonplace in the mid-1990s: to dismiss conclusions based on inadequate evidence and call for well-designed studies. Those who used inadequate or unpublished evidence to support their position were not called to account, and disputants could not agree on a policy for surrogate testing.

Discussions among the CDC's AIDS Working Group in early 1984 concluded that instituting anti-HBc testing would lead to exclusion of far more donors than would be expected to (or actually) have AIDS. If the test were implemented, its primary benefit would have been to allay patient's and physician's fear of AIDS, not to significantly reduce exposure to AIDS (OTA 1985). Thus during the early debates surrounding the issue of whether or not to use the test for anti-HBc as a means to reduce AIDS transmission, knowledge about the usefulness of the test was inconsistent and the value of the test was highly uncertain. The Committee found no evidence that an evaluation was ever undertaken to systematically examine these differences and to determine the utility of the test. In the Committee's view, evidence suggested there were differences geographically that may have made the test more useful in some areas of the United States than in others.

The disagreements about the benefits of surrogate testing resulted in the rejection of the recommendation to implement surrogate testing. There were several reasons behind this decision, including

- the cost of the test;
- the availability of the surrogate test;
- uncertainty as to the usefulness of the anti-HBc test as a screening measure for donors at risk of having AIDS; and
- the fact that the test was not an AIDS test, and that, as the cause and treatment of AIDS was not yet known, the notification of deferred donors as to why they were deferred would be difficult (Bove, Perkins interviews; FDA, BPAC 1983c).

The blood bank community believed that implementing surrogate testing while there was no specific test for AIDS would appear discriminatory and would result in discarding much noninfectious blood. Blood bank physicians raised doubts about the usefulness of the anti-core test for hepatitis B for three reasons. They questioned the validity of the CDC data on the correlation of anti-HBc to AIDS cases among a cohort of homosexuals who attended an STD clinic. They were concerned about donor attrition, which they estimated at over 5 percent among volunteer donors and up to 20 percent among commercial donors, which in turn could lead to serious blood shortages. Finally, some raised the concern that eliminating donors with the protective antibody for hepatitis B could endanger the blood supply, especially for plasma derivatives like gamma globulin (Perkins, Rodell, Sandler interviews). In addition, many believed that blood banks that performed surrogate testing (e.g., Stanford University in 1983) for HIV would attract high-risk donors who wanted to be tested to see if they were infected (Curran, Evatt, Francis, Perkins, Silvergleid interviews), which would decrease the safety of the blood supply (Bove, Sandler interviews; Doll, et al. 1991). At the time, there thus appeared to be within the blood bank community both many who feared for the safety of the blood supply if surrogate testing were implemented, and some who did not view the possibility of an infectious agent in the blood supply as great enough to warrant such testing. The FDA did not mandate screening for hepatitis B core antibody until the late 1980s as a surrogate test for non-A, non-B hepatitis (CCBC 1994; Evatt, Perkins interviews).

Criticism of the CDC's Data and Motives

Participants in the Atlanta meeting and others in key decisionmaking roles expressed reservations about the validity of the CDC data, as they did not believe the CDC to be a credible source of information regarding AIDS (Donohue, Gallo interviews). Some perceived the CDC's urgency regarding AIDS as a self-serving strategy to ensure its (CDC's) survival. A January 26, 1983, interoffice memo of the American Red Cross stated:

> CDC is likely to continue to play up AIDS—it has long been noted that CDC increasingly needs a major epidemic to justify its existence ... especially in light of Federal funding cuts ... AIDS probably played some positive role in CDC's successful battle with OMB to fund a new $15,000,000 virology lab. This CDC perspective is also obvious from the general "marketing nature" of the January 4, 1983 ... meeting. ... We can *not* depend on CDC to provide scientific, objective, unbiased leadership on the topic. ... Because CDC will continue to push for more action from the blood banking community, the public will believe there is a scientific basis and means for eliminating gays. ... To the extent the industry (ARC/CCBC/AABB) sticks together against CDC, it will appear to some segments of the public at least that we have a self interest which is in conflict with the public interest, unless we can clearly demonstrate that CDC is wrong [Cumming 1983].

In particular, as stated earlier, blood bank physicians questioned the validity of the CDC data on the correlation of anti-HBc to AIDS cases among a cohort of homosexual who attended an STD clinic.

Risk Assessment

Erroneous assumptions about the incubation period and the mortality rate for AIDS led to widely differing, inaccurate projections of the outcome of more vigorous donor screening. Some of the key decisionmakers relied upon their knowledge of the epidemiology of other viral disease to guide them in developing prevention and control measures. For example, it was believed that the incubation period for AIDS was one year, and at the maximum, two to three years (FDA, BPAC 1983b). A minority of persons proposed that AIDS was caused by a disease agent that had a much longer incubation period. In August 1982 *Medical World News* published a theory that AIDS was caused by a retrovirus; in 1982 Edgar Engleman, M.D., also proposed that AIDS was caused by a retrovirus (Engleman, Gallo interviews). The U.S. surveillance systems were ill-equipped to identify diseases with a long incubation period such as AIDS. Although 90 percent of AIDS cases were identified, it was difficult to identify those who were HIV infected but did not have AIDS (Francis interview).

The assumption by many decisionmakers that AIDS was similar to other viral agents in being caused by an agent with a short incubation period led to confusion regarding the incidence of AIDS in transfusion recipients or hemophiliacs, given the large number of blood units and blood products transfused annually (FDA, BPAC 1983b). At the time, there was insufficient information to state the mortality rate of AIDS; many believed it was approximately 40 percent or higher (FDA, BPAC 1983b). Decisionmakers did not know the high case fatality rate of AIDS and tended to deny the possibility of an infectious disease agent that could cause a devastating disease that would be fatal to most (if not all) of its victims. This information deficit, combined with incorrect assumptions regarding the natural history of AIDS, led to inaccurate analyses of targeted interventions for donor selection and donor blood testing. Thus, the known costs associated with donor screening interventions seemed to outweigh their benefits, which were unknown but depended on what were still incomplete scientific data.

If decisionmakers had known that AIDS had a long asymptomatic period during which people were infectious, they would have had to admit that the risk of AIDS transmission by transfusion was much higher than "one case per million patients transfused" (estimate of the American Association of Blood Banks, the American Red Cross, and the Council of Community Blood Centers, June 22, 1983; see Chapter 3). In addition, if they had known AIDS was virtually always fatal, decisionmakers might have been more aggressive about donor screening policies.

Lack of Leadership

The January 4, 1983, meeting in Atlanta was an opportunity for someone to take charge, but the meeting ended in disarray. The CDC had expected to leave the meeting with a consensus to draft recommendations to question donors, exclude all homosexuals, and implement surrogate testing (based on work done in their laboratories). The CDC had chosen Jeffrey Koplan, its assistant director for public health practice, to chair the meeting because he was believed to be a neutral figure in the AIDS effort (Curran, Evatt, Foege interviews). Whereas the CDC had hoped to pass the lead role over to FDA (Evatt interview), Dr. Bruce Evatt said he was stunned that the CDC "hit a brick wall" with the FDA. The CDC had been looking for overall agreement, but the crowded and raucous atmosphere made it impossible to achieve consensus (Curran, Evatt interviews).

The American Red Cross representative, Dr. Gerald Sandler, recalled that everyone at the meeting was "very frustrated" that the meeting did not reach a consensus on actions needed. He also noted that not one of Donald Francis' superiors had supported a recommendation to implement hepatitis B core testing. As a result, few in attendance accepted Francis' suggestions, as they assumed he did not have the support of CDC Director William Foege (Sandler interview). The FDA's role in implementing surrogate testing was not clear, as the FDA representatives believed that more research was needed before the FDA could issue a recommendation (Parkman interview). The lack of good interagency communication was a problem, and some participants believed that someone should have established an interagency, national task force (Sandler interview).

After the meeting, the sentiment at CDC was one of frustration that they had failed to convince others that the evidence supported their hypothesis that the disease was transmitted through blood and blood products (Curran, Foege interviews). Several CDC scientists recall that it was difficult to convince others of the potential for blood-borne transmission and to motivate them to respond (Curran, Evatt interviews).

In his summary report of the meeting, Dr. Foege recommended that each Public Health Service agency provide candidate sets of recommendations for the prevention of AIDS in patients with hemophilia and for other recipients of blood and blood products to Dr. Koplan, assistant director for public health practice, CDC, and the three agencies (CDC, NIH, FDA) should then develop a uniform set of recommendations on AIDS. In addition, Dr. Foege expressed his belief that the meeting had been successful in presenting the most recent data on AIDS and had served as a "forum" for different views to be expressed (Foege 1983).

Conclusions

Blood banks, government agencies, and manufacturers were unable to reach a consensus on how extensively to screen for high-risk donors in order to substantially reduce the risk of HIV transmission through the blood supply. There was no consensus at the January 4, 1983, meeting, and it appears that no individual or organization took the lead to develop a consensus in the months that followed. Lack of agreement on the interpretation of scientific data, pressure by special interest groups, organizational inertia, and the unwillingness of the regulatory agencies to take a lead role in the crisis resulted in a delay of more than one year in implementing strategies to screen donors for risk factors associated with AIDS.

December 1983 Blood Products Advisory Committee Meeting

Interim Local Efforts to Screen Aggressively

In early to mid-1983, studies had shown that AIDS patients had a low ratio of CD4 lymphocytes to CD8 lymphocytes when compared with healthy individuals (Evatt, Engleman interviews; Goedert 1989). On July 1, 1983, Stanford University Blood Bank became the first in the United States to screen donated blood with a surrogate test, which identified reversed T-cell ratios, to reduce transmission of AIDS. Between July 1983 and June 1985 at Stanford, a total of 33,831 blood donations were screened for CD4:CD8 ratios. Of those donations, 586 had CD4:CD8 ratios less than or equal to 0.85 and were discarded. However, serum samples from these donors were retained and later tested for HIV when the test became available. Dr. Edgar Engleman found that 1.9 percent of the 586 discarded donations were later found to be HIV positive (Galel, et al. 1995). The 1.9 percent of 586 donations translates to approximately 11 infected donations that were discarded. Each donation is usually divided into three components (red cells, platelets, and plasma), each of which is typically transfused into a different patient. Therefore, the removal of 11 infected units of blood may have protected 33 patients from acquiring HIV (Engleman interview; Galel, et al. 1995).

The test was relatively easy to implement at Stanford because the Stanford University Blood Bank was conducting immunological research at the time. Others interviewed stated that the CD4:CD8 ratio test would have been difficult to implement on a nationwide scale because the equipment required was costly and the test had to be performed manually (Perkins, Sandler, Osborn, Gompert interviews). It was believed that large-scale use of the CD4:CD8 ratio test required a flow cytometer, which was available only in research laboratory settings (Gompert interview).

In July 1983, NIH's National Heart, Lung, and Blood Institute released a request for application to develop tests to identify the AIDS carrier states and to measure the sensitivity of the tests. Shortly thereafter, Irwin Memorial Blood Bank in San Francisco, directed by Dr. Herbert Perkins, evaluated the anti-HBc test as a surrogate marker for HIV. The study took approximately three months, and the results were difficult to interpret, as the correlation between a positive anti-core test and selected areas of residence in San Francisco was more prominent by ethnic origin than sexual preference. Overall, 6 percent of donors tested positive for anti-HBc. The frequency of anti-HBc was higher in males than females, and the difference in frequency was larger between people of differing ethnic origins than between homosexuals and heterosexuals. The author concluded that implementing the test would not be of clear benefit and that the subsequent exclusion of 6 percent of donors could lead to blood shortages. In general, anti-core testing showed a 6 percent positive rate in blood donors, a 12 percent positive rate in blood donors who self-excluded, a 70 percent positive rate in gay men, and a 95 percent rate in AIDS patients in STD clinics (Pindyck interview). Irwin Memorial Blood Bank did implement the test in May 1984 to ease recipients' fears of receiving blood (Perkins interview).

Reliability of Surrogate Tests

On December 15-16, 1983, the FDA's Blood Products Advisory Committee (BPAC) held a two-day meeting to discuss the possible implementation of surrogate tests on blood donations to exclude high-risk donors. The objective of the BPAC meeting was to "review the results of research to define tests which could be applied to blood, plasma, or donors that would indicate an increased risk of the transmission of AIDS" (FDA, BPAC 1983).

Dr. Dennis Donohue, director of the FDA's Division of Blood and Blood Products, had recommended that hepatitis B anti-core testing be incorporated for routine plasma screening (in addition to current requirements) since it would identify 90 percent of all potentially infectious (or high-risk) donors (FDA, BPAC 1983c). In his opinion, the implementation of anti-core testing would add a further measure of confidence in product safety at a relatively low cost (Donohue interview; Ojala 1983). He stated, "Anti-core testing lends itself to the plasma situation," with only five to six central testing laboratories and one site responsible for product safety within each laboratory (CCBC 1983).

At the December BPAC meeting, industry representatives proposed the creation of a task force to deliberate the details of the recommendation and provide further information in three months (FDA, BPAC 1983c). According to CDC and FDA documents, industry proposed the task force in order to delay the implementation of surrogate testing (Donohue interview; Ojala 1983). An internal memorandum of one participant, Cutter Biological, stated that the proposal to convene a task force "was one that had been agreed upon by all the fractionators the previous evening" and that "the general thrust of the task force [was] to provide a delaying tactic for the implementation of further testing" (Ojala 1983). Although Dr. Donohue was not completely satisfied with the task force approach, he agreed to it; and thus the BPAC created an industry task force to consider the logistics of anti-HBc (core antibody) as an additional screening test.

Task Force Report on Surrogate Testing

The task force created at the December 15-16, 1983, BPAC meeting reported their findings on March 6, 1984. The members were divided as to "whether routine testing of potential blood and/or plasma donors for the presence of anti-HBc was an appropriate means of identifying members of high-risk groups associated with AIDS" (Rodell 1984). The report contained a majority position paper opposing the implementation of anti-HBc and a minority report favoring its implementation.

The task force reviewed several pilot tests performed at blood banks in high-risk areas. The pilot tests comprised four studies on anti-HBc; two studies on B2-microglobulins; and one each on Cytomegalovirus (CMV) and Epstein-Barr virus (EBV), immune complexes, Neopterin, T-cell ratio measurement, Thymosinal, and Alpha interferon. The discussion focused on the anti-HBc test.

Data showed that 5 percent to 18 percent of blood and plasma donors had a positive test for anti-core. The CDC data showed that 84 percent of homosexual males tested positive for anti-HBc and that 96 percent of IV drug users had a positive test for anti-core. The test itself was highly sensitive (98 percent) but not specific (70 percent).

The discussion at the December BPAC meeting had stipulated that "cost-benefit analysis and disease prevalence must be considered in the decision regarding whether or not to use the test" (FDA, BPAC 1983c). However, the task force could not agree upon the true cost of the test, with estimates as low as $2.50 per test for plasma collectors and as high as $12.00 per donation for whole blood collections (Rodell 1984). Additional costs were the blood that would be discarded and the recruitment and replacement of donors. The task force could not agree on the costs and the benefits of using the anti-core test as a surrogate for high-risk donors.

A contemporaneous internal Cutter memorandum indicated that industry believed core testing would eventually become a requirement. At that time, Cutter executives recommended that the company implement core testing as quickly as possible to "obtain a competitive advantage in the market place" and that they "[make] no mention of [their] plans to others" (Ojala 1983).

Support for the Implementation of Anti-HBc. The minority who favored implementation of the anti-HBc test presented the following arguments: 60-80 percent of homosexuals tested positive for anti-HBc; the test would reduce the need for recall of blood products (i.e., AHF concentrate); the test could help reduce the incidence of non-A, non-B hepatitis in recipients of blood products; and blood and plasma collectors had an obligation to do all that was possible to increase the safety of the blood supply.

Opposition to Surrogate Testing. The majority against using the test believed that the anti-HBc test was insufficiently specific for AIDS and would exclude excessive numbers of donors. In addition, some speculated that there would be a reduction in the availability of donations from groups such as Mexican, African, and Asian Americans, who have a higher prevalence of core antibody but whose rare blood types are needed in the blood supply to service that very population. Finally, the high proportion of positive sera from known homosexuals suggested that the test was not distinguishing homosexuals with multiple partners who may have been carriers of AIDS from homosexuals who were not at increased risk of having AIDS (FDA, BPAC 1983c; CCBC 1983). They argued that wide-scale implementation of core testing of donated blood would eliminate approximately 15 percent of plasma donors and 6–7 percent of whole blood donors (FDA, BPAC 1983c). Additional arguments were that the epidemic seemed somewhat contained within defined risk groups; the test would cause blood banks to incur high cost, and there would be a loss of the protective antibodies to hepatitis B in the blood supply.

Comment on the Blood Products Advisory Committee

The BPAC served in this instance as a forum through which the blood banks and plasma industry could, and did, influence the FDA to adopt policies that favored their interests at the expense of the public interest. The membership of BPAC included blood and plasma organization representatives, scientists, and physicians (FDA, BPAC 1983c). The group was not a monolith. Its members differed on the role of government agencies and actions to take regarding blood safety. There is also evidence from internal, nonpublic correspondence that some BPAC members deemphasized the risk to the blood supply in their public remarks but were very concerned in private. At a BPAC meeting in Washington in December 1982, Joseph Bove, M.D., committee chairman (and also chair of the American Association of Blood Bank's Committee on Transfusion Transmitted Diseases), said that there was not enough evidence that the blood supply could transmit AIDS to restrict donations from male homosexuals. However, in a contemporaneous report of the American Association of Blood Banks, Dr. Bove acknowledged the likelihood that AIDS was transmitted by blood. "I believe the most we can do is buy time," he stated, adding, "there is little doubt in my mind that additional transfusion-related cases and additional cases in patients with hemophilia will surface" (Bove 1983).

Informing the Public

The blood industry was concerned about providing information on AIDS to the public lest donors take fright and stop donating blood (Curran interview). In January 1983, Dr. Bove reported on behalf of the AABB's Committee on Transfusion Transmitted Diseases that "we do not want anything we do now to be interpreted by society (or by legal authorities) as agreeing with the concept— as yet unproven—that AIDS can be spread by blood" (Bove 1983).

AIDS Politics

Although many groups within the U.S. population had a stake in blood donations and blood transfusion, male homosexuals were well represented at the table where policymaking occurred, while other affected groups had minimal representation (e.g., patients with hemophilia were represented by the National Hemophilia Foundation) or no representation (e.g., future recipients of blood or blood products). The influence of special interest groups was reflected in the inconsistent recommendations about donor screening in the early 1980s. For example, as discussed earlier, prisoners could not donate blood even though their rate of hepatitis B infection was lower than the rate reported in male homosexuals. Haitians and tourists who had visited Haiti within the past three years could not donate (Katz 1983). There were no restrictions on donation, however, by the group with the highest prevalence of AIDS and hepatitis (homosexuals). Representatives of the homosexual groups demanded protection of gay rights to privacy or confidentiality. Moreover, there was a concern that homosexuals might lie about their sexual orientation and donate blood if blood banks implemented direct questions about sexual orientation (Evatt, Silvergleid interviews). Given the scientific uncertainties and lack of representation by other consumer groups, the demands of the gay groups exerted considerable force in the debates regarding donor screening (Rodell interview).

CONCLUSIONS

This review of the issues and central events concerning donor screening and deferral before the test for HIV (ELISA) became available in 1985 leads to several conclusions, the first of which follows:

- When confronted with a range of options for using donor screening and deferral to reduce the probability of spreading HIV through the blood supply, blood bank officials and federal authorities consistently chose the least aggressive option that was justifiable.

In adopting this limited approach, responsible officials rejected options that may have slowed the spread of HIV to individuals with hemophilia and other recipients of blood and blood products. Among these options were asking male donors about sexual activity with other men and screening donated blood for the anti-HBc antibody. The Committee believes that both of these activities were reasonable to require in January 1983. The question is, given that these options were reasonable and justifiable, why did public health authorities reject them?

Having reviewed the available documentary evidence and having interviewed many of the key participants, the Committee believes that two of its three hypotheses were powerful influences on decisionmaking about donor screening and deferral during 1983. The first hypothesis stated that lack of consensus about costs and benefits of screening and deferral resulted in decisions that took a limited approach to issues of donor safety. The second hypothesis stated that other constraints in the environment—which we categorize below as political, organizational, and historical—prevented decisionmakers from implementing screening for high-risk sexual practices and for anti-HBc. Though both of these hypotheses are supported by the facts, the first hypothesis explains rather different outcomes and events than the second. Their policy relevance differs widely as well.

Hypothesis One

There is little question that lack of consensus about the method of HIV transmission, the natural history of HIV-related disease, and the consequences of alternative modes of intervention to prevent its transmission was an important factor in decisionmaking on donor screening and deferral. There was, for example, uncertainty about the sensitivity and specificity of anti-HBc antibody screening as a method for identifying high-risk donors, and about the consequences of such screening for the safety of the blood supply. Some observers believed that the test was insensitive and would reduce the availability of naturally occurring antibody against hepatitis B infection. Others believed that the test was comparatively sensitive and that the benefits of its use would outweigh any possible costs. Lack of consensus also affected decisionmaking about using a history of homosexual encounters as a screening question. Though some observers, including most at the CDC, had concluded that HIV was spread in a manner analogous to hepatitis B (by exchange of bodily fluids, including blood), other reputable scientists continued to dispute this point of view or to argue that the probability of blood-borne transmission was very slight—a matter of one in a million, and therefore not a threat to those dependent on blood and blood products.

The absence of consensus on these basic matters of epidemiology led to second-order disagreements about the costs and benefits of alternative actions. These cost-benefit calculations were often hidden and unspoken. Indeed, the Committee suspects that many of those arguing alternative views would have been surprised and uncomfortable if told they were actually engaged in a dispute over cost-benefit calculations. However, as they projected the scenarios about what would happen if they undertook one strategy or another (e.g., the implementation of a screening test, the deferral of a high-risk group) and drew conclusions about the desirability of those scenarios, they were, in effect, tallying advantages and disadvantages of alternative courses of actions and reaching sums and totals that diverged from those advocating other approaches.

Uncertainty of this type is common in public decisionmaking, and it would be a mistake to relieve public health authorities of responsibility for their actions every time such legitimate disagreement occurred. When present, however, it has important implications for how decisions are made. Thus, when present, the forces postulated in the first hypothesis heighten the impact of the forces postulated in the second.

Hypothesis Two

It is worth dwelling at some length on the nature and manifestations of environmental influences on decisions concerning donor screening and deferral, for the working of these influences reveals the clearest opportunity for improving decisionmaking with respect to the safety of the blood supply. The environmental forces working on the process of deciding about donor screening and deferral fit the following general categories: political, ideological, organizational, and historical.

Political Factors

The political circumstances influencing the outcome of decisions on HIV/ AIDS took at least two general forms. First, interest group politics were at work in the efforts by homosexual groups to prevent the PHS from recognizing homosexuality as a risk factor in donor screening and deferral. The strong opposition of gay organizations undoubtedly had a major impact in heightening the sensitivity of FDA and CDC personnel to the potential negatives of taking a public health action—avoiding donation by men with a history of sex with other men—that would otherwise have made considerable sense. Interest group politics were also at work in the opposition of the blood products industry to screening for anti-HBc antibody. For the blood banks, and plasma fractionators, this was a matter of dollars and cents, and they used their access to FDA and to the BPAC to make their case.

- Gay groups, plasma fractionators and blood banks had more freedom to make their self-interested cases because the scientific information that would have clarified the nature of the calamity facing the United States was still in dispute.

Political influences took a second form as well in this debate, expressed in the general lack of sensitivity that the executive branch of government showed toward HIV and AIDS during the 1980s. The precise reason for this insensitivity is unclear, but it is clear that the administration was generally reluctant during the first half of the 1980s to treat AIDS as an urgent and serious public health threat. Thus, there was little potential political reward, and some political cost, associated with taking a leadership position in AIDS prevention, especially one that attracted political opposition from vocal and powerful groups that could argue that proposed actions were not required by scientific information.

Ideological Factors

An important ideological consideration at work during the period under review was a general antagonism or the part of the administration toward regulation. Even if AIDS had not been a topic of distaste for the Reagan administration, the issue of regulation itself made controlling the blood supply to prevent AIDS—in the absence of incontrovertible evidence of a public health crisis—an uphill battle.

- The ideological position of the executive branch with respect to regulation put the burden of proof on agencies that wanted to take leadership in regulatory affairs.

This consideration occasions the Committee's fourth conclusion about donor screening and deferral.

Organizational Factors

Interagency squabbling, lack of coordination, and miscommunication are part of the bureaucratic landscape in any governmental setting whether one is talking of towns, cities, states, or national governments, in this country or abroad. Such forces were clearly at work in the case of decisionmaking with regard to donor screening and deferral during the period under review. The Committee concluded:

- By far the most important organizational factor at work in explaining the cautious choices of public health authorities with regard to donor screening and deferral was mistrust and rivalry between the CDC and the FDA.

The Committee was particularly struck by comments made by FDA officials indicating a lack of confidence in the scientific capabilities of some of the CDC personnel. This lack of confidence seems to have reduced the credibility of CDC's early warnings and led FDA regulators, blood banks, and plasma fractionators to discount warnings presented at the January 4, 1983, meeting. The history of the CDC's handling of the swine flu episode less than a decade earlier (during 1976–1977) might have colored FDA perceptions, but the startling fact remains that key personnel in the agency primarily responsible for preventing epidemic transmission through the blood supply (namely, the FDA) harbored significant doubts regarding the competence of the primary U.S. agency responsible for warning of the threat of such an epidemic. It is hard to imagine an instance in which such interagency disagreement could have contributed to a more unfortunate outcome.

The Committee drew another conclusion about organizational influences:

- The structure and process of the FDA's Blood Products Advisory Committee (BPAC) lacked dimensions required to address nontechnical aspects of the controversy.

Because of the highly technical nature of many of its decisions, and the uncertainty that often accompanies them, the FDA has a history of relying on outside advisory groups to provide direction for many of its potentially controversial decisions. The area of blood policy and regulation was no exception. However, in this instance, the advisory system may have failed the FDA because the agency itself failed to understand the extent to which nontechnical issues, that is, issues of how to compare risks (such as the risk of HIV transmission versus the risk of further stigmatizing homosexuals), were actually at stake. The BPAC did not have the social, ethical, political, and economic expertise necessary to understand fully the ramifications of the decisions it was making. Furthermore, given how much authority FDA in effect has ceded to this advisory group, it did not sufficiently represent all potentially affected groups. In hindsight, such representation would have assured that all pertinent points of view would be considered during BPAC deliberations.

Historical Factors

Throughout the Committee's review of events concerning donor screening and deferral in the early 1980s, we were struck by how one historical event influenced the way in which individuals and organizations conducted themselves and interpreted the evidence they were presented regarding the HIV epidemic. This episode, already mentioned above, was the federal government's experience with the swine flu epidemic. In early 1976, at the urging of officials of the CDC, the federal government, with the visible participation of President Ford, engaged in a crash program to immunize every American against a disease that never materialized. Millions were vaccinated, however, and some died of complications attributed to the vaccine (Neustadt and Fineberg 1978).

- The swine flu episode seems simultaneously to have reduced the self-confidence of the agency and increased the skepticism with which its warnings have been regarded by other public health service groups.

It may be that CDC officials did not take a more forceful stand in urging their views out of fear of jeopardizing the CDC's remaining credibility. To what extent the lessons of the swine flu experience have positively influenced the behavior of the CDC, for example, by increasing the care with which it assesses the scientific evidence before issuing a warning of a new or threatening epidemic may never be known. However, the HIV case constitutes one clear example in which the experience and its lessons, however they were applied, led to disastrous results because of concern that being wrong on AIDS and the blood supply could destroy what remained of CDC's ability to see its warnings lead to public policy.

Although participants at the January 4, 1983, CDC meeting did not come to an agreement on actions regarding donor screening, there were several plasma fractionators and blood centers that initiated donor selection and screening interventions that surpassed the recommendations of the blood bank community and federal agencies. The decisionmakers could have defended wide-scale execution of these strategies in two ways: by obtaining information from a broader base of constituents, and by obtaining more information about possible consequences of action or nonaction from representatives of different theoretical premises regarding the epidemiology of AIDS. Instead, swine flu was used as a model by decisionmakers to illustrate the consequences of imprudent action. An important difference between swine flu and AIDS, however, was that swine flu was a threat that did not materialize, whereas AIDS cases were real, not theoretical, and were growing exponentially. Given the serious nature and devastating consequences of AIDS, all parties vested with the protection of the public health or the safety of the blood supply would have been justified in initiating both direct donor questioning and blood testing.

The Committee has not documented that any actions taken by decisionmakers were inconsistent with their responsibilities, but does believe that decisionmakers chose the least risky course (to them) throughout the events as they unfolded. A good example of this is that blood and plasma collection organizations failed to undertake anti-HBc testing and failed to recommend direct screening of homosexuals in 1983.

More stringent donor screening activities were not implemented in 1983 because of the limited scientific information related to AIDS and the influence of political, economic, and regulatory forces with different agendas. The lack of adequate scientific knowledge prevented the key actors from making an accurate (or reasonable) risk-benefit analysis of proposals to change the blood donor selection process. As a result of these uncertainties and pressures from the blood industry and special interest groups, options that would have reduced HIV infection were not chosen, and policies that resulted in minimal change to the blood donor selection process were implemented. These policies not only provided a minimum of political risk to the blood banks and regulatory agencies in 1983, they also provided a minimum of protection from HIV for recipients of blood or blood products.

AFTERWORD

Donor Screening 1985–1995

With the implementation of HIV testing in 1985, the extent of the problem of the HIV infectious agent in the blood supply was quickly understood. The perception of the safety of the blood supply changed both in the public's view and among the blood bank professionals. The era of HIV shifted the field of blood banking from one dominated by serology to one in which infectious disease transmission, donor concerns, and the quest for total safety have become paramount (Bove 1990). Several changes were introduced concerning donor screening, mainly the introduction of new laboratory tests.

Since 1985, donor screening has involved "lookback." Lookback is the tracing of a blood donor found to have anti-HIV (and who had donated in the past), to all recipients of the previous donation(s), who in turn are tested for HIV. Donor deferral lists have been used in the blood banks since the 1970s regarding donors positive for hepatitis B surface antigen (HBsAg), as well as donors linked with post-transfusion hepatitis. These lists have been extended to include donors found to be HIV positive and donors positive for other disease markers. Every donation is checked for previous donation by that donor to see if any unit from the donor has been rejected in the past.

The measures taken up to 1985 are still in effect: avoiding high-risk individuals, questions regarding HIV-associated symptoms, and confidential self-exclusion. Questions regarding foreign travel have been added in order to defer donors visiting areas endemic for malaria or those visiting central Africa, which has a high HIV prevalence. Questions regarding previous treatment with growth hormone have been added to defer previously treated donors because of the fear of transmission of Creutzfeldt-Jakob disease.

Additional screening tests for donated blood have been considered and were added after 1985, both for HIV and for hepatitis.

HIV

The anti-HIV test implemented in 1985 (ELISA) became more sensitive and specific following the first available kits. In spite of the improvement, a few post-transfusion HIV infections from donations in the "window" period (the time period between infection with the virus, but prior to a detectable antibody response in blood or plasma) continued to occur. In order to evaluate the effect of adding the p24 antigen test (a viral antigen that can be present in the window period), 500,000 donors in 10 different areas in the United States were tested for p24 (Alter, et al. 1990). As no cases of p24 positive blood donors were found, the test was not implemented on a wide-scale basis.

HIV-2 is a retrovirus that is distantly related to HIV-1 (HIV) that also causes AIDS in humans. Although it is prevalent in areas of West Africa and other parts of the world, it is only very rarely found in the United States. Despite its rarity in the United States, the FDA required that all blood donations be screened for HIV-2 in April 1992. A new variant, known as HIV subtype 0, has also been described and may also be included in the routine screening in the future.

Hepatitis

Post-transfusion non-A, non-B hepatitis cases continued to be reported. Without any evidence that the causative agent would soon be elucidated, surrogate tests were suggested. Based on previous studies and new evidence, the surrogate testing for non-A, non-B hepatitis was instituted during 1986–1987 by using both the ALT and Anti-HBc tests. In 1989, the genomic structure of a putative NANB virus (Hepatitis C virus [HCV]) was discovered. As a result, a test for antibodies to the HCV virus was licensed and implemented as a screening test for HCV in 1990.

In an NIH consensus conference held in January 1995 (there was no other consensus conference held earlier by the NIH), it was recommended that the ALT surrogate test be discontinued. However, anti-HBc was retained, not as a non-A, non-B surrogate marker, but as a second hepatitis B screening test for cases with low HBsAg titer.

HTLV-I and HTLV-II

In 1988 six positive HTLV-I cases were reported among 40,000 donors (Williams, et al. 1988). In November 1988, a screening test for HTLV-I (virus that causes leukemia and myelopathy) was instituted for all blood units. HTLV-I has been found in the United States, but HTLV-II has been seen more frequently. Not all blood donors with HTLV-II infection are effectively identified using the HTLV-I antibody tests; instances of transmission of HTLV-II by blood screened negative for HTLV-I have been reported.

Current Donor Screening Procedures

Currently, donor screening provides a potential donor with four opportunities to self-defer. Prior to donating blood, each donor is asked to read an introductory pamphlet about donating blood and about infections transmitted by blood, especially HIV. Those who think they are at risk are asked not to donate. This is the first opportunity to self-defer. A trained health professional then conducts a confidential interview with each donor, taking a health history and asking direct questions about high-risk behaviors, including drug use, sexual relations with drug users, and, for men, if they have had sexual relations with another man since 1977. Answering yes to one or more of these questions results in a temporary or indefinite deferral, in accordance with FDA recommendations and requirements. At this time the donor is asked to sign a release statement confirming that he or she has no risk for infection with HIV. This is the second opportunity to self-defer.

Donors are tested for anemia and checked for physical signs of intravenous drug use. Donors receive a "confidential unit exclusion" form and a call-back card. High-risk donors who may not wish to publicly acknowledge their risk behaviors may confidentially exclude their unit of blood by peeling a bar code sticker off the unit exclusion form and placing it on their donation record. A computer reads the bar code as "transfuse" or "do not transfuse" depending upon which sticker is used. This is the third opportunity to self-defer. The call-back card gives donors a telephone number to call within 24 hours and a special identification code to use if for any reason after leaving the donation site they decide their blood should not be used. This is the fourth opportunity to self-defer.

Any unit of blood found positive for any of the tests is destroyed and the donor is permanently deferred by being placed in a computer database (American Red Cross Blood Services 1994).

Current Infectious Risk Through Blood Transfusion

The current estimated risk (Dodd 1992, 1994; Busch, et al. 1995; Lackritz, et al. 1995) of becoming infected by the viruses being tested for is:

HIV (AIDS)	1:420,000
HCV (hepatitis C)	1:2,000 to 1:6,000
HBV (hepatitis B)	1:200,000
HTLV (leukemia and myelopathy)	1:50,000 to 1:70,000

Other infectious agents that are possible hazards are an additional hepatitis agent (non A,B,C), Chagas disease, Creutzfeldt-Jakob disease, Babbeiosis, new zoonotic infections, and new unknown agents. The problems associated with bacterial infection in blood units and especially in platelet concentrates have also not been completely resolved. Other issues concerning the safety of blood transfusion involve the long-term effects of lymphocytes transfused along with red blood cells, as well as with platelet transfusions.

REFERENCES

Allen, J. Garrott, et al. Blood Transfusion and Serum Hepatitis. *Annals of Surgery*, vol. 150; 1959.

Alpha Therapeutics. Statement submitted to Institute of Medicine; September 9, 1994.

Alter, Harvey, et al. Prevalence of HIV Type 1 p24 Antigen in U.S. Blood Donors—An Assessment of the Efficacy of Testing in Donor Screening. *New England Journal of Medicine*, vol. 323; 1990.

American Association of Blood Banks, American Red Cross and Council of Community Blood Centers. Joint Statement on AIDS Related to Transfusion. January 13, 1983.

American Association of Blood Banks. *Standards for Blood Banks and Transfusion Services*, Tenth Edition, Washington, D.C.; 1982.

American Blood Resources Association, Recommendations on AIDS and Plasma Donor Deferral. January 28, 1983.

American Red Cross Blood Services, Documents submitted to the Institute of Medicine; September 1, 1994.

Bensen, Paul B. Jaundice Occurring One to Four Months After Transfusion of Blood or Plasma. *Journal of the American Medical Association*, vol. 121: 1943.

Bove, Joseph, Chairman, Committee on Transfusion Transmitted Disease. Report to the Board, American Association of Blood Banks; January 24, 1983.

Bove, Joseph. Testing in the Years Ahead. *Transfusion*, Vol. 30; 1990.

Busch, Risk of Human Immunodeficiency Virus transmission by blood transfusions before the implementation of HIV-1 anti-body screening. *Transfusion*; 1991.

Busch, et al. Paper presented at the NIH Consensus Development Conference; January 1995.

Centers for Disease Control, *Morbidity and Mortality Weekly Report* , July 16, 1982

Centers for Disease Control, *Morbidity and Mortality Weekly Report* , December 10, 1982

Centers for Disease Control, *Morbidity and Mortality Weekly Report* , Prevention of Acquired Immune Deficiency Syndrome (AIDS): Report of Inter-Agency Recommendations; March 4, 1983.

Council of Community Blood Centers. *Blood Products Advisory Committee Recommends Fractionators Use Anti-core Screening Test*. Council of Community Blood Centers Newsletter; December 23, 1983.

Council of Community Blood Centers. Submission to the Institute of Medicine; 1994.

Cumming, American Red Cross. Memorandum to Mr. de Beaufort, American Red Cross National Headquarters; February 5, 1983.

Dodd, Roger, American Red Cross. Memorandum to Katz, Executive Director, Blood Services; July 9, 1982.

Dodd, Roger. "Adverse Consequences of Blood Transfusion: Quantitative Risk Estimates." in *Blood Supply: Risks, Perceptions, and Prospects for the Future*. American Association of Blood Banks; 1994.

Dodd, Roger. The Risk of Transfusion-Transmitted Infections. *New England Journal of Medicine*, vol. 327; 1992.

Doll, et al. Human Immunodeficiency Virus type 1 Infected Blood Donors: Behavioral Characteristics and Reasons for Donation. *Transfusion*; May 1991.

Eckert, R. AIDS and the Blood Bankers. *Regulation*; September 1986.

Food and Drug Administration. Blood Products Advisory Committee, July 19, 1983a.

Food and Drug Administration. Blood Products Advisory Committee, February 7, 1983b.

Food and Drug Administration. Blood Products Advisory Committee, December 15–16, 1983c.

Foege, William. *Summary Report of Workgroup to Identify Opportunities for Prevention of Acquired Immune Deficiency Syndrome (AIDS);* January 4, 1983.

Francis, Donald, CDC. Memorandum to Koplan, Jeffrey; January 6, 1983.

Galel, et al. Prevention of AIDS Transmission Through Screening of the Blood Supply. *Annual Reviews of Immunology*, Vol. 13; 1995.

Goedert, A Prospective Study of HIV Type 1 Infections and the Development of AIDS in Subjects with Hemophilia. *New England Journal of Medicine* , 1989.

Katz, American Red Cross. Information to Blood Service Regions, BSL 83-12; January 26, 1983.

Lackritz, et al. Paper presented at NIH Consensus Development Conference; January 1995.

McDougal, J.S., Martin, L.W., Cort, S.P., Mozen, M., Heldebrant, C.M., Evatt, B.L., "Thermal Inactivation of the Acquired Immunodeficiency Syndrome Virus, Human T Lymphotropic Virus-III/Lymphadenopathy-associated Virus, with Special Reference to Antihemophilic Factor," *The Journal of Clinical Investigation*, Vol. 76; August 1985.

National Hemophilia Foundation. Recommendations to Prevent AIDS in Patients with Hemophilia. January 14, 1983.

Neustadt, R. and Fineberg, H. The Swine Flu Affair: Decisionmaking on a Slippery Disease. U.S. Department of Health, Education, and Welfare; 1978

Ojala, S., Cutter. Memorandum to those listed; December 19, 1983.

Office of Technology Assessment. *Blood Policy and Technology*. U.S. Government Printing Office, Washington, D.C.; January 1985.

Petricciani, John, M.D., Food and Drug Administration, Office of Biologics. Letter to All establishments collecting human blood for transfusion. March 21, 1983a.

Petricciani, John, M.D., Food and Drug Administration, Office of Biologics. Letter to All establishments collecting source plasma. March 24, 1983b.

Petricciani, John, M.D. Food and Drug Administration, Office of Biologics. Letter to All licensed manufacturers of plasma derivatives. March 24, 1983c.

Pindyck J, et al. Measures to Decrease the Risk of Acquired Immune Deficiency Transmission by Blood Transfusion. Evidence of Volunteer Blood Donor Cooperation. Transfusion, vol. 25; 1985.

Rodell, Michael. Hepatitis B Core Antibody Testing Study Group. *Plasma Quarterly;* Fall 1984.

Seeff, Leonard. Transfusion Associated Hepatitis: Past and Present. *Transfusion Medicine Reviews*; December 1988.

U.S. Comptroller General. Report to the Congress, *Problems Carrying Out the National Blood Policy;* 1975.

Williams, Alan E., et al. Seroprevalence and Epidemiological Correlates of HTLV-1 Infection in U.S. Blood Donors. *Science*, vol. 240; 1988.

6

Regulations and Recall

INTRODUCTION

The Food and Drug Administration (FDA) is the principal regulatory agency with respect to blood and blood products, but it exercises its authority largely through informal action. For example, recall—the removal of a product from the market—exemplifies the relationship between the FDA's potent formal powers and its informal modus operandi. Recall is a voluntary act undertaken by the manufacturer but overseen by the FDA, which has authority to seize or delicense a product. Because the FDA's resources are quite limited, and because the regulation of blood and blood products is based on scientific consensus (much in the same way as the establishment of scientific facts generally), the agency relies upon the blood industry and others for advice. The FDA's Blood Products Advisory Committee (BPAC) is a venue for consensus building about blood regulatory policy. In an industry in which company and product reputation is critical to market success, the FDA's collegial and informed approach is usually effective.

This chapter presents an analysis of the FDA regulation of blood and blood products during the study period 1982-1986, when the HIV virus began to threaten the integrity of the blood supply and before tests and procedures were established and disseminated sufficiently to control, if not virtually eliminate, that threat. The analysis extends to consideration of a policy concerning the identification and notification of persons who may have received contaminated blood or blood products that was not formally put in place until 1991. In carrying out the analysis, the Committee examined the FDA's exercise of its regulatory powers and the actions it took during four critical events. For each of these events, the Committee posed a series of five hypotheses to explain the

FDA's actions. These hypotheses focused consideration on (1) the reach of the agency's legal powers, (2) the information available at the time in relation to relevant public health considerations, (3) the FDA's resources, (4) the FDA's institutional culture, and (5) the economic costs of particular actions and the prevailing political climate.

A later section of the chapter includes a short discussion of other federal agencies and of private organizations involved in the regulatory process. The section immediately below introduces the framework of analysis: critical events, related regulatory policy questions, and explanatory hypotheses.

FRAMEWORK OF ANALYSIS

Critical Events

The history of the threat that HIV infection posed to the safety of blood and blood products, and the eventual suppression of that threat through the combination of private and public actions, can be told from numerous perspectives. Any one perspective will to some degree falsify and distort a multifaceted narrative. This chapter structures the story in terms of the Committee's interest in the appropriate development of FDA recall and lookback (recipient tracing) policies. The Committee highlights a series of "choice points" (either events or nonevents) that were presented to the FDA as increments of information about AIDS as a disease—and about possible means of preventing its spread through blood and blood products—became available.[1] In particular we consider the following critical events and questions discussed in the following sections.

Critical Event 1

On March 24, 1983, the FDA issued letters to all blood banks, plasma centers, and plasma fractionators requiring particular practices related to donor

---

[1] Unfortunately, "information" in this context is not entirely separable from the very regulatory process under investigation. The information the FDA required of plasma fractionators and blood banks, and the points in time when the agency took certain "facts" to be established are also regulatory decisions. Hence, the Committee has been interested not only in whether the FDAappears to have acted appropriately given the information available to it, but also the degree to which the agency set appropriate thresholds for the determination of scientific facts and made appropriate demands upon others to investigate importantunknown variables that bore on it regulatory policies.

screening and the segregation of high-risk plasma supplies (Petricciani 1983a,b, c). Further regulatory action was possible at this time, although not necessarily prudent. The Committee sought to understand why, for example, manufacturers were not asked to withdraw and/or recall all existing products derived from donors who were not screened for AIDS on an orderly basis (i.e., on a schedule that would not seriously have affected the availability of blood and blood products)?

Critical Event 2

On July 19, 1983, the Blood Products Advisory Committee (BPAC) recommended to the FDA that recall of AHF concentrate and other plasma products not be "automatic" when those products had been linked to an individual donor that had been identified as having or as suspected of having AIDS (FDA, BPAC 1983). The FDA accepted this recommendation and, shortly thereafter, adopted a policy that a recall decision regarding AHF produced from a plasma pool that included material from a donor who was later found to have AIDS should be evaluated on a case-by-case basis, which would take into account for each suspected donor the accuracy of the diagnosis, the occurrence of the symptoms in relation to date of donation, and the impact of the recall on the supply of AHF (Novitch 1983). Was the FDA's acceptance of the BPAC recommendation a well-considered judgment? Even if it were, was the case-by-case recall policy sufficiently well specified and supported that it could be implemented effectively by the industry participants involved? Why was the policy applied only to AHF concentrate and not to cryoprecipitate, which when used can involve multiple infusions of single donor units that are stored before use?

Critical Event 3

Heat-treated AHF became available in 1983 (Persky pers. com. 1995), and by 1985 heat treatment had been accepted as effective in inactivating HIV (McDougal, et al. 1985). Why did the FDA wait until 1989 to require the recall and destruction of all untreated units?

Critical Event 4

By 1985, there was wide consensus that transfusion of HIV-infected blood products led to HIV infection in the transfusion recipient (Goedert and Gallo 1985; Curran, et al. 1984). Recipients became infective immediately but remained asymptomatic for approximately five years (Bove 1986) during which time their intimate contacts were at risk of acquiring HIV. In 1988, a presidential directive to the Department of Health and Human Services was issued on blood safety based on the report of the Presidential Commission on the Human Immunodeficiency Virus. The Department was instructed to formulate a policy for tracing recipients of possibly infected blood products ("lookback") and informing them of potential risks. However, the FDA did not issue recommendations until September 1991 (FDA, BPAC 1991a,b). Why were a presidential directive and six years of agency development (1985-1991) necessary to put such a policy into effect?

FDA Regulatory Authority and Practice

Since 1972, the FDA has been the principal regulatory agency with respect to blood and blood products. The FDA exercises its regulatory authority in an environment in which other agencies play important research, public information, and coordination roles. The agency clearly is dependent upon the information generated by these other federal agencies and by other public and private organizations. Nevertheless, the FDA's statutory regulatory authority is very extensive [federal Food, Drug and Cosmetics Act and the Public Health Services Act, codified at 42 U.S.C. § 262] (Hutt and Merrill 1991).

The FDA licenses all collectors and producers of blood and blood products; licenses those products themselves; and prescribes general regulations applicable to the production, testing, labeling, recordkeeping, and most other aspects of the blood collection, production, and distribution process. It is authorized to enforce its requirements in court by seizure, injunction, or criminal prosecution, and administratively by suspending or revoking the license of a producer of a blood product.

Interestingly enough, the formal powers of the FDA do not include mandatory recalls of products, although recall decisions loom large in the analysis in this chapter. Technically, all recalls of blood and blood products are voluntary [21 C.F.R. Subpart A and Subpart B, 1992]. The FDA has such broad authority under Section 262 of the Public Health Services Act that it could probably create a mandatory recall process by regulation (Falter 1994; FDA 1988). However, it has never adopted regulations of this type. Most recalls are manufacturer initiated, although some are undertaken at the urging of the FDA. Manufacturers recall their products in order to protect the public health, protect their own reputations, avoid civil litigation, and avoid the utilization of the FDA's formal powers of seizure, injunction, criminal prosecution, license suspension, or license revocation. Recalls are thus undertaken "in the shadow" of the FDA's formal powers. Moreover, the FDA has regulations and guidelines concerning how recalls will be conducted. Those documents describe a process in which manufacturers must notify the agency of all manufacturer-initiated recalls. The FDA works with manufacturers in every recall to determine the breadth and depth of the recall activity that is required [21 C.F.R. Subpart A and Subpart B, 1992] (FDA 1988).

The legal informality of the FDA recall process is emblematic of the agency's general approach to regulation. This informality is not necessarily evidence of a weak regulatory posture. Indeed, informal action by the FDA will often be more effective than formal action. The agency owes its ability to act informally in part to its extremely powerful statutory authority. An FDA action to suspend the license of a producer of blood products, for example, has the immediate effect of shutting down the manufacturer's business. Suspending a product license or instituting a proceeding to seize a product already distributed will almost surely destroy the market for that product. Given these formal possibilities, the FDA can expect significant cooperation from industry when it suggests or recommends changes in existing practices.

In addition, the plasma fractionation industry, like the pharmaceutical and food industries, is highly dependent upon the retention of public confidence. Reputational effects loom large and manufacturers generally have strong incentives to self-police and to be seen as "good citizens" who comply with all regulatory criteria. Manufacturers must also consider the costs of civil litigation should a violation of FDA requirements cause harm to persons using their products. It is perhaps worth noting that so-called "blood shield laws" protect those who supply certain blood products, such as whole blood, from civil responsibility for non-negligent injuries (see Chapter 2).

Perhaps most importantly, the regulation of blood and blood products is a scientific enterprise that operates within the broader norms of the scientific and medical communities. Those norms include broad-based cooperation in advancing scientific knowledge. Just as the establishment of most scientific fact is based on the development of a consensus view, so the appropriateness of regulatory action in relation to blood and blood products often operates by consensus. To the extent that the FDA can establish a collegial consensus on the state of scientific knowledge and on the appropriate actions to be taken to protect the public health given that knowledge, it can be assured both that its regulatory actions will be perceived to be well-considered and that they will be largely self-enforcing.

Effective, informal regulatory techniques also economize mightily on agency resources. Use of formal regulatory powers is often an extraordinarily costly and time-consuming process in the American legal system. That system's commitments to fairness, accuracy in the determination of facts, public participation, and political and legal accountability can make even the smallest, formal, legal task a bureaucratic nightmare.

Like any regulatory posture, the advantages of the collegial or cooperative approach to regulation that has characterized the FDA's regulation of the blood supply and blood products involve attendant disadvantages (Dubinsky, Meyer, Quinnan interviews). Collegiality can easily merge into coziness and lassitude. The perceived need to secure future cooperation can deter the timely exercise of power. The agency can become too dependent on regulated parties for voluntary submission of the information necessary for the agency's actions, as well as on industry self-regulation, as the first line of defense of the public health. Informal approaches may also have differential effects in a heterogeneous industry that includes large, centralized, and well-informed members as well as small, dispersed, and relatively under-informed participants.

Finally, consensus approaches may be inhibiting in the arena of regulating blood and blood products. These products are often lifesaving when administered, are critically necessary to certain groups of individuals (e.g., hemophiliacs), and are almost constantly in limited supply. Historically the "consensus" in the blood industry and those dependent upon its products has been to err in favor of maintaining product availability (FDA, BPAC 1983; Aledort, Rodell interviews).

Significant political will would be required, therefore, to take independent formal action given these long-standing informal understandings. In the primary period under study there is reason to believe that such political will would have been difficult to muster at the FDA. Not only was the general regulatory climate deregulatory in tone, the Reagan administration was slow to highlight AIDS as a public health crisis and the Centers for Disease Control and the FDA's Bureau of Biologics were still recovering from criticism that it had behaved much too aggressively in pursuing the swine flu vaccine.

Many of the questions that have been raised about the FDA's activities concerning the protection of the blood supply and blood products from contamination by HIV relate to the informality and tardiness of the FDA's regulatory actions (Donohue, Evatt, Feldman, Lipton, Rodell interviews). But even with 20/20 hindsight it is often difficult to determine whether the FDA utilized its powers—both formal and informal—appropriately. Evaluating whether actions were timely or appropriately formal depends upon recreating the historical context of those actions, including the knowledge base available to the FDA and the contemporaneous actions of private parties that would make public action appear either necessary or unnecessary under the circumstances. Because confident re-creation of the contemporaneous context is often impossible, and because interpretation of events in the light of subsequent knowledge might be misleading and unfair, the Committee has often been led to conclude that while actions may not have been optimal, they cannot be said to have been unreasonable.

Nevertheless, in retrospect we can learn lessons that suggest changes to the blood regulatory system that might produce better outcomes in relation to some future threat. In other words, while the Committee is uncertain how many regulatory decisions would have been *specifically* altered by changes in regulatory approach, it is reasonably confident that certain process changes would have given the FDA a better chance *in general* of producing improved public health results.

Explanatory Hypotheses

The Committee developed operating hypotheses that attempt to take account of the legal authority of relevant actors, the information available in particular time periods, the countervailing public health considerations that bore on particular decisions, the resource limitations that constrained particular actors, the institutional culture and structure within which decisions were made, and the economic and political incentives that bore on decisionmaking. Our general working hypotheses are captured in the following five explanatory propositions that—at least in theory—can be "applied to" or "tested against" particular regulatory actions or inactions:

1. Available information had not reached the necessary threshold for action given the legal authority of the relevant actor(s).
2. Information was legally sufficient for a relevant action, but that action was not clearly warranted by the facts given countervailing public health considerations.
3. Action was legally warranted and justifiable in the interest of public health, but was delayed or aborted by resource limitations.
4. Action was legally warranted and considered to be justifiable in the interest of public health, but was delayed or aborted because of the existing institutional structures, relationships, or standard operating procedures within which action was taken.
5. Action was legally warranted and considered to be justifiable in the interest of public health, but was delayed or aborted because of fears of either the economic or the political consequences of taking the action in question.

Each one of these general hypotheses has been restructured in specific terms in relation to the critical events scrutinized. These hypotheses are not necessarily exhaustive and are not mutually exclusive. Moreover, because questions concerning legal authority and public health policy (Hypotheses 1 and 2) are more easily analyzed than the indirect effects of resource constraints, standard operating procedure, and economic or political concerns (Hypotheses 3, 4, and 5), these latter hypotheses are often somewhat underdeveloped. The Committee often concluded that the influence of the factors that Hypotheses 3 to 5 test cannot be ruled out—indeed these factors are ever-present aspects of human decisionmaking, but that should not be confused with a finding that these factors have been shown to have had a determinate impact on the specific decisions analyzed.

FINDINGS AND CONCLUSIONS

FDA Letters of March 1983

On March 24, 1983, Joseph Petricciani, Director of the FDA Bureau of Biologics, issued three letters recommending steps to take to reduce the risk of transmission of AIDS through blood and blood products. These letters went to whole blood collection centers, plasma collection centers and plasma fractionators. Common to all these letters is a request that measures be taken to institute appropriate donor screening practices and procedures for individual donors and donor groups known to be at increased risk for transmitting AIDS (Petricciani, 1983a,b,c). (See also Chapter 3, Chapter 5, and Appendix D).

The letters sent by Dr. Petricciani (1983a,b,c) are interesting from three different perspectives. The letters recommend slightly different requirements. The requirements recognize the differing positions of whole blood collection centers, plasma collection centers and plasma fractionators in the collection and distribution of blood and blood products. The letter to plasma fractionators seems to have imposed a higher standard of donor education on source plasma collectors than for blood banks that collect blood for transfusion. For example, both blood banks and plasma collection centers were instructed to revise their standard operating procedures to include the quarantine and disposal of blood and/or plasma collected from a donor known or suspected to have AIDS (i.e., an individual with a history of night sweats, unexplained fevers, unexpected weight loss, or signs of lymphadenopathy or Kaposi's sarcoma). In addition to these requirements, plasma collection centers were required to label each unit of plasma if it was collected from a high-risk donor, to examine donors for lymphadenopathy, and to record the donor's weight prior to each donation. The American Blood Resources Association (ABRA) complained of this disparity and questioned its scientific and public health rationale (Reilly 1983). ABRA suggested that the plasma center protocol be applied to blood banks as well. Dr. Petricciani responded (on August 22, 1983) by saying only that there was concern that more demanding requirements might adversely affect the supply of whole blood.

The letters did not specify what was to be done about plasma or derivatives that had been collected from unscreened donors (i.e., individuals who had not been specifically questioned about early signs and symptoms of AIDS or whether they were members of high-risk groups) and had not yet been used. None of the letters required, by its terms, that collection centers or plasma fractionators segregate or destroy products collected or manufactured prior to the date of the letters. The Committee believes, however, that collection centers or plasma fractionators could have interpreted these recommendations as requiring that they withdraw or at least segregate all products that they had collected from unscreened donors and were currently in their stocks. Because these letters asserted that they were based upon a consensus of the collection centers and the plasma fractionators, the Committee believes that the letters suggested that these practices were ongoing at most, if not all, blood collection centers and blood products manufacturers at the time that the letters were issued.

Analysis

The Committee has not been able to determine definitively what the intended legal effect of these letters was or precisely how the letters were understood by their recipients. There are reports, both in testimony prepared for this Committee (McAuley interview; Gury 1982) and in the summary of the Public Health Service's Workshop to Identify Opportunities for Prevention of Acquired Immune Deficiency Syndrome (1983), suggesting that blood and plasma collection centers were engaging in some types of donor screening activities as early as December 1982 (Silvergleid interview; Gury 1982; see also Chapter 5). On December 17, 1982, Alpha Therapeutics began excluding the use of plasma from all donors who had been in Haiti, had used IV drugs, or, if male, had sexual contact with another man (Gury 1982). Alpha Therapeutics also adopted a policy effective December 26, 1982, that its affiliates should no longer send it any unscreened plasma (Gury 1982). There are, in addition, indications from the National Hemophilia Foundation's (NHF) Medical and Scientific Advisory Council (MASAC) (NHF 1983) and from recommendations of the ABRA issued on January 28, 1983, that most plasma fractionators and collection centers were moving toward donor screening and donor education programs in January 1983. Hence, it is impossible to know to what extent the stock of plasma or whole blood present in March 1983 contained blood or plasma that had not been subjected at least to some forms of donor screening.

On the other hand, donor screening practices may have varied substantially up to this point and may have been routine only in some organizations. Nor is there evidence that plasma fractionators were engaging in precisely the segregation and selective processing activities suggested by the Petricciani letters (1983a,b,c). Hence, it seems reasonable to suppose that there were substantial stocks of products in plasma fractionators' inventories and elsewhere that had not been screened in accordance with the FDA letters' directions.

The March 24, 1983, letters clearly did not impose a requirement that collection centers or plasma fractionators recall products that had not been collected or produced in accordance with the FDA's recommendations. The recall record that has been compiled by the Committee does not suggest that there was a rush to recall products following receipt of the FDA letters (Petricciani 1983a,b,c). Therefore, it seems unlikely that plasma fractionators interpreted these letters as requiring recalls. This in turn raises the question of why the FDA did not require a recall of unscreened and unsegregated (or selectively manufactured) products at this time.

The Committee failed to reject the first hypothesis; that the FDA lacked the legal authority or the resources to demand a recall seems unlikely. The FDA seems to take the position that it can request or require (by threat of seizure or of other action) a recall in any circumstance in which blood or a blood product fails to meet existing requirements or poses a risk to the public health [21 C.F.R. §7.11] (FDA 1988, 1994). The latter criterion seems clearly to fit this case and the former may as well. The Petricciani letters could be viewed as an official recognition of the existence of a good manufacturing practice rather than as a new requirement. And the FDA has taken the position (Falter 1994; Parkman, Quinnan interviews) that it can enforce good manufacturing practices that are or have become the industry standard even though they are not explicitly codified in any FDA issuances.

It seems unlikely that the FDA was influenced not to engage in recall activity because of resource constraints. Recalls put virtually all of the resource requirements on collectors or plasma fractionators. The FDA must monitor this process, but there is no suggestion that it did not have the resources to do that. (In the face of strong manufacturer resistance, the FDA would have had to engage in formal action, possibly a seizure. This could have been enormously resource intensive and probably could not have been carried through if attempted. But "massive resistance" is virtually unknown in this industry.)

On the basis of what the Committee currently knows, none of the other hypotheses can be rejected definitively. The March 21 and 24 letters (Petricciani 1983a,b,c) make clear that the FDA considered that contaminated blood or plasma (including AHF concentrate) might be a public health hazard. It is not clear, however, what the effect would have been on the availability of blood and blood products had the FDA required the recall of all stocks that had not been collected or manufactured in accordance with the requirements memorialized in the March 24 recommendations. There was grave concern in the whole blood collection and plasma fractionation industry, as well as in the medical profession and among patient groups, that sufficient blood and blood products remain available for necessary treatment. A recall of existing stocks could have seriously disrupted the availability of necessary therapeutic agents.

On the other hand, the Committee is puzzled why there is no evidence from any of the materials that it reviewed that a careful analysis was made of the availability issue or that thought was given to some form of "staged" recall that would replace unscreened inventories as soon as new screened and segregated products became available in requisite quantities (Novitch 1983; Petricciani interview). Hence it is not possible for the Committee to conclude that the FDA appropriately balanced the two public health concerns: risks of infection and availability of blood and blood products.

Although the Committee has found no direct evidence on this point, the FDA's approach to the possibility of a recall in this instance may well have been influenced by its standard, consensus-based approach to regulation of blood and blood products. The letters of John Petricciani (1983a,b,c) are suggestive of this. For example, they did not announce themselves as falling within any particular category of FDA issuance, which, under the FDA's contemporaneous organizational regulations, included "regulations," which had the force of law; "guidelines," which represented approved practices; and "recommendations," which were stated to be "matters authorized by but not involving direct regulatory action." The Petricciani letters (1983a,b,c) were clearly not regulations and they did not state that they were either guidelines or recommendations. Although the letters sometimes used language such as "we request" and asked manufacturers to "please advise the Office of Biologics" of the procedures that they had adopted, there were also sections that were written in the language of demand or requirement. The letters spoke, for example, of "compliance" with the notices and stated that if a producer was not following certain procedures that had been approved by the FDA's Center for Biologics Evaluation and Research for major organizations, its procedures must be submitted directly to the Office of Biologics for approval.

The ambiguity about whether the Office of Biologics was responding to consensus and officially recognizing good practices or was imposing requirements is emblematic of a consensual form of regulatory posture. The action was in the public health tradition of teamwork among multiple actors, both public and private. Moreover, because there was no consensus at this time, an appropriate trade-off between risk of infection and product availability with respect to blood and blood products that might possibly be contaminated with the AIDS virus, a recall may have seemed self-evidently premature.

The Committee simply has no record on the basis of which it could accept or reject the hypothesis that the FDA's failure to demand a recall at this point was motivated in part by considerations of economic loss to the manufacturers or political consequences. There is evidence in the general political and regulatory record, circa 1983, that might lend credence to the hypothesis that stronger action by the FDA would have run political risks. There was a strong deregulatory environment in the administration generally [Paperwork Reduction Act of 1980—P.L. 96-511; Executive Order on Federal Regulation, No. 12291, February 17, 1981] and at the FDA [DHHS response to Executive Order 12291—46 F.R. 26052] which, assuming industry opposition to recalls, might have put the Office of Biologics in a difficult position had it wielded its mandatory powers (or threatened to do so in order to assure "voluntary" recalls).[2] Moreover, as was mentioned earlier, these actions took place in a climate of White House skepticism concerning AIDS activism and the aftereffects of the swine flu incident.

Summary and Conclusions

The Committee is uncertain what public health consequence might have resulted from a more aggressive recall strategy circa March 1983. The uncertainties surrounding AIDS and its transmissibility may well have justified—certainly not rendered unreasonable—the modest approach of the Petriccianni letters (1983a,b,c). Nevertheless, with respect to transfused blood and nonpooled plasma products, small successes in screening out infective blood would almost necessarily have translated directly into lives saved. Hence, the FDA should have implemented its policy in a fashion designed to assure maximum efficacy. The Committee is concerned that the Petricciani letters failed to accomplish this goal in two respects.

First, the letters were difficult to interpret and did not reveal their own legal status. Such a tactic might be prudent from an agency operating at the margins of its regulatory authority, but that was hardly the situation here. Plasma fractionators and collection centers might thus easily have responded to them in quite different ways. Second, there is no indication that donor screening triggered serious analysis of what to do about a possible recall or withdrawal of already collected plasma or manufactured AHF concentrate. In the Committee's view, any action to increase the safety of new blood units or products should trigger systematic consideration of what to do concerning existing, and presumptively less safe, stocks. The Committee believes that this should be done even in situations such as this one, where the scientific uncertainties concerning AIDS and its transmission remained high.

---

[2] On the other hand, it is important to note that recall activity would not have embroiled the agency in an interagencyreview process, in particular the Office of Management and Budget regulatory review process. That process applied only toregulations, not to recall actions. And, of course, the FDA avoided the political and legal pitfalls of regulatory action by using its informal letter process to establish what appeared to be new, good manufacturing practices.

Nonautomatic Recalls

The question of what to do concerning the recall of AHF concentrate that might be contaminated with the pathogen that was the causative agent in AIDS seems to have come to a head in midsummer 1983. Virtually the entire meeting on July 19, 1983, of the FDA's Blood Products Advisory Committee (BPAC) was devoted to the question of what was known about AIDS and its transmission through the blood supply, and what BPAC should recommend to the FDA concerning recalls (FDA, BPAC 1983; see also Chapter 3).

The National Hemophilia Foundation seems to have been the only participant at the BPAC meeting that supported the automatic recall of any product that was found to have been manufactured with plasma taken from a person subsequently determined to have AIDS or to have had characteristics strongly suggestive of AIDS. Indeed, the BPAC recall agenda seems to have been set by an NHF Medical and Scientific Advisory Council (MASAC) position favoring automatic recall (FDA, BPAC 1983). However, that position had been formulated by the NHF prior to the BPAC meeting. At the meeting itself, NHF medical director, Louis Aledort, first stated the NHF position, then followed by stating his personal view that the NHF position had been formulated prior to the consideration of the Pharmaceutical Manufacturers Association assertions concerning the possible impact of automatic recalls on the availability of AHF concentrate (FDA, BPAC 1983).

The BPAC did not accept the automatic recall proposal. Instead, it recommended that product recall be handled on a "case-by-case" basis. The BPAC position was based on countervailing considerations. Distribution and use of "lots" of a product incorporating plasma from a donor with a definite diagnosis of AIDS was clearly undesirable. However, the BPAC was sufficiently concerned about the possibilities of misdiagnosis based on particular signs and symptoms, and about the effect of automatic recalls on the availability of AHF concentrate, that it was unwilling to recommend to the FDA that it demand automatic recall whenever a product was thought to contain plasma from an individual confirmed as or suspected of having AIDS.

The views presented to the BPAC were reviewed within the FDA (Donohue 1983). Based on that review it was decided that the "working policy" of the Office of Biologics would be to evaluate the desirability of a recall on a case-by-case basis whenever a batch of AHF concentrate was found to have been produced from a plasma pool that included material from a donor later found to have AIDS or strongly suspected to have AIDS (Novitch 1983). In each case the Office of Biologics was to take into account its judgment of the accuracy of the diagnosis, the timing of the occurrence of symptoms of AIDS in relation to the time of donation of the plasma, and the impact of a recall based on this particular donor's having had AIDS on the overall supply of AHF (Novitch 1983).

This case-by-case approach did not apply to whole blood or to plasma. Indeed, what to do concerning whole blood or nonfractionated plasma seems to have been missing from the discussion. Nor did the transcripts of the July 19, 1983, BPAC meeting or any of the internal FDA memoranda mention recall of any potentially contaminated units of cryoprecipitate (FDA, BPAC 1983).

Analysis

The Committee questioned whether the FDA was correct in focusing the discussion and recommendations on AHF concentrate. Clearly, AHF concentrate was the greatest threat to hemophiliacs. It was in far greater use than cryoprecipitate and large numbers of donors contributed to each lot of AHF concentrate. Nonetheless, once everyone recognized the danger of material collected from an infected donor before the discovery that he or she had AIDS, that lesson seems equally applicable to all products that could be stored before use. Why, then, did the FDA not instruct blood banks to search their inventory for cryoprecipitate derived from a donor with AIDS and destroy it?

The question also remains, Why did the FDA not demand the automatic recall of AHF concentrate where it was determined that the product had been manufactured with plasma from a known or suspected AIDS carrier? Indeed, an automatic recall requirement could have gone further to include the recall of AHF concentrate manufactured through the use of plasma from any of the high-risk groups identified in the March 1983 Petricciani letters.

The legal hypothesis is once again easily rejected. No one seems to have doubted FDA's authority to establish an automatic recall policy. Other hypotheses are not nearly so easy to accept or reject.

On the face of the record of the BPAC meeting (FDA, BPAC 1983) and background material that has been made available to the Committee, public health considerations were at the forefront of the agency's concerns (Bove, Curran, Donohue, Epstein interviews). One should remember that at this point the causative agent for AIDS had not been isolated. There were still disputes in the scientific community about whether AIDS was a specific disease and, if so, whether it was or could be transmitted through blood and blood products (Bove 1983; FDA, BPAC 1983; Osborn interview). All shades of opinion seem to have been represented at the BPAC meeting of July 1983. Moreover, these scientific disputes were in evidence elsewhere on the public record. For example, in testimony before the House Intergovernmental Relations Subcommittee in early August 1983, Assistant Secretary for Health Edward Brandt stated that AIDS was believed to be transmitted through blood and blood products (U.S. House of Representatives 1983). He further testified that evidence was strong that transmission was by a virus not yet identified and that the virus had a relatively long incubation period. Yet, at the same set of hearings Dr. Joseph Bove, then head of the Yale Blood Bank, chairman of BPAC, and a chair of the American Association of Blood Banks, testified that the scientific community did not know that AIDS could be transmitted by transfusion or through other blood products (U.S. House of Representatives 1983). Moreover, he emphasized that from what was known, the incidence of such transmission was likely to be less than one in one million transfusions (U.S. House of Representatives 1983).

The general tenor of the BPAC discussion on July 19, 1983, seems to have been that there was a strong possibility that a combination of inaccurate diagnosis, multiple donations by a suspected AIDS carrier, and the pooling process for the production of AHF concentrate could result in rapid elimination of all batches of Factor VIII should the FDA adopt an automatic recall policy. A worst-case scenario presented by Dr. Michael Rodell, who was representing the four member companies of the Pharmaceutical Manufacturers Association (PMA) involved with the manufacture of AHF concentrate, seems to have been particularly salient (FDA, BPAC 1983). In Dr. Rodell's scenario, under an automatic recall policy, the identification of a single donor as having or as suspected of having AIDS could result in the elimination of 25 million to 250 million units of AHF concentrate from existing inventories. Because the industry only produced 800 million units of AHF concentrate per year, three or four automatic recalls, based on identification of three or four suspect donors, who were each represented in 50 plasma pools in a given year, might completely eliminate the availability of AHF (FDA, BPAC 1983).

On the basis of discussion at the BPAC meeting, one view that could be taken of the contemporaneous public health situation might be something like this: The automatic recall of AHF concentrate whenever it was found to have been produced with plasma from a suspected AIDS carrier might easily have led to catastrophic shortages of a lifesaving and life-enhancing drug. Moreover, this policy would have been adopted in a situation in which the disease that it would prevent had not been firmly established to exist, the etiology of the disease was unknown, its transmissibility through blood and blood products was not established, and, if established, it suggested a risk of one infection in one million transfusions. Looked at in that light, public health clearly did not demand the adoption of an automatic recall policy. Indeed, it would seem to have demanded precisely the sort of cautious policy that the FDA adopted.

On the other hand, it is not obvious why the scientific information available to the BPAC or to the FDA should have been analyzed in precisely this way. The PMA's worst-case scenario involved a recall because of the discovery that plasma had been used from a very frequent plasma donor represented in as many as 50 plasma pools in a single year (FDA, BPAC 1983). No information (so far as the minutes reveal) was provided to suggest how often this worst-case scenario might occur. Nor was there serious consideration of how collection and pooling might be managed to avoid the realization of this doomsday scenario in the future. Moreover, while there was still disagreement in the scientific community about the existence, etiology, and transmissibility of AIDS, those who disagreed with Assistant Secretary Brandt's testimony to the Intergovernmental Relations Subcommittee were in a distinct minority (Bove 1983; Osborn interview).

Indeed, the working hypothesis of most people in the field seems to have been that AIDS was a disease that had an epidemiologic pattern and perhaps an etiological pattern very similar to hepatitis (Curran, et al. 1984, Goedert and Gallo 1985). On that assumption one would have predicted with considerable confidence that AIDS would be a blood-borne disease and that it might rapidly become ubiquitous in a population, such as hemophiliacs, who took large amounts of AHF concentrate. If the disease also had a long latency period, as Assistant Secretary Brandt had suggested, then it would also be the case that computation of risk factors based on the current number of identified AIDS sufferers would vastly understate the risk. Hence, there was an equally plausible scientific scenario that suggested that without a very strong policy designed to eliminate all infective AHF concentrate from the market, AIDS would become widespread in the hemophiliac community. This, indeed, had been the position of some scientists at CDC and elsewhere for several months (Curran, Evatt, Foege, Francis interviews; Foege 1983).

From the public record it appears that the FDA, in a climate of uncertainty, adopted a middle position (FDA, BPAC 1983). FDA sought a policy that would screen out AHF concentrate potentially contaminated with HIV while maintaining availability of the product.

Nevertheless, there are two unanswered questions concerning this superficially prudent approach. The first has to do with the effectiveness of the approach as implemented. In retrospect, the Committee realizes that the approach was not particularly effective and that large numbers of hemophiliacs were infected with HIV between July 1983 and 1985 (the time at which a high percentage of available AHF concentrate was heat-treated) (Hammes pers. com. 1995; Leahy pers. com. 1995 McAuley pers. com. 1995; Persky pers. com. 1995). Given the large plasma pools from which AHF concentrate was made, it seems doubtful that anyone could have viewed donor screening as likely to be 100 percent effective for this product. Second, it is not clear why the loss of AHF concentrate, or shortage of it, for some period was considered intolerable. Alternative treatment modalities—admittedly less convenient and effective— were available for hemophiliacs (see Chapter 7). The second issue is addressed first.

There is no indication from the public record that the FDA did a careful calculation of the risks and benefits involved in a recall policy that might have been criticized as "overreactive" given the state of scientific knowledge. In a brief letter to Dr. Petricciani, Dr. Dennis Donohue, director of the FDA's

Division of Blood and Blood Products, reported his interpretation of the BPAC review (Donohue 1983). Dr. Donohue concluded that it was clear that the benefits of the availability of AHF concentrate as a protection against life-threatening or disabling hemorrhage far exceeded the risks of acquiring AIDS from the administration of AHF (Donohue 1983; Novitch 1983). What is not clear is why Dr. Donohue came so firmly to that conclusion given the evidence that was presented to BPAC—that is, why the prospective loss or shortage of AHF concentrate appeared to eclipse the threat of AIDS. Nor is it clear why the BPAC evidence and recommendations became the sole basis for FDA's recall policy. There may have been independent investigations and analyses done within FDA that supported these conclusions, but they do not appear in the record that has survived and been made available to the Committee.

The Committee believes it is not possible to conclude that the FDA made a decision that was clearly in the interest of public health given available information as of July 19, 1983. A close reading of the data suggests that a policy, not only of automatic recall, but of delicensing AHF concentrate until further information was available concerning its role in the transmission of AIDS might have been justified on public health grounds. This would have included, of course, a recall of all stocks of AHF then on the market and withdrawal of all AHF concentrate in the inventory of producers. On the other hand, the Committee would like to reiterate that the facts clearly did not compel such an aggressive approach.

To return to the first unanswered question, how effective could the policy that was adopted have been expected to be? It appears to have been extremely poorly conceived—indeed, virtually a nonpolicy. The case-by-case review was to use three criteria: (1) the reliability of the diagnosis, (2) the time lapse between the donor's donation and the appearance of AIDS symptoms, and (3) the effect on the availability of AHF concentrate (Donohue 1983). None of these criteria has any operational content, and in some cases they seem to ask for information that would be very difficult to acquire or process. There are no standards for what is a "good" diagnosis, no time period is established as an appropriate interval between donation and diagnosis, and no quantitative or qualitative guidance is provided concerning how large an effect on availability would be too great to tolerate. Indeed, no latency period had been established for AIDS and it is not obvious how anyone could rapidly determine how much AHF concentrate from a particular donor was still in stock or what proportion of existing stocks it represented.

Because there was no established system of tracking the health of blood donors, the Committee is puzzled by how plasma fractionators were to learn that a donor had AIDS. There is no suggestion that the CDC would or could legally share its lists of AIDS cases with the manufacturers. It was difficult to diagnose AIDS, and AIDS was not, at this time, a notifiable disease except in a few states

(CDC, MMWR, June 1983).[3] Case-by-case recall thus seems to have been a nonsystematic approach that dealt with cases only if an individual was diagnosed with AIDS. However, there was certainly no assurance that most or even many of these diagnosed AIDS cases would come to the attention of the FDA, the CDC, or the plasma fractionators.

The hypothesis that the FDA lacked the resources to engage in stronger regulatory action cannot be rejected. On the one hand, the policy that the agency adopted was more resource-intensive from the agency's perspective than either an automatic recall policy or a blanket ban on further production and distribution of AHF concentrate. Indeed, the criteria established were so vague that the case-by-case approach required revisiting all the factual uncertainties present in the July BPAC meeting in every instance of a proposed recall. On the other hand, FDA may not have had the internal resources to develop an independent and more systematic recall policy. Hence, once BPAC made its recommendation, FDA had little choice but to follow it.

Given these circumstances it is not possible to reject hypotheses that feature the influence of institutional roles and of economic interests or political factors. The FDA's policy seems to have been very much influenced, if not wholly determined, by the advice that it received from the BPAC. That FDA committee included broad representation on this issue, but seems to have been strongly influenced by plasma fractionators. It was the manufacturers and their industry organization that had the important data related to availability and the technology of production. And those data seem to have been highly influential in molding the BPAC position. Moreover, this episode illustrates the potential weakness of consensus policymaking. In the absence of scientific consensus, FDA seemed to feel itself bound to craft a middle-of-the-road policy, which was remarkably vague and had unknown efficacy to protect the blood supply.

Because automatic recall might have virtually eliminated the market for AHF concentrate, the plasma fractionators had very strong economic interests in seeking to avoid that result. Their advice may well have been influenced by this economic interest. (Indeed, in their presentation they suggested that a

---

[3] The CDC reported in the MMWR (June 24, 1983): "During 1982 and early 1983, city and state health departments throughoutthe United States began assuming an increasingly active role in the surveillance and investigation of AIDS. At the annualConference of State and Territorial Epidemiologists in May 1983, the groug affirmed the urgency of AIDS as a public healthproblem and passed, as one part of a resolution on AIDS, the recommendation that AIDS be added to the list of notifiable diseases in all states. The method of making a disease notifiable varies markedly in different states, ranging from a changein state law to regulatory action by the Board of Health or executive decision by the health officer. Several states have alreadymade AIDS notifiable; other states are talking similar action."

general recall would cause them to rethink the continuation of AHF concentrate production.) When the BPAC recommendation is combined with the deregulatory political climate of the times, including the micro-politics of the strong demand by hemophiliacs and the hemophilia treatment community that AHF concentrate remain available, it becomes plausible to imagine that the FDA resolved scientific uncertainty in favor of inaction—or, more precisely, very limited action—when a more protective policy would have been justified in the interests of public health.

It seems important to stress once again that these conclusions are being offered with the benefit of 20/20 hindsight focused on an incomplete record of the events. Had AIDS turned out not to be a viral disease capable of transmission through blood products, an FDA that had eliminated the availability of AHF concentrate in midsummer 1983 would have been at least as politically vulnerable as the FDA that had banned saccharin on the basis of good scientific evidence and a mandatory legal requirement only a few years earlier, or that had moved rapidly to develop a swine flu vaccine.

Summary and Conclusions

Once again this episode seems to suggest weaknesses in the regulatory process related to blood and blood products. The weakness took three forms:

1. A reactive agency posture permitted views of outside parties to shape both the recall agenda and the ultimate policy choice. Apparently, one of the reasons that the recall question was put on the BPAC agenda was the position the NHF's Medical and Scientific Advisory Council was taking on automatic recalls. Then when industry raised seemingly decisive objections to that policy and offered the case-by-case alternatives, there were no other options on the table for discussion. Moreover, blood and blood products of no interest to NHF did not receive consideration.

2. There was an apparent inability to rethink, or gather the necessary factual basis for rethinking, advice from outside parties once it was offered.

3. An acute decision dilemma failed to provoke a search for broader alternatives. If widespread contamination of pooled blood was a legitimate bar to regulatory action, why was there no mandate to search for alternative methods for pooling plasma that would minimize the risk of widespread contamination and avoid the doomsday scenario offered by the PMA? For example, the FDA could have encouraged the plasma fractionation industry to devise methods that would make it economically feasible to reduce the number of donors to a lot of pooled plasma. (There has apparently been no change in this situation. In December 1994, Dr. Rodell posed a similar scenario at the BPAC during a

discussion on the possible recall of AHF thought to be contaminated with Creutzfeldt-Jakob Disease (CCBC 1994).

Heat-Treated AHF Concentrate and the FDA's Recall Policy

When Assistant Secretary Brandt testified before the U.S. Congress in August 1983, concerning FDA's decision to reject a blanket recall policy, he included as one of his reasons for that rejection the belief that safer AHF concentrate would soon be available (U.S. House of Representatives 1983). Leaving aside for a moment the question why this belief would not have justified a stronger rather than a weaker recall policy (e.g., a temporary ban or license suspension), it seems probable that Secretary Brandt's reference was to the emerging availability of heat-treated AHF concentrate.

By early 1984, all producers of AHF concentrate had been licensed to produce heat-treated AHF concentrate (Hammes pers. com. 1995; Leahy pers. com. 1995; McAuley pers. com. 1995; Persky pers. com. 1995). The FDA approved licenses of the heat-treated AHF on the basis of clinical trials demonstrating its biologic effectiveness to correct blood clotting problems (Fratatoni 1995). Testing revealed that heat treatment had substantial positive effects with respect to the elimination of hepatitis viruses, and it was conjectured by some that it would reduce the infectivity of AHF concentrate with respect to AIDS as well (Colombo, et al. 1985; McDougal, et al. 1985) (see Chapter 4 for complete discussion of the development of heat treatment methods for viral inactivation).

One must remember, of course, that these developments took place before the April 1984 isolation of the AIDS virus and at least 18 months prior to the development of a test (ELISA) that could detect the existence of HIV in blood and/or plasma prior to transfusion or the manufacture of AHF concentrate (Hammes pers. com. 1995; Leahy pers. com. 1995 McAuley pers. com. 1995; Persky pers. com. 1995). Hence, it was hoped that heat treatment would be useful against HIV, but it was not scientifically proven (Aronson interview). In fact, events later demonstrated that heat treatment was almost 100 percent effective with respect to the elimination of HIV (Levy, et al. 1984; McDougal, et al. 1985). Like most other strains of virus, the HIV virus was not resistant to the application of heat. In October 1984, the CDC announced that preliminary evidence concerning the effects of heat treatment on the viability of the AIDS virus was strongly supportive of the usefulness of heat treatment in reducing the potential for transmission of the AIDS virus in AHF concentrate and suggested that the use of non-heat-treated AHF concentrate should be limited (CDC, MMWR, October 1984). Most people accepted the model virus studies on inactivation of the AIDS virus by heat treatment by 1985 (Hammes 1995; Leahy 1995; McAuley 1995; Persky 1995).

Heat-treated AHF became available in 1983 (Persky pers. com. 1995), and by 1985 heat treatment was accepted as effective in deactivating HIV (McDougal, et al. 1985). Even though there was a reasonable supply of heat-treated products, the FDA waited until 1989 to require the recall of all untreated AHF concentrate. By the time the FDA required recall of untreated units of AHF, the manufacturers had acted on their own (Epstein interview).

Analysis

In this case, it is possible to construct a scenario in which the legal authority hypothesis cannot be so easily rejected. This may seem a strange conclusion given the argument above that the FDA might, in July 1983, have delicensed all AHF concentrate. However, the data necessary to delicense only untreated AHF concentrate, while leaving heat-treated AHF concentrate on the market, were not necessarily available for HIV. Removal of all AHF concentrate from the market might have been premised on a determination that, given the epidemiological evidence that was accumulating, AHF concentrate could no longer be determined to be safe under normal conditions of use. However, circa 1983, that same conclusion would have to be drawn with respect to heat-treated AHF concentrate as well. There was no test that would demonstrate definitively that heat-treated AHF concentrate was less infective with respect to HIV than non-heat-treated AHF concentrate until the mid-1984 studies by the CDC (CDC, MMWR, October 1984; McDougal, et. al. 1985). The CDC, in cooperation with Cutter Biological, conducted a study in which the AIDS virus was added to Factor VIII concentrate and was subsequently heat treated. The study showed that the virus was undetectable after 24 hours of heat treatment (CDC, MMWR, October 1984). Preliminary data were presented to NHF's Medical and Scientific Advisory Council in September 1984 and formed the scientific basis for NHF's subsequent October 1984 recommendations that heat-treated AHF concentrate be considered in the treatment of hemophilia.

On the other hand, the FDA could have decided that untreated AHF should be removed from the market because heat-treated AHF concentrate was safer with respect to the propagation of hepatitis. However, as is explained in Chapter 4, the FDA and others for many years had doubts about the utility of heat-treating AHF concentrate for hepatitis. Recipients of AHF concentrate were likely to be infected with hepatitis from exposure to numerous donors through multiple administrations of AHF concentrate (Aledort, Dietrich, Levine, Lusher interviews). This position itself may not have been well considered, but that seems to be the way that the FDA and others looked at the situation as of the end of 1983 (Aledort, Dietrich, Levine, Lusher interviews).

In this view, then, the situation from a legal and public health perspective might be summarized as follows: Because, prior to October 1984 at the earliest, the FDA could not demonstrate that heat-treated AHF concentrate was less infective for AIDS than untreated AHF concentrate—label inserts for heat-treated AHF concentrate could not say that it was a safer product [Baxter Product Insert, October 1983]—it had no legal basis upon which to demand that untreated AHF concentrate be recalled while leaving heat-treated AHF concentrate on the market. This is a situation in which the FDA's greater legal power (the probable authority to delicense all AHF concentrate owing to public health concerns) does not necessarily include the lesser (the power to eliminate untreated AHF concentrate on grounds of AIDS risk when it was not demonstrably less safe than heat-treated AHF concentrate). By contrast, the FDA might have required the expeditious elimination of untreated AHF concentrate on grounds of its demonstrated infectivity with respect to hepatitis by comparison with heat-treated AHF concentrate. Here, however, the public health benefits looked small (given the assumptions outlined above) in relation to the substantial economic costs involved in eliminating all untreated AHF concentrate from the market.

Moreover, there was some resistance in the medical community to the use of heat-treated AHF concentrate as it became available (Aledort, Dietrich, Levine, Lusher interviews). The reasons for this resistance included the problem of possible neoantigencity and subsequent inhibitor formation (which renders the patient untreatable with the AHF concentrates), the knowledge that heat treatment was developed to eliminate hepatitis virus, and the higher cost to the patient (Aledort, Dietrich, Lusher interviews). Physicians continued to prescribe non-heat-treated AHF to patients known to be infected with hepatitis (Aledort, Dietrich, Lusher interviews). Under these assumptions, the NHF and physicians treating hemophilia were reluctant to recommend the heat-treated product until there was more clinical evidence to prove that it was effective. Indeed, some manufacturers have suggested that the FDA's concerns about availability and resistance from the medical community probably influenced the FDA not to suspend licenses for untreated AHF concentrate when heat-treated AHF concentrate products were approved (Hammes pers. com. 1995; Leahy pers. com. 1995 McAuley pers. com. 1995; Persky pers. com. 1995).

It is worth noting, however, that there is another perspective on this story which might suggest that more aggressive action would have been warranted based wholly on the protection of individuals with hemophilia against the further spread of hepatitis. It is not clear, for example, exactly how great the economic or political costs would have been to plasma fractionators and to the FDA to remove untreated AHF concentrate from the market more rapidly. The Committee has only fragmentary information about how rapidly untreated AHF concentrate was removed through manufacturer's voluntary efforts or about what FDA action would have added to the rapidity of its removal. However, Alpha

Therapeutic reports that while licensed to produce heat-treated Factor VIII in February 1984, it was already processing 45 percent of its total Factor VIII output with the heat treatment step in anticipation of licensing and requested voluntary withdrawal of its license for untreated AHF concentrate in July 1985 (McAuley pers. com. 1995). Miles, Inc. reports that 40 percent of its shipped product (Factor VIII) was heat-treated in 1984 and 99 percent was treated during 1985 (Hammes pers. com. 1995). (The timing was somewhat later concerning Factor IX.) Moreover, by 1985 the unit prices to intermediate consumers for heat-treated Factor VIII were only slightly higher than the unit price of untreated Factor VIII in 1983 and 1984 (Hammes pers. com. 1995; Persky pers. com. 1995). However, it was reported to the Committee that the price to the final consumer was higher and this was one of the reasons why some in the medical community did not recommend heat-treated AHF concentrate earlier (Dietrich, Lusher interviews). From these data it would appear that supplies of treated AHF concentrate were rapidly becoming available and that the costs of eliminating untreated AHF concentrate in inventory would have been limited essentially to its production costs and the costs of retrieval.

Had the FDA demanded recall of all untreated AHF concentrate—based perhaps on an assumption that the AIDS virus would turn out to be more like the general run of viruses in its susceptibility to pasteurization—there might have been no legal contest from the industry. Once a retrovirus had been isolated as the causative agent in AIDS, most virologists would have presumed that it would be susceptible to heat inactivation. Moreover, by 1985 the medical and scientific community agreed that heat-treated AHF concentrate was less likely to infect humans with HIV (McDougal, et al. 1985). Hence, even if the FDA doubted its legal authority to press for a recall of untreated AHF concentrate, it might well have achieved that goal without any test of its legal authority. And, if tested, it might well have prevailed on one of several theories.

Summary and Conclusions

On the positive side, this series of events demonstrates some of the strengths of industry self-regulation. The plasma fractionation industry seems to have perceived clear advantages to developing a workable heat treatment process and to have rapidly secured approval for different processes (Hammes pers. com. 1995; Leahy pers. com. 1995; McAuley pers. com. 1995; Persky pers. com. 1995. Also, the FDA licensed heat-treated AHF concentrate with commendable speed using relaxed testing requirements.

On the other hand, the weaknesses of this approach are also evident. The industry is responsive to the demands of physicians and therefore was not particularly interested in the pursuit of heat treatment when the threat was hepatitis because, at the time, the hemophilia treatment community considered the risk of hepatitis to be an acceptable price to pay for the benefits of AHF concentrate. This delayed development for several years. Then, when heat treatment was coming into use there seems to have been no particular effort by the FDA to help overcome treater resistance to the new product. Any regulatory actions would have required careful attention to availability problems, but there seems to be no reason to believe that the transition from untreated to treated AHF concentrate could not have been accomplished faster with active agency leadership (see also discussion in Chapter 4).

Lookback and Notification of Individuals Transfused with Contaminated Blood Products

By 1985, it was known that recipients of HIV-infected blood products became infective immediately but remained asymptomatic for up to five years (Curran, et al. 1984; Bove 1986), during which time those with whom recipients had intimate contacts were at risk of acquiring HIV. The FDA did provide interim procedures to blood establishments to apply when a repeat donor had a positive (repeated reactive) test for HTLV-II antibody, which included lookback of all prior donations and notification of all consignees of possibly contaminated products (Esber 1985). However, despite a 1988 presidential directive to the Department of Health and Human Services to formulate a lookback and notification policy for tracing the recipients of possibly infected blood products, the FDA did not issue recommendations until September 1991 (FDA, BPAC 1991a,b). Why did it take the FDA from 1985-1991 to recommend tracing recipients of transfusions from a donor who was later found to have AIDS?

Analysis

One of the basic principles of infectious disease prevention is notifying infected individuals so that they can avoid infecting other people with whom they come into contact. Even as early as 1983, it was clear that AIDS had an incubation period of at least 18 months, and later it appeared that approximately 5 years was a common interval between exposure, infection, and developing the symptoms of AIDS (Bove 1986). In January 1983, there was evidence for transmission of AIDS by heterosexual contact (CDC, MMWR, January 1983). Thus, transfusion recipients are likely to transmit HIV infection without being aware that they are doing so. Neither the FDA recommendations about donor questioning and deferral nor the FDA working policy on recall strategy contained recommendations concerning recipients of blood products donated by individuals subsequently found to have HIV infection. Failure to develop such a policy is peculiar.

In 1988, the Department of Health and Human Services received a presidential directive to implement actions in response to blood safety issues raised by the report of the Presidential Commission on the Human Immunodeficiency Virus Epidemic. One issue was prompt notification of individuals who are at increased risk of HIV infection but are unaware of their increased risk (Presidential Commission on the Human Immunodeficiency Virus Epidemic 1988). In 1991, Jay Epstein, acting director of the FDA's Division of Transfusion Services, reported progress to the BPAC and solicited their advice about the wording of regulations (FDA, BPAC 1991a,b). The issues in question included lookback[4] and recipient notification.[5]

At the September 26–27, 1991, BPAC meeting, Dr. Epstein presented recommendations that were to be applied to product recalls and recipient tracing (lookback) related to components from prior collections. The BPAC unanimously approved the recommendations, which included the following: "When it is discovered that a donor is HIV-positive a blood center should search for recipients of any donations from that donor during the preceding five years and quarantine any suspect blood product. Blood centers must also notify the consignees of units for transfusion obtained from the donor's prior collections of the results of additional testing of the donor's current blood collection" (FDA, BPAC 1991b). Assuming that this policy is sufficient for the future, why did it take so long for the FDA to take action to protect the contacts of people who may have unknowingly become infected with HIV through a transfusion?

Did the FDA have insufficient information to justify legally a vigorous stance about lookback? To the contrary, there was an abundance of relevant biomedical evidence by 1985. In a memorandum from the FDA to blood establishments dated July 22, 1985, the FDA provided interim procedures to "apply when a repeat donor has a positive (repeated reactive) test for HTLV-II antibody," which included lookback of all prior donations with a maximum dating period of products and notifying all consignees of products so that products can be destroyed (Esber 1985). However, the Committee found no evidence on the record that the FDA formulated recommendations on lookback until January 18–19, 1991, when Dr. Epstein presented to the BPAC a draft of the recommendations the BPAC voted to adopt seven months later (FDA, BPAC

---

[4] The term "lookback" refers to checks for prior donations of current donors who test positive and tracking ofthose products to the recipients.

[5] The term "notification" refers to informing the hospital in which the transfusion occurred that the patient has received a potentially contaminated blood product. The hospital must then inform the physician, who is expectedto inform and monitor the patient and to caution the patient to behave in a way that minimizes risk to others.

1991b). The FDA had both legal justification and sufficient information for taking action on lookback and notification. Aggressive action by the FDA could have been justified legally and on public health grounds, because notifying an individual that they had HIV could have reduced the risk of secondary transmission to a loved one. Clearly, public health considerations strongly favored a policy of lookback and notification.

The Committee has found no evidence to suggest that resource constraints prevented action. A lookback and notification policy would primarily burden local blood centers, which would have responsibility for tracing recipients of blood or blood products that had been transfused any time within five years of the donor becoming aware of his or her HIV infection. The FDA may have been sensitive to the resource limitations of blood centers, but the Committee has found no evidence to suggest that anyone sought to influence the FDA to delay instituting a policy of lookbacks.

Summary and Conclusions

The FDA's delayed approach to lookbacks is similar to its general approach to patient information detailed elsewhere in this report (see Chapter 7). Providing information in such circumstances as those attending the HIV invasion of the blood supply seems to have a particularly strong justification. Information would have permitted protective action concerning others as well as possible benefits for the infected, or potentially infected, individuals.

INFLUENCE AND RESPONSIBILITIES OF OTHER ORGANIZATIONS

While the FDA had primary regulatory responsibility for blood and blood products, it acted in an environment populated by other organizations having both responsibilities and influence. Other than the FDA, the primary governmental agencies were the Centers for Disease Control and the National Institutes of Health. The primary nongovernmental organizations were the not-for-profit blood bank community, the commercial collectors of plasma and producers of plasma fractionated products, and the National Hemophilia Foundation.

Governmental Organizations

The National Institutes of Health has responsibilities for intramural and extramural biologic and biomedical research. The NIH has a scientific role in sponsoring the advance of biological and biomedical knowledge and in ensuring the integrity of research findings. It also has a public health responsibility that is discharged, in part, through its allocations of research funds in relation to public health needs (U.S. Government Manual 1994).

In connection with the AIDS contamination of the blood supply, there was little basic biomedical knowledge on HIV and AIDS and the rapid development of new knowledge was extremely valuable. Once the AIDS virus had been isolated, events moved very rapidly toward effective screening and treatment of blood and blood products. The Reagan administration and the NIH itself have been criticized for their failure to make AIDS research an urgent matter (Alter, Gallo, Perkins interviews). While it is clear that scientific uncertainty had a great impact on the regulatory process, we do not know what extent the devotion of greater research resources at earlier stages would have sped the resolution of some of the basic mysteries concerning AIDS as a disease and its transmission through the blood supply. It seems safe to assume that there would have been some effect; the magnitude is what is in doubt.

The Centers for Disease Control has responsibility for epidemiological research and monitoring, as well as for the dissemination of information concerning public health markers. In many ways the CDC seems to have played its early warning role quite well in this crisis. Certain CDC officials were extremely active very early in the critical period that we are discussing. They offered hypotheses about the etiology of the disease and its potential transmissions through the blood supply, which turned out to be quite accurate (Curran, Evatt, Foege, Francis interviews). Other governmental agencies seemed rather slow-moving by comparison with the CDC. However, it should be remembered that the CDC's role is to collect and disseminate information that it believes to have public health significance. It is not responsible for regulating other parties' behavior. Hence, it can responsibly use a much lower threshold of certainty in sounding alarms and pressing data on others. By contrast, it was sensible for other public health agencies to act cautiously considering that the CDC's concerns were based on a small number of cases and on hypotheses about those cases that appear more plausible in retrospect than they did at the time (Foege interview).

Nongovernmental Organizations

With respect to nongovernmental organizations, it seems clear that there was a presumption that the blood bank industry, and perhaps to a lesser degree the commercial plasma and plasma fractionation industry, would be substantially self-regulating. Moreover, there was considerable concern throughout the critical period reviewed to take into account the desires and knowledge of affected producer, patient, and physician constituencies, particularly when they were highly organized and active. Moreover, these same parties were given a substantial role in providing technical advice to the FDA concerning the exercise of its regulatory responsibilities (Aledort, Bove, Rodell interviews).

In normal times these close working relationships between the FDA and the nongovernmental sector have major advantages, as we point out at the beginning of this chapter. Indeed, it would appear that self-regulation and advice-giving played important positive roles in mitigating and ultimately limiting the tragedy of blood-borne HIV virus. Certain blood banks acted early to institute screening programs. Alpha Therapeutic acted with great dispatch in eliminating unscreened components from its AHF concentrate (Gury 1982). And the plasma fractionation industry adopted a strong screening policy that was urged on all its members (ABRA 1983) well before the March 1983 FDA letters that recommended screening (Petricciani 1983a,b,c). Ironically and tragically, plasma fractionators were not encouraged by government to aggressively produce and market heat-treated AHF concentrate a year before scientific proof that heat treatment killed HIV, but they moved rapidly to provide that product once it became plausible to believe that heat treatment was effective against HIV. Although many may now think that its advice was myopic, the National Hemophilia Foundation was very active in attempting to balance the risks of HIV infection against the risks of uncontrolled bleeding and in informing its member units concerning what it believed to be the proper course of action [e.g., NHF Chapter Advisories #4-12; NHF Medical Bulletins #3-11].

Nevertheless, we have noted many worrisome aspects of the FDA's reliance on both self-regulation and information development and dissemination in the nongovernmental sector. Because the FDA did not demand information and monitor action, it had no way of knowing whether either self-regulation or implementation of its recommendations would be effectively carried out by regulated parties. The FDA and others may have been overly influenced by the concerns of the NHF and other treaters that AHF concentrates remain fully available (in some cases, in a non-heat-treated form) (FDA, BPAC 1983). Information about availability and the effects of regulation on availability seems to have come almost exclusively from the industry and to have had major impacts on FDA decisionmaking (FDA, BPAC 1983). Actions were not taken in the absence of consensus among nongovernmental parties, when stronger action to manage uncertainty in the interest of public health may have been warranted. Reliance seems to have been placed on the ordinary processes of the market in substituting higher for lower quality products, when it is uncertain whether those processes were effective or were as effective as would have been optimal.

Implications

The divided specialized responsibilities of governmental agencies and close association with and reliance upon nongovernmental organizations may work well in routine regulatory situations. In situations where uncertainty is great, there is a need to change regulatory routines to closely monitor potentially catastrophic health threats more closely. The ordinary routines of the regulatory system may too strongly favor the status quo. The difficult institutional design problem is how to develop a set of "triggers" that would force regulatory action, or the careful consideration of actions, without simultaneously overburdening the blood regulatory process as it deals with routine matters. Achieving this sort of balance in the system motivates the Committee's recommendations for restructuring the blood regulatory process (see Chapter 8).

THE ADVANTAGES OF MARGINAL THINKING

The FDA had several opportunities to take actions that appear to have had little or no risk for causing net harm and some possibility of reducing the number of people who contracted HIV infection through blood or blood products. None of these activities would necessarily have had large effects, which may explain why they were overlooked. The important strategy that these instances highlight, however, is a strategy of opportunistic, marginal improvements in safety in the absence of sufficient information or opportunities to make larger improvements. Consider the following examples that appear from the previous discussion.

Lookback and Notification

The FDA instituted the "lookback" recommendation in 1991, at least six years after it was clear that AIDS had a long incubation period during which the patient could transmit HIV through sexual contact or contact with blood (FDA, BPAC 1991b). Lookback required blood banks to contact recipients of blood from infected donors and notify them that they might be a HIV carrier and should be tested for HIV antibodies. To be sure, blood banks instituted their own partial lookback systems. But there is no reason to believe that these practices were universal, uniform, or fully effective.

Removal of Untreated AHF Concentrate

When heat-treated AHF concentrate became available, there was an opportunity to reduce the amount of untreated AHF concentrate in the treatment centers' stocks. The number of potentially infectious vials would have decreased if, for example, the FDA had required a staged withdrawal of a vial of untreated AHF concentrate for every vial of treated AHF concentrate that was distributed. The success of this strategy presupposes that demand for treated AHF concentrate could be influenced by the FDA's policies. But clearly the agency could have been more aggressive in its removal efforts once more information was known about the efficacy and safety of heat-treated concentrate.

Use of Screened Whole Blood

Blood banks discard whole blood after about three weeks of storage. The Petricciani letters of March 1983 (Petricciani 1983a,b,c), among other things, required blood banks to screen potential donors for some high-risk behaviors and to quarantine or discard blood collected from these people. Blood collected from screened donors had a lower probability of being infectious. The Petricciani directive could have required blood banks to institute a policy of using blood from screened donors whenever possible. With this policy, the chance of receiving infected blood would have decreased, at no risk to the overall supply of blood. Once again the likely effects would have been small. Nevertheless, every substitution of a safe unit for a contaminated unit of blood would have prevented an infection and subsequent death.

Destruction of Potentially Contaminated Cryoprecipitate

Blood banks freeze cryoprecipitate from single donors and store it until the time of use. The FDA could have required blood banks to check their stores of frozen cryoprecipitate and destroy units obtained from donors subsequently found to have AIDS. This would have been an unpopular move, given the short supplies of cryoprecipitate, and of marginal benefit. Yet once again it would have been a low-cost option and would have provided a chance of saving some lives.

Innovative Techniques for Pooling Plasma

The smaller the number of donors to a lot of pooled plasma, the smaller the chance that the pool would contain HIV or other contaminants. The FDA could have encouraged the plasma fractionation industry to devise methods to reduce the number of donors to a lot of pooled plasma. For example, storing units obtained from repeat donors and using material from a donor only when a preset number of units had accumulated would reduce the number of donors to a given lot of pooled plasma. Other techniques might also have been available or developed.

Reducing risk by smaller pools would not eliminate risk. Indeed, a substantial pool is necessary to assure the efficacy of some plasma derivatives and reduce certain risks in others. But maintaining these levels could be accomplished while reducing pool sizes by a factor of 20. The critical point to this example is that because FDA promoted no changes in pooling practices, it faces in 1995 the same dilemma concerning Creutzfeldt-Jakob disease that it faced in 1983–1984 concerning AIDS (FDA, BPAC 1984; CCBC 1994). Recall of all tainted products might severely compromise the availability of AHF concentrate.

Testing Previously Untested Blood and Plasma for HIV

When blood and plasma collection centers first began to use the ELISA HIV test on blood donors (see Chapter 3), they began to face the problem of having two classes of blood and plasma: tested, which was presumably "safe," and untested, which had a higher risk of containing HIV. The FDA could have required blood and plasma collection centers as well as plasma fractionators to test each unused unit for HIV and discard positive units. The FDA did not issue such a directive, although there may have been testing carried out by some blood banks and others may have discarded untested units (Fratantoni 1995).

*****

In summary, there were several opportunities for the FDA to specify practices that would have reduced the chance that blood or a blood product would transmit HIV, or that might have improved the FDA's chances to exercise regulatory control over future threats in the interests of public health. The Committee believes that there was enough knowledge at the time to be confident that these practices would have caused little or no harm. These practices were no guarantee, either individually or collectively, of a risk-free blood supply, but each would have made a marginal improvement in reducing the chances for immediate or future harm from blood or blood products.

SUMMARY

The analysis of these four critical events led the Committee to identify several weaknesses in the FDA's regulatory approach to blood safety issues. Most importantly, they reveal the lack of a systematic approach to safety in which events serve as triggers for careful consideration of options, including safer, but not zero risk, actions. In the absence of such an approach, uncertainty strongly reinforces the status quo as the agency waits for a consensus to crystallize and for the normal processes of FDA informal action and industry self-regulation to solve new problems.

REFERENCES

American Blood Resources Association. Recommendations on AIDS and Plasma Donor Deferral; January 28, 1983.

Bove, Joseph. Statement before the U.S. Congress, Committee on Government Operations; August 1, 1983.

Bove, Joseph. Transfusion-Transmitted Diseases: Current Problems and Challenges. Progress in Hematology; 1986.

Centers for Disease Control, *Morbidity and Mortality Weekly Report*, June 24, 1983.

Centers for Disease Control, *Morbidity and Mortality Weekly Report*, October 26, 1984.

Centers for Disease Control, *Morbidity and Mortality Weekly Report*, January 7, 1983.

Colombo, et al. Transmission of non-A, non-B Hepatitis by Heat Treated Factor VIII Concentrate. *Lancet;* July 6, 1985.

Council of Community Blood Centers, FDA Committee Recommends Some Blood Recalls for Rare Neurological Disease. *CCBC Newsletter;* December 23/30, 1994.

Curran, et al. Acquired Immune Deficiency Syndrome (AIDS) Associated with Transfusion. *New England Journal of Medicine*, Volume 310; January 12, 1984.

Donohue, Dennis. Memorandum to Petricciani, John, FDA, Director, Office of Biologics; July 21, 1983.

Esber, Elaine, M.D., Director, Office of Biologics and Review, Food and Drug Administration. Memorandum to all registered blood establishments; July 22, 1985.

Falter, Steven, Director, Division of Bioresearch Monitoring and Regulations, Food and Drug Administration. Memorandum to Don Fowler; October 19, 1994.

Foege, William. Summary Report of Workgroup to Identify Opportunities for Prevention of Acquired Immune Deficiency Syndrome (AIDS); January 4, 1983.

Food and Drug Administration. Blood Products Advisory Committee, July 19, 1983.

Food and Drug Administration. Blood Products Advisory Committee, January 18, 1991a.

Food and Drug Administration. Blood Products Advisory Committee, September 26–27, 1991b.

Food and Drug Administration. Blood Products Advisory Committee, December 13, 1984.

Food and Drug Administration. Memorandum from Chief, Recalls and Administrative Actions Branch, to Don Fowler, Chief Freedom of Information Branch; November 8, 1994.

Food and Drug Administration. Regulatory Procedures Manual. U.S. Government Printing Office, Washington, D.C.; 1988.

Fratatoni, Joseph, M.D., Director, Division of Hematology, Food and Drug Administration. Letter to the Institute of Medicine; May 8, 1995.

Goedert and Gallo. Epidemiological Evidence that HTLV-III is the AIDS Agent. *European Journal of Epidemiology,* Volume 1; September 1985.

Gury, David, Vice President, Plasma Supply, Alpha Therapeutics. Letter to all source affiliates; December 17, 1982.

Hammes, William J., Associate Counsel, Miles, Inc. Letter to Institute of Medicine; February 13, 1995.

Hutt, Peter and Merrill, Richard. *Food and Drug Law: Cases and Materials* . The Foundation Press, Inc. Westbury, New York; 1991.

Leahy, Beth, Director Public Affairs, Armour Pharmaceutical. Letter to Institute of Medicine; March 17, 1995.

Levy, et al. Recovery and Inactivation of Infectious Retroviruses froFactor VIII Concentration. *Lancet;* September 29, 1984.

McAuley, Clyde, M.D., Medical Director, Alpha Therapeutic. Letter to Institute of Medicine; February 8, 1995.

McDougal, J.S., Martin, L.W., Cort, S.P., Mozen, M., Heldebrant, C.M., and Evatt, B.L. "Thermal Inactivation of the Acquired Immunodeficiency Syndrome Virus, Human T Lymphotropic Virus-III/Lymphadenopathy-associated Virus, with Special Reference to Antihemophilic Factor." *The Journal of Clinical Investigation*, Vol. 76; August 1985

National Hemophilia Foundation. Recommendations on the Prevention of AIDS in Patients with Hemophilia. January 14, 1983.

Novitch, FDA, Deputy Commissioner, Food and Drugs. Memorandum to Assistant Secretary of Health; July 23, 1983.

Persky, Marla, Associate General Counsel, Biotech Group Baxter Healthcare, letter to Institute of Medicine; February 24, 1995.

Petricciani, John, M.D., Food and Drug Administration, Office of Biologics. Letter to All establishments collecting human blood for transfusion. March 21, 1983a.

Petricciani, John, M.D., Director, Food and Drug Administration, Office of Biologics. Letter to All establishments collecting source plasma. March 24, 1983b.

Petricciani, John, M.D., Food and Drug Administration, Office of Biologics. Letter to All licensed manufacturers of plasma derivatives. March 24, 1983c.

Presidential Commission on the Human Immunodeficiency Virus Epidemic. Report of the Presidential Commission on the Human Immunodeficiency Virus Epidemic. U.S. Government Printing Office, Washington, D.C.; 1988.

Reilly, Robert, American Blood Resources Association. Letter to Petricciani, John, Food and Drug Administration; July 27, 1983.

U.S. Government Printing Office. *U.S. Government Manual*. Washington, D.C.; 1993–1994.

U.S. House of Representatives. Committee on Government Operations, Subcommittee on Intergovernmental Relations Hearing: The Federal Response to AIDS. U.S. Government Printing Office, Washington, D.C.; August 1, 1983.

7

Risk Communication to Physicians and Patients

INTRODUCTION

The introduction of HIV into the blood supply posed powerful dangers to those individuals with hemophilia and recipients of blood transfusions during the early years of the epidemic. During the period from 1982 to 1984, before the AIDS virus was finally identified and a test developed to determine its presence, there was considerable speculation about whether the blood supply could be a vector for this new, fatal infection. As evidence about risk developed, consumers of blood and blood products—as well as their physicians—found themselves in a complex dilemma. Continued use of blood and blood products might heighten the risk of acquiring a new disease. Reducing or discouraging the use of blood products might increase the morbidity and mortality associated with hemophilia. Approximately half of the 16,000 hemophiliacs and over 12,000 recipients of blood transfusions became infected with HIV during this period (CDC, MMWR, July 23, 1993). More effective communication of the risks associated with blood and blood products and the opportunity to choose from a wide spectrum of clinical options might have averted some of these infections.

To explore these questions, the Committee analyzed how the risks associated with using blood and blood products as well as clinical options were communicated to relevant physicians and patients by examining the content and process of the communications from 1982 through 1985. The Committee focused on the information available to decisionmakers and analyzed the institutional, social, and cultural obstacles to effective risk communication. The analysis includes an examination of the information about the risks associated with blood and blood products and possible risk reduction options that were available during this period of uncertainty. The chapter also considers the role of a voluntary health organization, the National Hemophilia Foundation (NHF), in the communication of information to physicians and individuals with hemophilia.

FRAMEWORK FOR ANALYSIS

Critical Questions

The Committee addressed four fundamental questions about the content and process of risk communication:

1. What clinical options for risk reduction, even if marginally effective, were available and could have been communicated?
2. What information was actually communicated to patients?
3. What were the institutional obstacles to risk communication?
4. What were the social and cultural obstacles that influenced physician-patient relationships and risk communication?

To better understand how information about the risks associated with blood and blood products was actually perceived and responded to at the clinical level, the Committee utilized a case study approach. This approach provided the means for the Committee to gain an in-depth familiarization with the context and culture of hemophilia treatment. It also helped illuminate the range of possible clinical options that existed during this period of uncertainty, and to assess their impact in these instances. Finally, the Committee evaluated the institutional, social, and cultural obstacles to communication about the risk of using blood and blood products.

Critical Factors

Three critical factors in the environment for individuals who are dependent on blood products help explain risk communication patterns: (1) progress in the treatment of hemophilia; (2) the development of a national network of hemophilia treatment centers; and (3) the medical community's consideration of hepatitis as an "acceptable risk." These factors shaped the decisionmaking process as the AIDS epidemic emerged.

The advent of antihemophilic factor (AHF) concentrate in the early 1970s brought a remarkably effective means to treat a disease characterized by spontaneous bleeding, pain, crippling, and early death (Jones and Ratnoff 1991). AHF concentrates significantly altered the morbidity and mortality associated with hemophilia, dramatically improving the quality of life of those affected. In

1972, the major cause of death for individuals with hemophilia was cerebral hemorrhage. The mean life expectancy was approximately 40 years between 1941 and 1960 and approximately 54 years between 1961 and 1970; it increased to 60 years between 1971 and 1980 (Jones and Ratnoff 1991). By the early 1980s, hemorrhage was no longer the major cause of death (Levine interview). To the extent that the pain and the visible signs of a crippling disease were reduced, the stigma of hemophilia was also significantly reduced (Jones and Ratnoff 1991; Resnik 1994).

While the development of the AHF concentrate products revolutionized the treatment of hemophilia, the development of hemophilia treatment centers provided a nationwide system of care and treatment. In 1975, the federal government established funding for 20 regional centers, representing approximately 100 local treatment centers, to provide hemophilia care (Department of Health and Human Services 1994). The treatment centers ensured comprehensive medical care and early application of treatment as well as fostering a sense of community for individuals with hemophilia and their families (Smith and Levine 1984).

In the setting of the treatment center both physicians and patients were able to see the advantages of treating bleeding episodes early. This observation translated into advocating home care therapy; hemophiliac patients and their families quickly became proficient in self-infusion (Smith and Levine 1984). The results were significant—home care therapy nearly eliminated the crippling associated with the disease and led to significant improvements in the health and quality of life for the individual with hemophilia (Eyster, et al. 1980; Brinkhous 1981; Smith and Levine 1984; Rosendaal, et al. 1991; Chorba, et al. 1994).

In this context of progress in the treatment and care of hemophilia, the physicians treating hemophilia and their patients shared in a rather unique and close relationship. In part, this stemmed from the somewhat insular care network for individuals with hemophilia at the hemophilia treatment centers, and in part, it developed from sharing in the significant medical progress in hemophilia treatment. Hemophiliac patients and their families generally held their physicians in high regard and trusted them implicitly (Kasper interview). The third important factor in the treatment of the hemophilia patient in the years before the AIDS epidemic was the recognition that infection with hepatitis B as well as non-A, non-B hepatitis was a frequent risk associated with use of AHF concentrates (Aronson 1979; Johnson et al. 1985; Chorba et al. 1994; Hoyer 1994; Goldfinger, Kasper, Louvrein, Roberts interviews). This observation can be traced to the early 1970s when hepatitis emerged as a frequent complication in patients receiving blood and blood products (Seeff 1988). During this era, it came to be expected that most hemophiliac patients would develop hepatitis (Chorba, et al. 1994; Hoyer interview). Although hepatitis infections were occasionally severe, leading to liver failure and death (Aronson 1979; Johnson, et al. 1985), the benefits of treatment seemed to outweigh the risks from such infections (Hoyer interview). In the context of the dramatic improvements in the care and treatment of hemophilia offered by AHF concentrates, infection associated with the use of these blood products came to be deemed an "acceptable risk" (Aledort 1982; Aronson 1979; Hoyer 1994; Furie, Roberts interviews).

It was against this background that the initial reports began to surface that individuals with hemophilia and transfusion recipients might be at risk for a new disease, called AIDS. There was considerable uncertainty and disagreement among medical, scientific, and public health decisionmakers about whether AIDS was a new disease, and if it could be transmitted via a blood-borne agent (Public Health Service 1982; FDA, BPAC 1983). If AIDS was a new, blood-borne disease, the implications for individuals with hemophilia —as well as other consumers of blood and blood products—could be dire.

The Role of the National Hemophilia Foundation

In the early 1980s, there was no organization that assumed specific responsibility for communicating directly with physicians and patients about the risks associated with blood and blood products. Although the hemophilia treatment centers received federal funding, the basis of information about the nature of the risk of AIDS associated with blood and blood products came from the National Hemophilia Foundation (NHF) and its Medical and Scientific Advisory Council (MASAC), whose membership included medical directors of hemophilia treatment centers. Immediately upon hearing directly from the CDC about three cases of AIDS in individuals with hemophilia (CDC, MMWR, July 1982), the NHF took on the responsibility of communicating to physicians and patients about the epidemic and the risks associated with use of blood products. In this role, NHF served a crucial function as an intermediary between the sources of scientific and medical information (i.e., CDC, FDA, plasma fractionation industry) and the consumers of that information—the physicians and users of blood products who had to make daily decisions about hemophilia treatment.

Founded in 1948, the NHF was committed to advancing the care and treatment of persons with hemophilia and strengthening the community. During the mid-1970s, NHF helped to successfully lobby for major changes in the care and treatment of hemophilia (Aledort, McPherson interviews; Brownstein 1994). But in 1982, it stepped into a new role for which it had little preparation and experience and limited resources. First, in the early 1980s, the NHF was recovering from bankruptcy and had a small staff (Brownstein 1994; Bias, Carman interviews). In addition, it had limited funding and expertise for developing a system for communicating information until it obtained additional support from Human Resources and Services Administration's Office of Maternal and Child Health (HRSA/OMCH) in October 1983 (NHF 1983). The decisions about what to communicate and the process for communication, however, remained the primary responsibility of the NHF.

The leadership of NHF was comprised of individuals who were committed to the advancement of medical care and services for individuals with hemophilia. The NHF had established close relationships with the plasma fractionation industry (pharmaceutical companies) which provided badly needed financial support for some of the NHF's activities, including its communication programs (Aledort interview; Hammes pers. com. 1995; Brownstein, 1994). NHF, with the help of its newly reconstituted Medical and Scientific Advisory Council (MASAC), established itself as the primary source of information for the consumers of blood products (Brownstein 1994). Given the heated tenor of the discussions of the AIDS crisis, and the complex scientific, medical, and social questions that it would raise, the NHF's assumption of responsibility for communicating expert advice was without precedent in its history.

The NHF utilized two modes of communication, medical bulletins and chapter advisories, for educating and advising physicians and patients concerning what was and was not known at the time. (Appendix C summarizes these communications.) Medical bulletins formulated by members of the NHF AIDS Task Force and some of the members from MASAC (referred to as *Hemophilia Newsnotes*) were sent directly to treating physicians (primarily at the hemophilia treatment centers); chapter advisories were sent to the local chapters of the NHF. From July 1982 through December 1985, the NHF issued 32 medical bulletins and 37 chapter advisories. Both forms of communication came from the leadership of the NHF rather than directly from MASAC (Aledort, Carman interviews).

The information developed for the recommendations came from the interactions of the NHF AIDS Task Force with government and private organizations. The communications were written by the members of the NHF AIDS Task Force, with review and approval of MASAC members. The AIDS Task Force was an ad hoc group comprised of the MASAC chair (Dr. Leon Hoyer), the NHF officers including the executive director (Mr. Alan Brownstein), the medical director (Dr. Louis Aledort), and the president (Dr. Charles Carman). The NHF AIDS Task Force had the primary role of collecting information, interacting with the various federal and private organizations about the risks associated with blood products, and developing recommendations and advising the NHF leadership about the HIV risks. The NHF executive director and board had the final authority over the AIDS Task Force and MASAC recommendations (Aledort, Carman interviews). The process of developing recommendations and providing information also included a review by CDC scientist Bruce Evatt to ensure accuracy (Aledort, Carman, Evatt interviews).

The October 22, 1983, meeting of MASAC was the occasion to learn that the Office of Maternal and Child Health (OMCH), the source of federal funding for the hemophilia treatment centers, would provide practical support for the establishment of a hemophilia information exchange network. Dr. Jeanne Lusher, a member of MASAC, was designated to be the project director for the hemophilia information exchange (HIE) (NHF 1982a). OMCH worked with MASAC and the NHF to set up a process for information exchange. The NHF, however, took the primary responsibility for developing the information and disseminating it to the treatment centers and chapters (McPherson interview). The purpose of the information exchange network was to provide paid subscribers with "preprints" (manuscripts not yet published in scientific journals) concerning various aspects of hemophilia, including, orthopedic management, genetic analysis, inhibitors, and infectious complications such as AIDS. A bibliography of articles of interest to the hemophilia community was included in each distribution.

Although MASAC had committed itself in October 1982 to provide the same information to patients that was provided to physicians, the primary recipients of NHF communications were the physicians and chapter leaders (NHF 1982b). Indeed, a cover letter, dated July 19, 1982, from Charles Carman to NHF chapter presidents, accompanying Chapter Advisory #2, explicitly recommended that the Advisory be kept in the chapter files to answer questions about *Pneumocystis carinii* pneumonia (PCP) and that mass mailings were not necessary.

Although some specific messages changed over time, the recommendation to continue to use AHF concentrate for severe hemophiliacs remained constant from January 1983 to October 1984, when the NHF first recommended using heat-treated concentrates. The communication issued on July 14, 1982 (Patient Alert No. 1), was the first of many NHF communications that stressed that "the CDC was not advising a change in treatment regimen at this time." Although some specific recommendations changed over time, one message remained constant throughout the entire period: "Patients [should] maintain the use of concentrate or cryoprecipitate as prescribed by their physicians. The life and health of hemophiliacs depends on the appropriate use of blood products." The NHF reaffirmed this message in medical bulletins and chapter advisories on many occasions, six of which, between May 11, 1983, and October 5, 1984, were within days of recalls (i.e., industry's voluntary withdrawal) of AHF concentrate due to the diagnosis of AIDS in individuals donors. Many of the communications contained messages to encourage patients to maintain current treatments and to reassure them that the risk was remote despite the possibility that the patients may be using vials of AHF concentrate from lots recalled by industry's voluntary withdrawal of the product [Medical Bulletin #7, May 1983; Chapter Advisory #8, May 1983; Chapter Advisory #9, September 1983; Chapter Advisory #11, November 1983; Chapter Advisory #13, January 1984; Chapter

Advisory #19, October 1984; Chapter Advisory #24, December 1984; Medical Bulletin #20, December 1984].

RISK REDUCTION OPTIONS

Many of the debates and discussions that occurred during the MASAC and NHF meetings concerned clinical options to reduce the risk of AIDS transmission for individuals who were using blood products or were in need of receiving blood transfusion. Although these options to reduce the risk of AIDS transmission through blood products were not appropriate to every patient's circumstances, there was a range of clinical approaches for physicians and their patients to consider. The full list of these options is shown in Table 7.1. The Committee found that, for the most part, there was little systematic communication and assessment of the full range of these options for reducing the risk of infection.

Specific Options

The primary clinical option for mild, moderate, and previously untreated hemophiliacs was to use cryoprecipitate rather than AHF concentrate. Because cryoprecipitate is derived from single donors or small pools of 10–15 donors, some physicians believed that it was less likely to be infected with AIDS (Roberts interview; Ratnoff 1994). There were several rationales for not recommending cryoprecipitate, including issues of adequate supply, requirements for storage, and unfavorable attitudes (Aledort, Dietrich, Kasper, Levine, Lusher interviews). In addition, blood bank officials were concerned about the burden of extra work for the blood banks (Barker, Sandler interviews). A minority of MASAC members advocated cryoprecipitate for treating mild, moderate, and severe hemophilia, but it was never an official recommendation of MASAC or the NHF. The Committee is not aware of any systematic studies of cryoprecipitate, and it seems that this option was discarded as infeasible without a thorough analysis.

The NHF communications reflected inconsistency, or at least some degree of ambivalence, in the presentation of information about this option. Communications as early as December 21, 1982, and again on January 14, 1983, cautioned against introduction of AHF concentrates to individuals who had never used them before and recommended the use of cryoprecipitate instead [Chapter Advisory #5 and Medical Bulletin #4, December 1982]. Chapter Advisory #12 (December 21, 1983) said that the potential advantages of cryoprecipitate over AHF concentrates were unknown. Most of the adult hemophiliacs had used cryoprecipitate or fresh frozen plasma to treat their

Table 7.1 Summary of Clinical Options, Status and Sources of Recommendations, and Recommended

Clinical Options and Date Recommended	Status and Sources of Recommendations	Date Recommended
Use of Cryoprecipitate Newborn infants and children under four; newly diagnosed and previously untreated hemophiliacs	Provided as "advice" to physicians and NHF chapters by NHF AIDS Task Force	December 21, 1982
Mild hemophiliacs who require infrequent treatment	Provided as recommendations to physicians and patients by NHF/MASAC	January 14, 1983
For severe hemophilia A, or patients who require frequent treatment	Not recommended	
Patients under treatment with AHF concentrate should be reevaluated to see if it would be possible to switch to directed donor cryo program	Minority opinion of several MASAC members; option recommended by small number of individual physicians and adopted by some hemophiliac patients and physicians	Not officially recommended by NHF/ MASAC
Discourage prophylactic treatment	Not an official recommendation of MASAC; several treatment center physicians implement and some patients reduce their use	Not officially recommended by NHF/ MASAC
DDAVP (desmopressin acetate) Should be used for mild and moderate hemophilia A whenever possible	MASAC; some physicians implement this early and encourage FDA to expedite licensing	January 14, 1983 (DDAVP licensed by FDA in April 1984)

Clinical Options	Status and Sources of Recommendations	Date Recommended
Surgical Procedures Elective surgical procedures should be evaluated for possible delay	MASAC	January 14, 1983
Physicians should strictly adhere to medical implications for transfusions, and autologous blood transfusions are encouraged	PHS	March 4, 1983
Heat-Treated Products Expedite the development of processing methods to inactivate viruses potentially present in AHF concentrate	MASAC	December 2, 1983
Physicians should strongly consider changing to heat-treated AHF concentrate	MASAC	October 13, 1984 (FDA licensed first heat-treated product March 1983; all four companies licensed by October 1984)
Secondary Transmission Warnings		
Use condoms or practice safe sex	Not recommended	
Open discussion between sexual partners and advice from physicians	NHF no recommendation by MASAC	February 3, 1984

disease before AHF concentrate became the standard treatment in the mid- to late 1970s. It is more difficult to treat adults who have severe hemophilia with the cryoprecipitate or fresh frozen plasma because of the large amount that is required. To go back to cryoprecipitate or fresh frozen plasma presented several obstacles in terms of logistics, amount needed, and the time involved in this type of infusion.

That the NHF and MASAC did not recommend some clinical options to prevent AIDS in hemophiliac patients did not discourage some patients and their physicians from improvising. The Committee found several instances of physicians implementing risk-reduction strategies such as discouraging prophylactic treatment and reevaluating the frequency of using AHF concentrate. Physicians who implemented these options instructed their patients about what types of bleeds to treat, when, and how often. Personal circumstances and fears about not treating serious bleeds made some physicians apprehensive about instructing patients to not treat bleeding episodes (Aledort, Dietrich, Levine interviews).

The NHF recommended the use of DDAVP (desmopressin acetate) to treat mild and moderate cases of hemophilia A, an option implemented by several physicians, initially for mild cases and later for moderate individuals (Dietrich, Kasper interviews). The availability of this experimental product came at the urging of the medical community, both to plasma fractionators for development and to FDA expeditious licensing of the product, which occurred by April 1984 [Medical Bulletin #5, January 1983; Chapter Advisory #15, April 1984].

In many cases, physicians treating individuals with hemophilia decided to delay elective surgical procedures on their patients (Dietrich, Kasper interviews), only to abandon this strategy after none of their patients developed symptoms of AIDS and individual patients insisted upon having the corrective surgery without delay (Dietrich interview; see also Case Study Two below).

Neither the NHF and MASAC nor individual physicians appear to have devoted much effort to communicating the possibility of the risk of secondary transmission of HIV to their sexually active, and possibly HIV-infected, hemophilia patients. The NHF did not communicate information about the risk of secondary transmission until it issued Chapter Advisory #14 on February 3, 1984. The communication discussed the risk of secondary transmission through sexual activity or other forms of intimate contact, but characterized the risk as remote. The NHF bulletin encouraged open communication between patients and physicians (NHF 1984). The MASAC never issued official recommendations about sexual transmission of AIDS.

The February 4, 1984, NHF medical bulletin communication about secondary transmission of AIDS provided information on the death of a 70-year-old hemophiliac who had died from AIDS in May 1983. The NHF communication stated that the wife was not known to be a member of a high-risk group, but it was still possible that she developed AIDS first and spread it to her husband, and that the patient's vulnerability may have been a function of age, rather than sexual contact. The communication stated there was still controversy about whether secondary transmission of AIDS could occur but that all agreed that if sexual partners of hemophiliacs were at increased risk of contracting AIDS, the risk was small: "Individual patients and their treaters need to consider whether or not they wish to employ prophylactic methods (e.g., condoms) in continuing their sexual relations as a strictly precautionary and temporary measure until more is learned about AIDS." The Committee learned that some physicians were frightened by the possibility of secondary transmission of AIDS (Hoyer interview). MASAC acknowledged its limitations in dealing with AIDS transmission. According to Brownstein (1994), MASAC members were hematologists and did not have expertise in the area of sexual disease transmission. The NHF transmitted information about sexual transmission of AIDS from the CDC to treating physicians as they were informed.

The NHF did not always fully communicate information. The NHF and MASAC did not communicate information about the availability of heat-treated products until October 1984, when it recommended using them after all four companies had received FDA license approval for their heat-treated products. The rationale for not prescribing heat-treated products included the absence of clinical trials to prove their effectiveness for viral inactivation, a belief that use of these products could lead to the development of inhibitors, their higher costs to the patient, and that these products were developed for eliminating hepatitis and therefore not necessary for those who were known to be infected with hepatitis (Aledort, Dietrich, Lusher interviews) (see Chapters 4 and 6). The NHF communications did not include information to help patients better understand product treatment methods, such as heat treatment, and other possible risk-reduction options.

The Process for Developing NHF Guidelines

After reviewing specific clinical options, the Committee examined the process by which the NHF developed its recommendations. While information about potential consequences for large-scale infection within the hemophilia community alerted members of the NHF to recommend several alternative treatment options, the NHF did not provide full information about potential risk reduction options. The NHF also did not say that there were debates within MASAC regarding some of the potential treatment options (Carman, Roberts interviews). Although the evidence that AIDS could be blood-borne was not conclusive in the earliest stages of the epidemic, the sense of urgency with which meetings were called and conducted, the early discussions of the potential needs for increased production of cryoprecipitate, and the explicit consideration of other possible changes in the treatment and management of hemophilia provide evidence that the NHF leadership was aware of a range of clinical alternatives and their implications for individual risk reduction (Carman, Levine interviews; NHF 1982a,b, 1983).

The initial discussions between the NHF leadership and experts from CDC, FDA, and PHS, and industry about the report of three immune-suppressed hemophiliacs resulted in immediate concern and specific recommendations [Medical Bulletin #4 and Chapter Advisory #5, December 1982] from the NHF to the commercial and voluntary blood community (NHF 1982a,b). These recommendations included implementing donor screening and testing measures as well as expediting efforts in viral inactivation methods. Even as early as November 2, 1982, an NHF letter to manufacturers of AHF concentrate urged the exclusion of high-risk donors of plasma (Carman and Aledort, 1982). The timing, range, and advocacy of these recommendations on behalf of instituting these risk-reducing changes in the blood industry is evidence that NHF officials had access to information and did appreciate and take seriously the warnings from the CDC. The MASAC was well aware of the alternative approaches to treatment as early as January 1983 and in some instances made recommendations for their use. On January 14, 1983, MASAC officially recommended a range of clinical options for reducing the risk of HIV exposure for mild or moderate hemophiliacs and previously untreated cases.

As indicated in Appendix C, the communication strategy of the NHF did reveal incremental modification of several recommendations as new information became available (e.g., avoiding sexual contact, considering heat treatment), but provided it relatively late and did not provide physicians with further information on how to switch severe hemophiliac patients to cryoprecipitate.

When plasma fractionators began to withdraw suspected lots of AHF concentrate found to be associated with a donor known to have or suspected of having AIDS (see Chapter 6), physicians had to intensify their efforts to communicate the risks associated with blood and blood products to patients and to notify patients who may have been using, or have in their possession, contaminated lots of AHF concentrate. Dr. Jenne Lusher stated, "It made it much more apparent to our patients; even if they were not involved in the recall, a particular recall, they would hear all about it. ... They all interacted with each other, knew each other. They began to fear that if one of us from the [treatment] center called them, it was because the product was being recalled (Lusher interview). On May 11, 1983, the *Hemophilia Newsnotes* referred to the recent recall by Baxter [Chapter Advisory #8, May 1983]. In August 1983, the NHF noted two additional recalls of contaminated lots, one by Baxter (Hyland Therapeutics) and one by the American Red Cross. The NHF sent a notification within days of learning of a recall. However, the NHF communications did not always reach the patient, and in some instances the information about the recalled product came from the pharmacy or the physician (Jason interview) and in some cases not at all (Kuhn interview).

In the case of individuals receiving blood transfusions, possible clinical options included autologous or directed donor programs. In the early years of the AIDS epidemic, patients were not always informed of the risks associated with blood transfusions (Alter, Crispen, Goldfinger, Silvergleid, interviews). In some cases, particularly in geographic areas known to be associated with a large number of high-risk individuals, patients were told that if they were going to have surgery to have blood drawn ahead of time if possible, or have a relative donate blood for them (Amman interview). However, directed donor and autologous donations were viewed with considerable skepticism in the blood bank community. Further, blood bank leaders have often viewed discussions of the risks of the blood supply as having a detrimental effect on donation and availability (see Chapter 5).

CASE STUDIES

The following case studies are presented to illuminate what was communicated about the risks associated with the use of blood and blood products from the perspective of specific patients and physicians. They also provide information about the individual perceptions of possible clinical options that existed during this period of uncertainty.

Case Study One: Conviction and Change

The particular patient-physician relationship described here serves as an example of how important it was that both the individual with hemophilia and the treating physician arrive early at the belief that the risk of AIDS from using AHF concentrate was high and that cryoprecipitate was a feasible option.

Dr. Melvin Simonson[1] is a psychiatrist living in the Southeastern United States. He has severe hemophilia with a Factor IX deficiency. Dr. Simonson first became aware of the potential risk of exposure to AIDS from use of blood and blood products in October 1982. He remembered a particular news story as well as an article on T4/T8 reversed cell ratios in AIDS cases that appeared in the *New England Journal of Medicine* in 1982. Dr. Simonson's immediate response was one of panic, in all senses of the word. Dr. Simonson believed that the theories about AIDS (e.g., associated with the use of amyl nitrates, homosexual promiscuity) were wrong. He was convinced that if hemophiliacs were getting the disease, it had to be from use of the AHF

---

[1] The names used in the case studies one to four are pseudonyms to protect confidentiality.

concentrate products. Therefore it had to be in the blood supply and it had to be infectious.

Dr. Simonson went to speak with his physician, Dr. Arnold Schmal, who was serving on the Medical and Scientific Advisory Council of the National Hemophilia Foundation. Dr. Simonson discussed his beliefs about the risk of AIDS from AHF concentrate, and asked to be treated with fresh frozen plasma. When Dr. Simonson discussed the risk with other physicians at the same treatment center, he was told he was "overreacting, the risk was not that bad, there are always risks, and finally, let's wait and see what happens." However, his physician concurred with his concerns about the risk and believed that his request for an alternative treatment was rational. Furthermore, before AHF concentrate became standard treatment, Dr. Simonson had treated his disease with fresh frozen plasma successfully for 18 years. His physician was supportive and helped him to set up a directed donor plasma program. If he had a life threatening bleed during this time, Dr. Simonson believes that he probably would have used the AHF concentrate treatment.

Setting up a directed plasma donor program was not an easy task at the end of 1982. Dr. Simonson's initial attempts to work with the American Red Cross (ARC) were futile, as they were not receptive to the idea of such a program. He also tried to work with two universities' hemophilia treatment centers, however, both universities told him they only used donations for research projects and blood for clinical use was obtained from the Red Cross. In early 1983 Dr. Simonson located a private blood bank that agreed to assist him. To do this, he approached 20-30 personal friends and wrote a letter to colleagues in his professional society asking them to donate plasma necessary for his treatment. He started this program in February 1983. Dr. Simonson relied on this same group of individuals until February 1995 when he enrolled in a clinical trial for recombinant Factor IX. He remains HIV negative.

Case Study Two: Reduction in Use of AHF Concentrate

Dr. Eugene Baker is an example of a person who, because of his own concerns and unease about AIDS, sought out the advice of the medical community and received continual reassurances about the safety of the product he was using. His eventual change in behavior to reduce his use of AHF concentrate, and to later switch to cryoprecipitate, was actually self-initiated and subsequently reinforced by a physician who did believe that the AHF concentrate was contaminated with AIDS.

Dr. Baker came of age during the time when the world was changing for individuals with hemophilia. He is from Wisconsin, born in 1959, and is the second of two sons with severe hemophilia. For the first 10 years of his life he was treated with fresh frozen plasma. In 1969, his family physician prescribed a new product, cryoprecipitate, which he continued to use on an in-patient basis until 1974. In 1974, he was introduced to the AHF concentrates. His physician told him that there was a minimal risk of hepatitis. For Dr. Baker, the use of AHF concentrate made home infusion possible, and hospital stays were a thing of the past.

In 1976, Dr. Baker's older brother developed acute hepatitis. His brother survived, but at the age of 17 he was left with a lasting impression and growing fear about the possible transmission of hepatitis from using these blood products. When he queried various individuals in the medical community about the risk of hepatitis from the use of AHF concentrate, he was told that the hepatitis problem was due to the pooling of blood from thousands of paid donors, who were themselves at high risk for hepatitis.

In January 1981, Dr. Baker was told that he was negative for hepatitis A antibody and hepatitis B surface antigen, and positive for hepatitis B core antibody. His physician also told him that he should not be concerned about these findings. When he graduated from college in 1981, his bleeds were minor and easily treated with AHF concentrate. In the fall of 1981, he began graduate school.

He first became aware of a possible risk of AIDS from using blood products in the spring of 1982, when he read a scientific article that described an immune disorder diagnosed in a severe hemophiliac. The disease was predominantly associated with homosexual behavior, but he became concerned of the risk of this new disease being transmitted via the AHF products, because he knew how the product was manufactured. He made an appointment immediately with one of the hematologists at his university's hospital. The physician told him there were as many as 10 cases in hemophilia patients. He was told not to worry, that the National Hemophilia Foundation was advising hemophiliac patients not to change their treatment regimen.

In early 1983, Dr. Baker learned that the CDC had reported 11 additional cases of AIDS in hemophiliacs (CDC, MMWR, March 4, 1983). Again he questioned the hematologists at his school, and was told only a small fraction (1 percent) of the hemophiliacs were contracting the disease and that the etiology was not yet known. His physicians reassured him that it was the position of the NHF, as well as the plasma fractionators, not to withhold or reduce treatment. Dr. Baker made the decision to use the product sparingly. In August 1983, he discussed his decision with his older brother and learned that he was not reducing his use, and in fact had even planned elective surgery for early the next year.

In September 1983, Dr. Baker began to have digestive problems involving bouts of diarrhea; he knew this was one of the symptoms of AIDS and became quite fearful. He also knew that as a severe hemophiliac he was now a member of a high-risk group for developing AIDS. His physician conducted some initial tests that proved inconclusive, and antibiotics prescribed by his physician had no effect. His physician administered an immunological test, and one week later he received a letter from his physician saying that he had a very low T4 count and an inverted T4/T8 ratio. His physician told him that he may have a mild case of AIDS, but not to worry because there were many new experimental treatments.

Later the same month, Dr. Baker made an appointment with another physician for a second opinion. This physician did not agree with the initial diagnosis of AIDS because of the absence of any of the symptoms usually associated with AIDS (i.e., PCP, Kaposi's sarcoma). He queried his physician about the possibility that AHF concentrates were infected with the AIDS virus. The physician stated that he believed that they were, but expressed caution that this was not the position of the NHF or the plasma fractionation companies. Dr. Baker demanded an alternative treatment that would reduce his risk; the physician told him the best thing would be to go back to cryoprecipitate obtained from voluntary donors.

It was not the physician, but Dr. Baker himself, who had to try to make these arrangements. He contacted the American Red Cross and was not given much help with his specific request. He was told that cryoprecipitate was made only in small quantities for special needs and that it would not be possible to accommodate the needs of all hemophiliacs.

In October 1983, Baker scheduled appointments with several other physicians at the university (this included a longtime family hematologist). At this juncture, he was told that the risk of AIDS was small and that he should neither reduce therapy nor return to cryoprecipitate (he was told that this was the position of the NHF and plasmapheresis companies). He was adamant and persistent; finally someone at the local chapter of the ARC agreed to supply him with the necessary cryoprecipitate. He infused himself at home and stored the cryoprecipitate in his freezer. During this time his T4 cell count remained abnormal, and he continued to have frequent digestive problems.

In March 1984, Dr. Baker's brother underwent his scheduled elective surgery. His brother was told that the risk of AIDS was almost nonexistent. Three weeks after the surgery, his brother developed night sweats, fever, and unexplained weight loss. In March 1985, his brother started to develop serious health problems, which were a result of AIDS and an acute brain infection. The new HIV antibody test revealed that his brother was HIV positive. His brother died in June 1985.

In August 1986, Dr. Baker began to pursue a Ph.D. He treated his hemophilia with heat-treated AHF concentrate at first, and then switched to monoclonal antibody products when they became available. Despite his low T4 count, he was in good health. In October and November of 1986, he participated in clinical trials of AZT therapy, which initially, but only temporarily, increased his low T4 cell counts. In November 1989, Dr. Baker tested positive for HIV. In December 1990, he was awarded his Ph.D. and became a nutritional consultant. He also continued to participate in clinical trials. At this time, his T4 cell count had dropped below 50.

By December 1994, his physician told him to take full and permanent leave from his employer for reasons of declining health. He disclosed his HIV status to his friends and colleagues. Currently he is on an array of antiviral and other medications. He also suffers from liver disease from a hepatitis C infection.

Dr. Baker believes that erroneous and misleading information was provided to patients from the pharmaceutical companies. He believes that the NHF neglected its responsibilities to the people they were supposed to be serving by inadequately warning patients of the risks involved with using the concentrates. He is convinced that treatment options to reduce the risk of infections were not discussed or disclosed to the hemophiliac community, and that the physicians treating hemophiliacs either were not told of the risks or were misled into believing that the risks were low.

Case Study Three: Continue AHF Concentrate Treatment

This case study illuminates the influence of situational factors, or personal experience, on the perception of risk and changes in behavior. It is from the perspective of a physician of one of the larger hemophilia treatment centers where 400–500 active patients are seen at least once per year.

Dr. Susan David first became aware of the possible risk of AIDS sometime in 1981, primarily through the media attention. She believed AIDS, known then as "GRID" (gay-related immunodeficiency disease) was a problem in the homosexual population. Dr. David remembers receiving the CDC's *Morbidity and Mortality Weekly Report* (MMWR) in July 1982, the first report of AIDS in three people with hemophilia.

In November 1982, the CDC sent a very detailed survey to the treatment center requesting information on the number of patients with enlarged nodes and the causes of death in hemophilia patients over the past 10 years. Completing the survey was an administrative burden, and Dr. David phoned CDC to see why the information was required. She was told that they were investigating whether AIDS was a real problem in the hemophilia population. Sometime close to Thanksgiving, Dr. David remembered a 12-year-old boy who had a bleed and enlarged lymph nodes. The child was not sick and she recalled wondering if the child's enlarged lymph nodes were relevant to the reports in the *MMWR* and the information that the CDC was requesting.

In early December, Dr. David learned of the case of the baby in San Francisco who had possibly gotten AIDS from a transfusion (see Chapter 3). At this point, the staff among the treatment center began to talk about the new disorder. In December, one of the physicians suggested arranging directed donor programs for patients who were put on cryoprecipitate, but this suggestion was not implemented; nor was another suggestion to use a preparation of only female-donated AHF concentrate prepared by one of the plasma fractionation companies.

On January 3, 1983, the treatment center held a meeting for all of the center's patients, families, and other interested persons. Its purpose was to discuss the risk of blood and plasma transfusion therapy to hemophiliacs, and it was attended by approximately 100 people. At this point, the staff told the patients and families that they were cooperating with the CDC survey, they saw no reason to change treatment at this time, and they were trying to get more information. The message to the patients was to keep in touch with the treatment center.

On January 4, 1983, Dr. David attended the CDC meeting in Atlanta (see Chapter 3 and Chapter 5). She did not agree with the blood bank community's decision not to implement direct questioning of donors, but did agree about not implementing surrogate testing (i.e., the hepatitis anti-core test) for AIDS. As a physician at a major hospital, she was concerned about maintaining an adequate blood supply for transfusions and the surgical work that was done at the hospital. Clinical care continued as usual, although a bulletin describing what was known about AIDS was issued by the treatment center to patients following the January 4, 1983, meeting.

In the latter half of 1983, the treatment center held another meeting with patients and their families. At this time, according to Dr. David, the center was following the advice of the NHF, "not word for word, but in accord with their recommendations." In addition, by the first half of 1983 the treatment center's pediatrician changed the younger children's treatment to cryoprecipitate. By April 1983, the first heat-treated product had been licensed by the FDA and the center debated its use, weighing the expense of the new product with the unknown potential problem of inhibitor formation. According to Dr. David, heat treatment was originally developed for hepatitis inactivation. Dr. David stated that hepatitis did not seem like a terrible risk in 1983, so the benefit of heat treatment for reducing hepatitis risks was not an impressive safety feature. The physicians decided to selectively use the heat-treated products; heat-treated AHF concentrate was given to patients who were known to not have been exposed to hepatitis. The center's staff also decided that patients should treat bleeds promptly, but to have them reduce use of AHF concentrate whenever possible. Dr. David personally believed that patients significantly overused AHF concentrate. At this time, the treatment center, with its large number of patients, had still not seen a single case. They were convinced that the risk was small. They also decided to resume elective surgeries because of the many requests that were made by the patients and because of the organization of a prospective surgery study of the immune system.

According to Dr. David, there were lengthy discussions about AIDS among the scientists and physicians at the Stockholm meeting of the World Hemophilia Federation in May 1983. The final conclusions were that no one knew what to do; there was no indication to change treatment. After the meeting, she talked to the head of the local chapter of the American Red Cross about producing more cryoprecipitate. This official was not receptive because an increase in production would have placed a tremendous burden on the system. Dr. David stated that she did give her patients the option of using cryoprecipitate, but not many patients decided to use it. One theory was that because that area had a high prevalence of AIDS in homosexual men, who had been donating to the blood supply, it was likely that HIV was in the donor pool and that cryoprecipitate would transmit AIDS as well. Logistically, the treatment center could not possibly have switched everyone to cryoprecipitate; but patients were given the option.

By the end of 1983, everyone at the center realized that there was likely an infectious agent in AHF concentrate and that both blood and cryoprecipitate were transmitting it. The only options were to offer cryoprecipitate (which no one took), to suspend surgeries, and try to get the patients to reduce their consumption of AHF concentrate.

In January 1984, the center diagnosed their first case of clinical AIDS in a young man, who died within a week of his diagnosis. This was soon followed by a second case. Dr. David phoned Bruce Evatt, a scientist at CDC, who remarked, "It is really happening now." The response, according to Dr. David, however, was not dramatic: "We still did not make any change. Each doctor at the treatment center prescribed AHF concentrate according to his or her best judgment. I did not use a lot of heat-treated AHF concentrate because at this point I believed that everyone who had received a lot of AHF concentrate was already exposed, the cost of heat-treated products was very high, and I was still worried about the side effects [inhibitors]."

In May of 1984, one of Dr. David's patients, a teenage boy, died from an untreated head bleed. He had hit his head in an accident at home, resulting in an intracranial bleed. He did not treat his injury with AHF concentrate and he subsequently died. According to Dr. David, everyone at the treatment center was shocked. It was evident to her that if you told patients to cut down on AHF concentrate use, it could be a catastrophic event for all hemophilic patients. According to Dr. David, "this one case influenced our thinking."

The center had an influential role in transmitting information to physicians about what to do. According to Dr. David, "We got phone call after phone call. We knew that it was transmissible, but to translate that to a plan of action was difficult, as there was not any plan of action that seemed coherent. A huge change in treatment may have endangered lives. The patients knew basically what we knew."

In reflecting on lessons learned, Dr. David perceived the FDA and the NIH as remote entities that had no influence on daily practice. In addition, Dr. David stated that most of the information on AIDS came from the NHF and their bulletins, and personal contacts. She said, "The FDA did not realize that the NHF and from MASAC represented a certain small group of doctors and how much was getting out to the hemophilia community was a little bit questionable. The grassroots level was really doing its own thing. Our group was more in the middle, and I think that I was more advanced because I had many informal contacts."

Case Study Four: Prescribing Cryoprecipitate for a Newborn and Continuing AHF Concentrate Treatment for a Four-Year-Old

This case study is about a father who relied on and trusted the medical experts (i.e., MASAC and other physicians) and did not question the NHF recommendations made on January 14, 1983 (i.e., to treat newborns, newly diagnosed hemophiliacs, children under four, and mild hemophiliacs with cryoprecipitate, and to continue to treat others with AHF concentrate).

Robert Thomas is a father of two sons with severe hemophilia, both born during the period when HIV was entering the blood supply. His older son, John, born in 1979, is HIV positive; his younger son Steven, born in 1982, is not.

When Mr. Thomas's first son was born, the new father did not know anything about hemophilia. His son had his first bleed in March 1980, when he was eight months old. The physician tested him and Mr. Thomas was told that his son was a hemophiliac. Initially, he was not concerned about the risk of hepatitis, because he was overwhelmed with learning how to deal with hemophilia. He soon learned to "roll with it" and became comfortable with the treatment recommended by his physician. He learned that hemophilia could be easily treated through the use of AHF concentrate, which was infused by the staff at the hospital. Reflecting on this, Mr. Thomas stated that "he did not know enough to ask a lot of intelligent questions, and did not understand enough to be assertive." After this, his son did not receive many infusions until he was 15 months old. On October 31, 1980, his son had surgery for a blot clot in his spinal cord that had left him paralyzed. During surgery he received thousands of units of AHF concentrate. The surgery was not successful; his son remained paralyzed. At some point, his son contracted post-transfusion chronic hepatitis infection.

In 1981, Mr. Thomas decided to join his local chapter of the National Hemophilia Foundation, and he became its president. The active membership of the chapter, at the time, consisted of five members: an individual with hemophilia, Mr. Thomas, and three other parents of individuals with hemophilia. There was one chapter in the state. While there were several hundred individuals with hemophilia in the state, most of the adults had their own physicians or were affiliated with either one of the two major hospitals serving the population at that time. According to Mr. Thomas, the other reason for the low membership in the chapter was a "general lack of interest by most of the hemophiliac community at that time."

Mr. Thomas's second son, Steven, born in early 1982, had severe hemophilia. Mr. Thomas first became aware of a possible risk of AIDS from using blood products in July 1982, when he received the first patient alert from the NHF (July 14, 1982). In October 1982, Steven had a bleed. He went to the hospital and was told by the hematologist, "There are just too many unknowns about Factor VIII concentrate right now; we need to treat your son with cryoprecipitate." Mr. Thomas asked, "What about my other son?" The physician told him that since he was already on the AHF concentrate, he should continue to use it, and that the NHF was recommending that treatment with concentrate be continued, except when indicated by overriding medical concerns. In October 1982, Mr. Thomas's older son, John, was only three years old.

As president of the local NHF chapter, Mr. Thomas said, he sent out the NHF alerts to 90 percent of the hemophiliacs in the state. Mr. Thomas said that he did not discuss the decision to put his younger son on cryoprecipitate with other chapter members. He remembers that most people (himself included) were occupied learning how to home infuse.

Mr. Thomas continued to have the hospital medical staff infuse his older son with the AHF concentrate. He states he was led to believe that if he did not adhere to this treatment, his son would die from a bleed. Mr. Thomas recalls that, "the potential of a life-threatening bleed was a message reiterated in every NHF alert and bulletin and physician/patient discussions."

In August of 1983, Mr. Thomas received a booklet from Alpha Therapeutic Corporation that contained information about what was known from the AIDS cases that had recently been diagnosed in a small number of hemophiliacs. The following is a synopsis of the information put together by the medical director of Alpha Therapeutic to inform the patients using AHF concentrate.

Alpha was concerned about what it referred to as, "a newly-recognized— and apparently new—disorder." It told its readers that in cases of AIDS, the body's immune system was altered and functioned less efficiently. Its victims "may be afflicted with severe infections, including a rare and deadly form of pneumonia, and other illnesses which their bodies would normally be able to resist. Many AIDS victims die as a result of immune deficiency. The commonest causes of death have been Pneumocystis carinii pneumonia and an unusual cancer, Kaposi sarcoma." The booklet also stated that "AIDS was discovered in, and is still largely confined to, bi-sexual or male homosexuals," and also occurred in IV drug users, and Haitian immigrants. The reader was informed that AIDS was found in a hemophilia patient who did not belong in any of the high-risk groups in March 1982. As of March 1983, there were 11 additional cases in hemophiliacs, 9 of 12 had died. According to the booklet, "hemophilia patients now constitute about one percent of AIDS victims. More importantly, only about one in every thousand hemophilia patients has developed AIDS." The readers were informed that the cause was unknown, but it was possible that it was transmissible.

Mr. Thomas looks back and does not understand how the recommendation could have been made to treat his newborn with cryoprecipitate, but continue to treat his three-year-old with concentrate. He believes there was a clear double standard in this recommendation derived from the manufacturer's desire to sell their factor concentrate. Mr. Thomas' three-year-old son weighed less than 40 pounds. Therefore, the reason given that only young children, because of low body weight, could be effectively treated with cryoprecipitate to stop bleeds was inapplicable to Mr. Thomas' three-year-old. Furthermore, Mr. Thomas believes that both his sons should have been using cryoprecipitate unless a life-threatening situation necessitated the use of concentrate. He asks, "How could any medical professional or anyone in the blood industry logically come up with these recommendations? Were hemophiliacs who contracted HIV from AHF concentrate an acceptable loss from a business standpoint?"

Case Study Five: A Transfusion Case

In 1980, Elizabeth Glaser,[2] when she was six months pregnant, began hemorrhaging. She was rushed to the hospital, where after the delivery of her daughter, Ariel, she was transfused with seven pints of blood. In 1984, Glaser gave birth to her son, Jake. In September 1985, Ariel became ill with serious and baffling stomach pain and fatigue. From January to April 1986, a series of tests revealed nothing. The belief at the time was that an individual needed direct contact with blood or semen to get AIDS. Mrs. Glaser recalled that, "There was nothing about breast milk as a source of transmission." One of the physicians wanted Ariel tested for AIDS because of Elizabeth's transfusions. The test came back positive and the family learned that Ariel had a disease called AIDS. "I screamed as loud as I could. My life was over ... my daughter is going to die" (Glaser and Palmer 1991).

Mrs. Glaser's physicians determined that she had received contaminated blood and had unknowingly passed on the HIV infection to her daughter Ariel through breastfeeding and in utero to her son Jake. For the family "It was our worst nightmare ... It was too much to comprehend." The family learned that there were no drugs or treatments that could make Ariel well. Elizabeth, her

---

[2] This case study uses the real name of the individual.

husband Paul, and their son Jake, were also tested for HIV in 1986. Mrs. Glaser learned that she and her son were HIV positive, but her husband was not. Although Mrs. Glaser had unknowingly passed on the HIV infection to her son, her husband remained HIV negative.

Elizabeth and her family struggled with the isolation that they experienced after they disclosed their problem to their friends, at a time when "there were no assurances to give them that this was not a risk for their children, unlike now." Ariel had to be taken out of summer camp because no AIDS children were allowed there, and when they did tell more people, some would not let their children play with Ariel and Jake.

Elizabeth Glaser's daughter continued to grow weak and frail. In February 1988, Ariel stopped walking. In March she was hospitalized for pneumonia and her physician said her brain was severely atrophied; she lost her ability to speak. Ariel recovered briefly from the pneumonia, was put on AZT, and died in August, shortly after her seventh birthday.

Elizabeth Glaser became a public symbol of the AIDS tragedy in this country. She became active in policy for increased funding for pediatric AIDS research. In 1989, she helped to establish the nonprofit Pediatric AIDS Foundation. On December 3, 1994, at the age of 47, Mrs. Glaser lost her battle against AIDS (McCormick 1993).

Summary of the Case Studies

In the course of the Committee's investigation, many individuals were interviewed about how clinical options were evaluated and in some instances implemented. The case studies indicate how certain options were evaluated by physicians and patients. In some instances options were considered and discarded; in others, clinical options were never fully assessed and discussed between physicians and patients. In yet other instances there were potential inconsistencies in the clinical options. The case studies provide a window into the risk/benefit calculus as physicians and patients confronted the increasing risks of blood and blood products.

The case studies help demonstrate how individuals pursued, or failed to pursue, various clinical options. In the first case, the individual was acutely aware early on in the AIDS epidemic of the risks posed by using blood and blood products. This individual aggressively pursued an alternative option (i.e., a directed donor cryoprecipitate program) with the support of his physician. In the second case, the individual also became apprehensive about the potential risks at an early date, but physicians reassured him that the AHF treatment was safe, the risk of infection was small, and the treatment regimen should be maintained. The third case reveals the difficulties of weighing treatment options, in particular the reduced use of the AHF concentrate and the possible consequences if the patient decides not to treat certain bleeds. The fourth case demonstrates the inconsistencies in the manner in which treatment options were sometimes portrayed. A father was confronted with the decision to treat his newborn son with cryoprecipitate and to maintain AHF concentrate treatment for his older son. Finally, the fifth case illustrates how the options for a transfusion recipient were not communicated even though the assessments of the risk of contracting AIDS through blood transfusions were increasing.

OBSTACLES TO COMMUNICATION

Institutional Obstacles

In its examination of institutional obstacles to communication of risks the Committee has three major findings. These concern: (1) the resources and expertise of the NHF and MASAC; (2) the relationship of the NHF with the plasma fractionators, which ultimately cast doubts on the ability of the NHF to produce authoritative, objective recommendations in the absence of any governmental authority; and (3) the style that the NHF assumed in communicating with both the providers of hemophilia treatment and the individuals who had hemophilia.

Resources and Expertise of the NHF

As the AIDS crisis emerged, the NHF stepped into an institutional vacuum, taking on the critical responsibility for communicating to individuals with hemophilia about the risks associated with the use of blood and blood products. Serving as a liaison between government agencies and the hemophilia community, the NHF (with the help of MASAC), established itself as the primary source of information for individuals who used blood products (Brownstein 1994; Aledort, Carman, Levine interviews). At that time, the NHF was the only national organization enjoying a combination of expertise (through MASAC) in treating individuals with bleeding disorders, the confidence of hemophiliac patients and their physicians, and a reputation among government and industry leaders as representing the interests of individuals with hemophilia. While the federally funded hemophilia treatment centers disseminated information to their patients, the NHF communications provided the basis for assessment of the risk and the development of treatment options. In addition, most members of MASAC were associated with individual treatment centers.

Despite the system of federally funded treatment centers, there was no universal system for notifying patients about risks associated with blood and blood products, and consequently not all individuals in the hemophilia community were informed. In 1982, 50–70 percent of the hemophiliac patients in the United States were members of local NHF chapters or received treatment through the hemophilia treatment centers (Evatt pers. comm., 1995; Smith and Levine, 1984; Aledort, Kasper, Hoyer interviews). In addition, patients in geographically remote areas were especially likely to have less access to treatment and risk information, and some areas had no treatment centers. In these instances, hemophiliac patients were apt to receive AHF concentrates through their local hospital's pharmaceutical dispensation centers (Jason, Reumke interviews). The NHF's early involvement in policy debates and its vigilance in tracking the trajectory of the disease were not matched by comparable efforts to communicate directly with patients. Local chapters owned their own mailing lists, as did the treatment centers, and the NHF left to individual chapters and treatment centers any decision to mail or otherwise distribute information received from the NHF to members (Brownstein 1994; Bias, Carman interviews). The Committee learned that in some instances chapters and treatment centers had insufficient resources for dissemination of NHF mailings (Bias interview). Hence, information sent by the NHF to the treatment centers of NHF chapters did not reach many of the hemophiliacs. Moreover, there was no national registry of hemophiliac patients or treating physicians that the NHF or government agencies could use to communicate directly with hemophiliacs (Bias, Hoyer interviews; Brownstein 1994). In 1981, the NHF tried to compile a registry of all hemophiliac patients but failed owing to confidentiality concerns. The NHF tried again in 1992 but listed only 7,000–8,000 out of as many of 16,000, indicating the problem with reaching the total hemophilia population (Brownstein 1994). Some chapters had low memberships at the time because of a general lack of interest, and most hemophiliacs were on home infusion programs and were not dependent on the chapters and treatment centers. In addition, many hemophiliac patients had private physicians who were not associated with the treatment centers. In one state that had several hundred residents with hemophilia, only five were members of the chapter (Reumke interview).

In the early 1980s, the NHF and MASAC had neither the experience nor adequate expertise to provide specific recommendations to reduce the risk of HIV infection. The NHF had been a nonprofit health organization with interests specifically focused on maintaining federal funding for treatment centers and responding to more general needs of the hemophilia community through local chapter affiliation. When the NHF reactivated MASAC in October 1982, it was comprised of experts in the physical and psychological aspects of the disease and its treatment. These individuals were, by and large, elected to MASAC through the regional treatment centers. Thus, although they had the respect, trust, and support of many in the hemophilia community (Bias, Carman, Hoyer, interviews), their expertise did not extend to all aspects of HIV and its putative transmission through blood products. In addition, the NHF leadership could appoint several members to MASAC (Carman interview). In the early 1980s, however, there was no expertise within MASAC in such areas as infectious disease, epidemiology, or decision analysis. The Committee concluded that the MASAC or NHF leadership did not have all the expertise required to assess the information about the nature and severity of risk as it became available and to understand the possible ramifications of the transmission.

One caveat, however, is necessary. Although the NHF, and MASAC in particular, may have lacked expertise in the critical areas, it did include among its membership some of the nation's most respected physicians involved with treatment of hemophiliac patients. In this respect, at least, the NHF arguably was in a unique position to give careful and informed consideration to the range of possible clinical options that patients and their physicians should consider.

The NHF and the Plasma Fractionation Industry

A second important finding of the Committee was that the NHF and the plasma fractionators had developed close ties that may have compromised the independence of the NHF treatment recommendations. Over the years, the NHF and treatment center physicians had worked closely with the plasma fractionators to develop AHF concentrate. Leaders in the hemophilia field described the relationship to the Committee as synergistic (Hammes pers. com. 1995; Aledort, Carman, Levine interviews). Physicians participated in industry's clinical trials of AHF product, they assisted in the development of information brochures produced by the plasma fractionators about the product, and NHF benefited from industry's financial support of its various committees (e.g., the Nursing Committee) and program meetings (Brownstein 1994; Carman interview). In the Committee's judgment, this close and interdependent relationship led to the perception that the recommendations provided by the NHF and MASAC reflected conflicts of interest, were not adequately objective, and seriously compromised NHF's credibility.

Communication Style of the NHF

The Committee's third finding is that the leadership of the NHF, until October 1984, adopted a generally paternalistic style of communicating information to physicians and patients in which, instead of presenting the rationale for their conclusions and the range of treatment options which they themselves considered in private meetings, the NHF disseminated only their conclusions. These conclusions were accompanied by strongly worded admonishments against reduced use of AHF concentrate. As a group composed of blood disorder specialists, MASAC exhibited a strong tendency to maintain existing treatment regimens and to make only incremental modifications in clinical practice. Until October 1984, NHF communications minimized the potential risk and the extent of possible infection within the hemophilia community and avoided publishing information that individuals with hemophilia and their physicians could utilize to make their own risk assessments and medical decisions.

A more general institutional concern is the fact that the NHF exhibited some tension in the ways in which it defined and carried out its own mission. Executive Director Alan Brownstein, expressing his views about the role of directors of hemophilia societies in an address to the World Hemophilia Federation Conference in June 1983, emphasized the aim of becoming "the source" of information about AIDS and hemophilia. To that end, according to Brownstein, the NHF had decided to retain tight control of the flow of information, to impose strict discipline on who would speak for the NHF, to allay public fears exacerbated by media reports, and "to spread the message throughout the land that clotting factor use should be maintained" (Brownstein 1983). The possible difficulty with the vision of NHF expressed by Brownstein is that goals with respect to institution-building may have been in conflict with and have even overshadowed the commitment to meeting the informational needs of the organization's constituency. One consequence of the NHF's efforts, in the Committee's view, was to restrict rather than to increase the flow of information that patients and their physicians could have used in their own individual medical decisionmaking.

Social and Cultural Obstacles

Several social and cultural impediments in the relationships between patients and physicians interfered with the communication of information about the risks associated with using blood and blood products. These included the tendency of physicians to not discuss, or to downplay and deny, the risk of AIDS; the confidence of physicians and patients in the benefits of AHF concentrate; the context of hepatitis as a medically acceptable risk; the difficulties of communicating dire news to patients; and the problems associated with communicating uncertainty.

With reports of the Committee's finding that physicians tended to avoid, downplay, or deny the possible risk associated with the use of blood and blood products, one of the case studies revealed that physicians often responded to the initial questions of patients with reassurances that the risk was not serious, that the patient was overreacting, that "there are always risks," and that patients and doctors should wait and see what happens (see Case Study One). Or, the physician conveyed the impression that the risk was a problem associated with homosexual behavior and therefore not a problem for individuals with hemophilia (see Case Study One; Bias, Dietrich interviews). In addition, physicians downplayed the size of the risk, saying, for example, "that the patient need to be concerned because only one percent of hemophiliacs were contracting the disease" (see Case Study Two). Information from the NHF and the treatment centers repeated these messages. For example, in a February 1983 newsletter one hemophilia treatment center [Regional Comprehensive Hemophilia Center of Central and Northern Illinois] told patients that "out of some 20,000 hemophiliacs in the U.S., about 10,000 with severe hemophilia A, who have been transfusing some 500 million units of factor VIII each year, only eight or ten have developed AIDS." Similar estimates appeared in information sent to individuals with hemophilia by the plasma fractionation industry.

In assessing the risks associated with using blood and blood products, physicians emphasized the known benefits of AHF concentrate and underweighted the risks of AIDS, which were still uncertain. The NHF and MASAC assessment weighed the benefits of AHF concentrates against what it perceived as "small numbers of AIDS cases in hemophiliacs," and recommended a firm policy to adhere to AHF concentrate therapy rather than cryoprecipitate. Some physicians believed that any change in treatment would endanger the lives of their patients and that the good quality of life with AHF concentrate outweighed the uncertainties of AIDS risk and prognosis (Aledort, Dietrich interviews). In their risk-benefit analysis, physicians believed that the probability of getting AIDS was lower than the probability of morbidity from nontreatment (Aledort interview). Whereas many in the hemophilia treatment community knew the morbidity and mortality attributable to decreased use of AHF concentrate, the morbidity and mortality from AIDS was unknown (Aledort, Carman, Dietrich, Kasper, Levine, Lusher interviews).

Individuals with hemophilia had similar perspectives (Bias, Wadleigh, Dubin, Botelho interviews). According to Bias, "One theory was that hemophiliacs would develop antibodies, like hepatitis, and would not be infected. This was coupled with the desire to lead a normal life" (Bias interview). In one case study (Case Study Four), the father of two sons with hemophilia believed that if he stopped using the AHF concentrate treatment prescribed by his son's physician, the boy would bleed to death.

Some of the attitudes of the patients and their physicians originated in the 1970s when hepatitis emerged as an infectious complication in patients receiving blood and blood products (see Chapter 4). In the context of hemophilia treatment, hepatitis became a medically acceptable risk. In the beginning, HIV engendered analogous attitudes (Lusher interview). Although hepatitis infections were occasionally severe, leading to liver failure and death, it was clear to many physicians that the benefits of the AHF concentrate treatment or the blood transfusion outweighed the disability from the hepatitis (Aledort, Alter, Goldfinger, Hoyer, Johnson, Levine, Lusher interviews). Hepatitis was seen as well understood and manageable: "We used to deal with hepatitis, you get it from blood, it was well established. No one got sick right away ... and it was not life-threatening" (Alter interview). Individuals with hemophilia knew that hepatitis was a problem associated with using AHF concentrate derived from pooled plasma from thousands of individuals (see Case Study Four; Aledort interview). Hepatitis was "acceptable," and individuals with hemophilia were told not to be concerned about it (case study four; Bias interview). When AIDS appeared in the early 1980s, the first reaction of both physicians and individuals was that this new problem would also be manageable (Case Study Three; Bias, Botelho, Louvrein interviews; Pierce 1983). "The response of the patients was not one of fear, and the parents of hemophiliacs were getting used to the risks involved with hemophilia" (Louvrein interview).

As late as the end of 1984, the number of hemophiliacs with AIDS was small compared to the number of patients who received AHF concentrate, and some MASAC members doubted that the infection would become widespread among hemophiliacs (Aledort, Carman, Lusher interviews). Their judgment was due to the then widespread misunderstanding of the length of the latency period in HIV infection and thus what was assessed as the small number of patients with AIDS relative to the number with HIV infection.

As the recognition of the risks of infection with AIDS grew during the period between early 1983 and mid-1984, physicians and other providers of hemophilia care began to assume that most of their patients might already be infected. This assumption also contributed to the rationale to maintain treatment regimens with AHF concentrate. If patients were already infected, changing to cryoprecipitate would only lead to suboptimal treatment for the symptoms of hemophilia; it would no longer reduce the risk of infection. Therefore, many physicians decided not to change their approaches to treatment. The Committee believes that these explanations do not provide sufficient justification for the NHF's decision to communicate only its conclusions rather than provide patients and physicians with the information needed for them to reach their own conclusions.

The doctrine of informed consent—communication of information and discussion of treatment alternatives and risks by physicians to their patients—has long been recognized as a central moral and legal tenet of medical practice in the United States (Katz 1986; Faden and Beauchamp 1985). While it had entered clinical practice by the early 1920s, by the late 1950s, the legal duty to obtain consent had evolved to include an explicit duty of physicians to disclose to patients medical information relevant to making a decision about treatment [*Salgo et al.* v *Leland Stanford, Jr.*, 1957]. However, in some special medical practices, such as hemophilia and transfusion medicine, it was not fully adhered to until the early 1980s. However, court opinions during this era qualified the duty of disclosure by permitting physicians to exercise discretion when full disclosure was deemed medically inappropriate. As Jay Katz has observed, both law and society more generally reflected a fundamental ambivalence between a commitment to patient self-determination and traditional practices of medical paternalism (Katz 1986).

By the early 1970s, however, the ambivalence was replaced by a more stringent conception of the duty of physicians to disclose all relevant information to patients. In *Canterbury* v. *Spence*, the first and most influential of a series of court cases in the 1970s, the court held: "[T]he patient's right of self-determination shapes the boundaries of the duty to reveal. That right can be effectively exercised only if the patient possesses enough information to enable an intelligent choice" [464 F. 2d 772, 786 (D.C. Cir 1972)]. Faden and Beauchamp, in their authoritative treatise *A History and Theory of Informed Consent*, summarize the impact of *Canterbury* and other cases from this period as follows: "[These cases] recognized that although professional expertise is necessary in identifying the nature and consequences of the procedure, the feasibility of alternatives, and the severity of risks, once the physician has exercised medical judgment in developing and presenting this information to the patient, further deference to the physician's judgment is unnecessarily in derogation of the patient's decisionmaking right" (Faden and Beauchamp 1985). An influential 1980 California Supreme Court case, *Truman* v. *Thomas*, represented the logical culmination of the changes in judicial attitude about matters requiring disclosure. The *Truman* decision made it clear that a physician's duty of disclosure encompasses discussions of all relevant treatment options, including the option of nontreatment and its attendant risks and benefits [165 Cal. Rpter, 308, 611 P 2d902 (Cal. 1980)].

The decade of the 1970s thus closed with a legacy of litigation that fundamentally changed the common law of informed consent in most states, and in half of the states newly enacted legislation replaced the remnants of the common law with explicit requirements for adequate disclosures (President's Commission for the Study of Ethical Problems in Medicine and Behavioral Research, 1983). These changes in the law reflected an emerging social consensus on the importance of full disclosure of information to patients for the exercise of the patient's right of self-determination. This new consensus also rested on grounds other than the rationale embodied in the law. Medical ethicists such as Robert Veatch (1982) of the Hastings Institute argued that informing patients of treatment alternatives so that they can participate in or control the decisionmaking process increases the likelihood that benefits to individual patients will be maximized and other social objectives such as improved medical decisionmaking would be achieved [DHEW Publication No. 78-0014, 1982]. Indeed, a substantial body of empirical literature demonstrates that enhanced communication and discussion of treatment alternatives and risks improves patient satisfaction, understanding and deliberation, adherence to treatment, and medical outcomes (Levine, et al. 1979; Eraker, et al. 1988; Hall, et al. 1988).

The norms of full disclosure of the benefits and risks of alternative treatment options had become deeply entrenched in clinical practice by the early 1980s. The best evidence of how pervasive these norms had become can be found in a 1981 statement of the Judicial Council of the American Medical Association:

> The patient's right of self-decision can be effectively exercised only if the patient possesses enough information to enable an intelligent choice. The patient should make his own determination on treatment. Informed consent is a basic social policy for which exceptions are permitted: (1) where the patient is unconscious or otherwise incapable of consenting and harm from failure to treat is imminent; or (2) when the risk-disclosure poses such a serious psychological threat of detriment to the patient as to be medically contraindicated. *Social policy does not accept the paternalistic view that the physicians may remain silent because divulgence might prompt the patient to forego needed therapy.* Rational, informed patients should not be expected to act uniformly, even under similar circumstances, in agreeing to or refusing treatment [emphasis added] [Judicial Council of the American Medical Association, 1984].

This review of the history of informed consent illuminates how the practice of hemophilia and transfusion medicine was somewhat removed from recognized medical norms.

The Committee also found that some physicians were reluctant to discuss bad news, including a prognosis with dire implications, once symptoms of AIDS began to occur in their patients. Even when confronted with initial symptoms of AIDS, the physician's message to his patient sometimes was to not worry (see Case Study Four). The appearance of AIDS in a previously healthy individual with hemophilia became a frightening experience for physicians (Hoyer interview). Once physicians realized that the majority of individuals with severe hemophilia were infected with HIV, they became uncomfortable with discussing the implications of the widespread infection with their patients (Dietrich, Dubin, Levine, Kasper, Lusher, Wadleigh interviews).

In addition, medical uncertainty about the incidence of the infection caused difficulties in communications between physicians and their patients (Aledort, Carman, Crispen, Dietrich, Kasper, Louvrein, Lusher, Silvergleid interviews). According to one physician, "somehow there were enough different things being conveyed, different theories, and a lot of opposition to the idea that all of the clotting factor was contaminated. And, [there was] a lot of unknown[s] about whether or not we did have any alternative; whether or not heat treatment would kill the virus or whatever was causing AIDS, so that really nothing was done" (Lusher interview).

Under the uncertainty posed by the risk of blood-borne transmission of AIDS, many physicians attempted to communicate risks to their patients using strategies to present information gently [*The Hemophilia Bulletin*, Orthopedic Hospital, January 1983; Regional Comprehensive Hemophilia Center of Central and Northern Illinois, February 1983] as if to counter the effect of information that patients had heard from more alarmist sources, such as the public media (Levine interview).

The public media played an important role in raising the consciousness of hemophilia patients about their risk of AIDS. Physicians became concerned because many of the patients were reducing their use of AHF concentrate (Dietrich, Levine interviews). In some instances, physicians believed that one of the reasons patients were reducing their use was because of the public media: "You couldn't open a newspaper or magazine without seeing an AIDS patient along with language linking it to hemophilia. So we went through late 1983 and early 1984 seeing many patients withholding treatment. You had people come in with horrible lesions that you had gotten used to not seeing anymore" (Levine interview). Counteracting media attention was one reason for the NHF policy of urging treatment physicians to reassure patients that the risk of AIDS was low and to maintain their use of AHF treatment (Carman interview). In the early days of AIDS in hemophilia patients, there were many examples of ill effects of reducing use of AHF concentrate and few patients with symptoms and signs of AIDS. By the end of 1983, one of the largest hemophilia treatment hospitals had not yet seen a case of AIDS in their patients but they did have a young child die from intracranial bleeding because the person was afraid of the treatment (Dietrich interview). The death of the young hemophiliac from an intracranial bleed reinforced physicians' fears and beliefs of how important it was to maintain treatment. Soon, AIDS would appear in hemophilia patients, and there would be second thoughts about the balance of risk and benefit from AHF concentrate treatment.

The uncertainty of the AIDS epidemic bred difficulty in communication between physicians and their patients. In response to the medical uncertainty, physicians had difficulty deciding to change, especially when the experience of both the physicians and patients was based on the success of AHF concentrate (Aledort, Dietrich, Levine, Lusher interviews). For example, several physicians reported that patients and families resisted MASAC's cryoprecipitate option if they had experience with AHF concentrate. But some individuals with hemophilia believed that single donor cryoprecipitate was a way to buy time (see Case Study Two). In several instances, physicians or patients who contacted the American Red Cross to obtain cryoprecipitate were told that it was not available (see Case Study Two; Dietrich, Louvrein interviews). But even when cryoprecipitate was available, patients were resistant to using it (Dietrich, Lusher interviews). Patients and their families seemed unwilling to "go back" to the previous era of dependence on cryoprecipitate (Aledort, Dietrich, Kasper, Levine, Lusher interviews). Patients and physicians both seemed to want to maintain the status quo, perhaps believing that in the face of uncertainty, the best option was inaction.

CONCLUSIONS

In its analysis of risk communication, the Committee sought to identify the clinical options that would have reduced the risk of AIDS and to understand what information was actually communicated to patients. In those instances in which information seems not to have been communicated, the Committee explored the institutional, social, and cultural obstacles to communication. The Committee drew the following conclusions:

- Individuals who were dependent on blood and blood products during the AIDS epidemic faced difficult decisions and desperately needed information.

  Physicians and patients who had become accustomed to making few decisions suddenly found themselves in complex clinical situations in which the risks and benefits of treatment were now uncertain. Restricting or abandoning the use of blood and blood products could lead to increased mortality and morbidity. On the other hand, continued use of these products apparently increased the risk of AIDS.
- The NHF stepped into a critical communication role.

As often happens in times of intense scientific and medical uncertainty, communication to individuals with hemophilia and to transfusion recipients about the use of blood and blood products was limited in the early years of the epidemic. The NHF acted during these years as an intermediary between federal agencies and the hemophilia community. There was no single government agency responsible for providing information about the risks associated with blood products directly to the consumers of those services. The NHF was able to do this because it was the only national organization with the expertise (through MASAC) in treating individuals with bleeding disorders.

In contrast to the situation for hemophiliacs, no organization stepped forward to communicate the risks of blood transfusions to potential recipients. Many blood bank officials during this period publicly denied that there were any significant risks of AIDS to blood recipients. In this context, because many transfusions occurred on an emergency basis, patients were often not apprised of the growing concerns about the contamination of the blood supply. For both individuals with hemophilia and transfusion recipients, concern that they might refuse care deemed a "medical necessity" further contributed to failures to apprise them fully of the risks.

- There were many clinical options for responding to the potential risk, but patients did not actively consider many of them.

The Committee documented that a range of clinical options might, in some instances, have reduced or eliminated dependence on AHF concentrate, thereby reducing the risks of HIV infection in the early years of the AIDS epidemic. While it listed some of these options, the NHF never encouraged thorough discussion of these options by patients with severe hemophilia. Rather, the NHF advocated continued use of AHF concentrates for these patients. While members of MASAC were concerned that alternative treatments were unproven, nonetheless, discussion of full range of options with patients should have occurred.

The dramatic successes in the 1970s of treatment with AHF concentrate provided a context in which it was very difficult to abandon, or radically restrict, use of these products for severe hemophiliacs. In their effort to find the right balance between the risks and benefits of AHF concentrate, the NHF, MASAC, and physicians tended to overweight the known risks (i.e., bleeding due to inadequate treatment) and underweight the risks that were still uncertain (i.e., infection with a new, unidentified infectious agent).

Given that so few hemophiliacs had actually manifested symptoms of AIDS, and with no intuition that AIDS has a long asymptomatic incubation period, many concluded that it would be inappropriate to "overreact" to reports of possible blood-borne transmission of the disease. Concerns that patients would respond irrationally to reports of the epidemic led to attempts to "reassure" the hemophiliac community about the use of blood products.

- The NHF had serious institutional shortcomings as it tried to assume its self-designated role as the source of information about AIDS and its treatment options. These included inadequate resources and experience; possible conflicts of interest problems; and a generally paternalistic communication style that did not accommodate itself to the uncertainties and complexities attendant upon the emergence of AIDS.

Institutional barriers to patient-physician communications and complex relationships between relevant organizations impeded the flow of information. If the NHF had received input from a wider group of experts and consumers, it might have communicated a more explicit and systematic list of clinical options. In addition, in the Committee's opinion, financial and other relationships between the NHF and the blood products industry presented a conflict of interest that ultimately compromised the perceived independence and credibility of NHF's recommendations.

The NHF undertook a mission that now clearly corresponds to the task of advising patients and physicians about the benefits and risks associated with alternative treatment options. The NHF mission was to give treatment advice, but the advice was conclusory. It was offered without discussion of the range of options, the benefits and risks associated with each option, the medical or scientific rationales for its conclusions, or the areas in which uncertainty or scientific disagreement existed. Given the level of uncertainty engendered by the early years of the epidemic, the NHF should have more fully appraised its constituents of the process and logic of its recommendations, and should have done more at an earlier date to publish information patients and physicians might have used in only their assessments and decisions.

- There were serious social and cultural obstacles to communicating clinical options to reduce the risk of HIV infection for users of blood and blood products. These include the inability of some physicians to accept the implications and their preference for the status quo; misplaced confidence in AHF concentrate; a context in which some severe risks were medically acceptable; and the difficulty of talking about a dire prognosis and communicating uncertainty.

Physicians tended to not discuss all clinical options since their relative merits were so difficult to evaluate in the context of the powerful uncertainties of the AIDS epidemic. During this period, the knowledge base of AIDS was changing rapidly. Buffeted by news and rumor, with no consistent sources of information, many physicians opted to maintain the status quo in their treatment recommendations. In the Committee's view, once the NHF and physicians embarked on a course in which disclosure was constrained, it became much more difficult to move toward disclosure of risk. As physicians began to recognize that many hemophiliacs were infected, the difficulty of discussing the dire implications of the epidemic also compromised candid discussion between patients and physicians.

In addition, the Committee found that the NHF did not perceive the need to let the patients themselves decide matters that were far too complex for simple recommendations. The prevailing assumptions in the hemophilia community about the medically acceptable risks of hepatitis virus infection led to complacency and failure to react to reports of a new infectious risk with sufficient concern. Paternalistic assumptions about medical decisionmaking led to failures to adequately disclose the risks of continuing to use AHF concentrate and enable individuals to make informed decisions for themselves. Failures to develop opportunities for communicating the possibility of widespread infection in the hemophiliac community led to ancillary failures to warn possibly infected individuals of the risks they might pose to others through sexual contact.

- These obstacles resulted in poor communication of information.

The Committee believes that the need for communication of information actually increased as the dimensions of the epidemic became more apparent. Medical uncertainty increases the need for communication of information about risks associated with blood and blood products and risk reduction options.

- Better recognition of obstacles to communication of options and a deeper commitment to present patients with a range of possible clinical options might have reduced the powerful sense of betrayal and guilt experienced by many hemophilia patients and their families.

In instances of great uncertainty, it becomes more important for patients to become active participants in the evaluation of the risks and benefits of alternative treatments. Active participation requires knowledge of options. The failure to adequately and fully communicate these options led to a powerful sense of betrayal that exacerbated the tragedy of the epidemic for many patients and their families.

- The Committee concluded that there were serious shortcomings in effective communication of risks associated with the use of blood and blood products.

Uncertain circumstances warrant increased communication of information about risks associated with blood and blood products and risk-reduction options. As often happens in times of intense scientific and medical uncertainty, communication about risks, benefits, and clinical options was limited.

REFERENCES

Aledort, Louis. Current Concepts in Diagnosis and Management of Hemophilia. *Hospital Practice*; October, 1982.

Aronson, David. Factor VIII (Antihemophilic Globulin). *Seminars in Thrombosis and Hemostasis*, Vol. VI, No. 1; 1979.

Brinkhous, Kenneth. "Hemophilia and Hemostasis: An Overview." In *Progress in Clinical and Biological Research, Vol. 72: Hemophilia and Hemostasis*, Menache, et al. editors, New York: Alan R. Liss, Inc., 1981.

Brownstein, Alan. U.S. District Court Northern District of Illinois, Eastern Division, Wadleigh, et al. vs Rhone Poulenc-Rorer, et al. Case No. 93C 5969; June 20, 1994.

Brownstein, Alan. Presentation to the World Federation of Hemophilia; June 28, 1983.

Carman, Charles and Aledort, Louis. The National Hemophilia Foundation. Letter to Cutter Laboratories, Inc., November 2, 1982.

Centers for Disease Control, *Morbidity and Mortality Weekly Report* , July 16, 1982.

Centers for Disease Control, *Morbidity and Mortality Weekly Report* , March 4, 1983.

Centers for Disease Control, *Morbidity and Mortality Weekly Report* , July 23, 1993.

Centers for Disease Control, *Morbidity and Mortality Weekly Report* , January 1984.

Chorba, et al. Changes in Longevity and Causes of Death among Persons with Hemophilia A. *American Journal of Hematology*, Vol. 45; 1994.

Department of Health and Human Services Public Health Service, Maternal and Child Health Bureau Fact Sheet; January 1994.

Eraker, S. et al. "Understanding and Improving Patient Compliance," *Annals of Internal Medicine*, Vol. 100; 1988.

Evatt, Bruce. Personal communication to the IOM, 1995.

Eyster et al. The Pennsylvania Hemophilia Program 1973 to 1978. *American Journal of Hematology*, Vol. 9; 1980.

Faden, Ruth R., Beauchamp, Tom L., *A History and Theory of Informed Consent*, (New York: Oxford University Press; 1985.

Food and Drug Administration, Blood Products Advisory Committee Meeting; February 7, 1983.

Glaser, Elizabeth and Palmer, L. *In the Absence of Angels: A Hollywood Family's Courageous Story*. G.P. Putnam's Sons, New York, New York; 1991.

Hall, J., et al. "Meta-analysis of Correlates of Provider Behavior in Medical Encounters," *Medical Care*, vol. 26; 1988.

Hammes, William J., Associate Counsel, Miles, Inc. Letter to Institute of Medicine. February 13, 1995.

Hoyer, Leon. Medical Progress: Hemophilia A. *New England Journal of Medicine*; January 6, 1994.

Johnson, et al. Acquired Immune Deficiency Syndrome Among Patients Attending Hemophilia Treatment Centers and Mortality Experience of Hemophiliacs in the United States. *American Journal of Epidemiology* , Vol. 121; 1985.

Jones, Paul and Ratnoff, Oscar. The Changing Prognosis of Classic Hemophilia (Factor VIII deficient). *Annals of Internal Medicine*, Vol. 114; 1991.

Judicial Council of the American Medical Association, *Current Opinions of the Judicial Council of the American Medical Association* (Chicago, IL: American Medical Association, 1984), 29–30 (the opinion quoted was first published in 1981).

Katz, Jay, "Informed consent: a fairy tale? Law's Vision," *University of Pittsburgh Law Review* 39 (1977); 1986.

Levine, D. et al., "Health Education for Hypertensive Patients," *Journal of the American Medical Association*, vol. 241; 1979.

McCormick, Patricia. Living with AIDS. *Parents' Magazine*, vol. 68; November 1993.

National Hemophilia Foundation. Hemophilia Information Exchange: AIDS Update; February 3, 1984.

National Hemophilia Foundation. Medical and Scientific Advisory Council Minutes; January 14, 1982a.

National Hemophilia Foundation. Medical and Scientific Advisory Council Minutes; October 2, 1982b.

National Hemophilia Foundation. Medical and Scientific Advisory Council Minutes; October 22, 1983.

Public Health Service. Summary Minutes "Opportunistic Infections in Hemophiliacs." July 27, 1982.

Ratnoff, Oscar. Testimony Provided to Committee. September 12, 1994.

Resnik, Susan. The Social History of Hemophilia in the United States (1948–1988): The emergence and empowerment of a community. Columbia University, School of Public Health; 1994.

Rosendaal, F.R., Smit, C., and Briet, E. Hemophilia Treatment in Historical Perspective: A Review of Medical and Social Developments. *Annals of Hematology*, Vol. 62; 1991.

Seeff, Leonard. Transfusion Associated Hepatitis: Past and Present. *Transfusion Medicine Reviews*; December 1988.

Smith, Peter and Levine, Peter. The Benefits of Comprehensive Care of Hemophilia: A Five Year Study of Outcomes. *American Journal of Public Health*, Vol. 74; June 1984.

Veatch, Robert, "Three Theories of Informed Consent: Philosophical Foundations and Policy Implications," *The Belmont Report* (DHEW Publication No. 78–0014, 1982).

8

Conclusions and Recommendations

The HIV epidemic has taught scientists, clinicians, public health officials, and the public that new infectious agents can still emerge. The nation must be prepared to deal with a fatal illness whose cause is initially unknown but whose epidemiology suggests it is an infectious disease. The AIDS epidemic has also taught us another powerful and tragic lesson: that the nation's blood supply—because it is derived from humans—is highly vulnerable to contamination with an infectious agent. A nation's blood supply is a unique, essential, life-giving resource. Whole blood and many blood products are lifesaving for many people. As a whole, our nation's system works effectively to supply the nation with necessary blood and blood products and its quality control mechanisms check most human safety threats. The events of the early 1980s, however, revealed an important weakness in the system—in its ability to deal with a new threat that was characterized by substantial uncertainty. The potential for recurring threats to the blood supply led this Committee to reappraise the processes, policies, and resources through which our society attempts to preserve its supply of safe blood and blood products.

GENERAL CONCLUSIONS

The events and decisions that the Committee has analyzed underscore the difficulty of decisionmaking when the stakes are high, when decisionmakers may have personal or institutional biases, and when knowledge is imprecise and incomplete. The Committee attempted to understand the complexities of the decisionmaking process during the period analyzed in this report and develop lessons to protect the blood supply in the future. In retrospect, the system was not dealing well with contemporaneous blood safety issues such as hepatitis, and was not prepared to deal with the far greater challenge of AIDS.

By January 1983, the Centers for Disease Control (CDC) had accumulated enough epidemiological evidence to conclude that the agent causing AIDS was almost certainly transmitted through blood and blood products and could be sexually transmitted to sexual partners. The conclusion that the AIDS agent was blood-borne rested on two findings. First, AIDS was occurring in transfusion recipients and individuals with hemophilia who had received AHF concentrate; these AIDS patients did not belong to any other known high-risk group for contracting AIDS. Second, the epidemiologic pattern of AIDS was similar to hepatitis B, another blood-borne disease. However, the magnitude and consequences of the risk for transfusion and blood product recipients was not known at this time. Furthermore, the epidemiological pattern of the new disease was difficult to interpret because, unlike most infectious diseases, there seemed to be several years between exposure leading to infection and the development of symptoms. As a result, physicians and public health officials underestimated the large number of infectious people who had no symptoms of AIDS but could transmit the disease to others and therefore substantially understated the risk of infection.

Compared to the pace of many regulatory and public health decision processes, the federal government responded relatively swiftly to the early warnings that AIDS might be transmitted through blood and blood products. Public and private sector officials considered a range of clinical and public health interventions for reducing the risk of AIDS transmission through blood and blood products. This period, however, was characterized by a great deal of scientific uncertainty about the risks of HIV infection through blood and blood products and about the costs and benefits of the available options. The result, the Committee found, was a pattern of responses which, while not in conflict with the available scientific information, was very cautious and exposed the decisionmakers and their organizations to a minimum of criticism. This limited response can be seen in the refusal of blood banks in 1983 and 1984 to screen for and defer homosexuals or use surrogate tests (Chapter 5), in the Food and Drug Administration's (FDA) cautious and inadequate regulatory approach to the recall of potentially contaminated AHF concentrate (Chapter 6), and in the failure of physicians and the National Hemophilia Foundation to disclose completely the risks of using AHF concentrate and the alternatives to its use (Chapter 7).

Blood safety is a shared responsibility of many diverse organizations. They include U.S. Public Health Service agencies such as the CDC, the FDA, and the National Institutes of Health (NIH), and private-sector organizations such as community blood banks and the American Red Cross, blood and plasma collection agencies, blood product manufacturers, groups such as the National Hemophilia Foundation (NHF), and others. The problems the Committee found were inadequate leadership and inadequate institutional decisionmaking processes in 1983 and 1984. No person or agency was able to coordinate all of the organizations sharing the public health responsibility for achieving a safe blood supply.

Decisionmaking Under Uncertainty

The management of a public health risk requires an evolving process of decisionmaking under uncertainty. It includes interpretive judgment in the presence of scientific uncertainty and disagreement about values. Public health officials must characterize and estimate the magnitude of the risk, which involves considering both the likelihood that infection might occur in various circumstances, and the costs and benefits associated with each of the possible uncertain outcomes. They must also develop and test public health and clinical care strategies, and communicate with the public about the risk and strategies for reducing it. When confronted with a poorly understood and anomalous public health threat, inertia often influences decisions. It is often easier to maintain the status quo than to make a change. In fact, regulatory policymakers, health scientists, and medical experts often require substantial scientific evidence before informing the public and adopting remedial action. Lack of scientific consensus becomes a kind of amplifier for the usual discord and conflict that can be expected whenever an important science-based public policy decision—one profoundly affecting lives and economic interests—must be made. First, uncertainty creates opportunities for advocates of self-interested and ideological viewpoints to advance plausible arguments that favor their desired outcome. Second, uncertainty intensifies bureaucrat cautiousness.

In the course of its investigations, the Committee learned several lessons about decisionmaking under uncertainty. These are set out here both as general lessons and to provide a framework for the recommendations that follow.

Risk Perception

Risk perception is shaped by social tensions, and cultural, political, and economic biases (Douglas 1985). It is important to understand the different contexts in which risk is perceived and the complex system of beliefs, values, and ideals that shape risk perception (Nelkin 1989). There are several other factors that influence risk perception, including locus of control, the type of risk posed by the threat, and the time interval involved in evaluating the risk. For example, people tend to underestimate risks that they perceive to be under their control, risks associated with a familiar situation, and low probability events (Douglas 1985). People have difficulty accepting estimates of a risk that is involuntary, uncertain, unfamiliar, and potentially catastrophic (Fischoff 1987). The epidemic caused by HIV in the blood supply illustrates these patterns of perception and behavior with respect to risk.

Risk Assessment Versus Risk Management

A central precept of risk management is to separate the assessment of risk from the management of its consequences (NRC 1983). Otherwise, risk managers tend to bias their estimates of the magnitude of the risk in favor of their preconceived notions about appropriate or desirable policy choices. The events that the Committee studied provide examples of what can happen when this precept is not followed. When there is uncertainty, it may be necessary to assess risk by making subjective estimates rather than by obtaining objective measures. Such was the case in 1983 when, as part of implicit risk-benefit calculations about donor screening and deferral, blood banks and blood product manufacturers had to make judgments about the risk that their products could transmit AIDS (see Chapter 5). Anticipating the consequences of taking action, which is in the domain of risk management, may bias risk estimates toward values that support risk-averse action. When blood bank officials estimated the risk of transmitting AIDS as "one per million" transfusions, they chose a rate that was low enough to justify their reluctance to take further action. Despite mounting evidence that the risk was much higher, they maintained their original estimate throughout 1983. If the CDC had made numeric estimates of the risk, and the blood banks, blood product manufacturers, or the FDA had used these estimates in a formal analysis of the decision problem, they might have reached different conclusions about, for example, surrogate testing for AIDS.

Consider the Full Range of Possibilities

When there is uncertainty about the facts that will determine the consequences of a decision, a systematic approach is usually best (NRC 1994). One important principle is to consider the full range of assumptions and alternative actions, not only worst-case scenarios. In the events studied by the Committee, systematic denial of worst-case scenarios was a recurring theme, as can be seen in the way that the NHF and the FDA discussed the CDC's warnings in 1982 and early 1983. The plasma fractionators introduced a worst case scenario of their own at the July 1983 Blood Products Advisory Committee (BPAC) meeting, when they estimated that three or four suspect donors and an automatic recall policy could lead to recall of all of the nation's supply of AHF concentrate (Chapter 6). A closely related principle is to scrutinize the evidence to ascertain what is based on fact, what is a "best-guess" estimate, and what is simply untested conventional wisdom.

One approach to such an analysis would be to use a formal group process to systematically sample expert opinion on relevant factors such as the probability of infection and the economic and noneconomic costs and benefits of each of the possible outcomes. Often these officials should use decision analysis, which takes into account the likelihood of events and the magnitude of their outcomes, as a tool to compare the expected value of the outcome of the policy alternatives under consideration. Two somewhat analogous models to consider include those used in Institute of Medicine studies to establish priorities for the development of new vaccines (IOM 1985) and to evaluate the artificial heart program of the National Heart, Lung, and Blood Institute (IOM 1991). The book *Acceptable Risk* (Fischoff, et al. 1981) also offers sensible approaches to dealing with this kind of situation.

Risk Reduction Versus Zero Risk

Decisionmakers tend to seek zero-risk solutions even when they are unattainable or unrealistically costly (NRC 1994). In doing so, they may run the risk of failing to implement solutions that are less effective but are certain to reduce illness. The failure to adopt risk-reduction strategies can be seen in the resistance of blood banks to screening for homosexual activity or using surrogate tests for AIDS (Chapter 5) and in FDA's limited approach to product recall decisions (Chapter 6). Chapter 7 also points out that many risk-reduction strategies for individuals with hemophilia were available but not fully disclosed or recommended. The perfect should not be the enemy of the good.

Risk Communication

Risk communication is a sensitive area because of its influence on the perceptions and behaviors of health professionals and consumers, regulatory policies, and public decisionmaking (Nelkin 1989). Many public health officials and physicians wish to appear in command and infallible. When uncertain, they remain silent rather than disclose their ambivalence (NRC 1989). In the Committee's view, however, the greater the uncertainty, the greater the need for communication. The Committee's analysis of physician–patient communications at the beginning of the AIDS era illustrates the tragedies that can accompany silence about risks (Chapter 7). Risk-communication skills are equally important when presenting information to the general public. The blood banks' reluctance to acknowledge the risk of transfusion-associated AIDS (Chapter 5) seems to have been due in part to the difficulties that they foresaw in presenting this information to potential donors and recipients.

Other important principles of risk communication are that the source of the information must be credible, the process should be open and two-way, and the message should be balanced and accurate (NRC 1989). When there was no other sources of information for physicians treating people with hemophilia and for their patients, the NHF and its Medical and Scientific Advisory Council (MASAC) took on an important risk-communication role—providing what would now be called "clinical practice guidelines." The NHF's credibility in this area was eventually seriously compromised by its financial connections to the plasma fractionation industry.

Bureaucratic Management of Potential Crises

Federal agencies had the primary responsibility for dealing with the national emergency posed by the AIDS epidemic. The Committee scrutinized bureaucratic function closely, and came to the following conclusions about the management of potential crises.

Coordination and Leadership

A crisis calls for extraordinary leadership. Legal and competitive concerns may inhibit effective action by agencies of the federal government. Similarly, when policymaking occurs against a backdrop of a great deal of scientific uncertainty, bureaucratic standard operating procedures designed for routine circumstances seem to take over unless there is a clear-cut decisionmaking hierarchy. An effective leader will insist upon coordinated planning and execution. Focusing efforts and responsibilities, setting timetables and agendas, and assuming accountability for expeditious action cannot be left to ordinary standard operating procedures. These actions are the responsibilities of the highest levels of the public health establishment.

The Public Health Service failed to bring these leadership functions to bear when CDC scientists raised concerns about the blood supply at the January 4, 1983 meeting but received no public support from the director of the CDC or the office of the Assistant Secretary for Health. Similarly, the record does not indicate that the highest levels of the FDA or the PHS were involved in responding to advice from the BPAC regarding donor deferral or product recall. Part of this leadership problem may stem from major changes in the PHS leadership that took place during this period: the leadership of the FDA, the

CDC, and the NIH, and the person serving as the Assistant Secretary for Health all changed between 1982 and 1984.

Advisory Mechanisms

In the early 1980s, the FDA and other agencies did not have a systematic approach to conducting advisory committee proceedings. Such an approach requires that agencies tell their advisory committees what is expected of them, keep attention focused on high-priority topics, and independently evaluate the advice offered. No regulatory process should have its information base effectively controlled by an advisory panel. Public agencies must be able to generate and analyze the information that they need to assure that decisions serve the needs of the public. The FDA failed to observe this principle when it allowed statements and recommendations of the BPAC to go unchallenged, apparently because it could not independently analyze the information (Chapter 6).

Because mistakes will always be made and opportunities sometimes missed, regulatory structures must be organized and managed to assure both the reality and the continuous appearance of propriety. The prominence of representatives from blood banks and blood product manufacturers on the BPAC, with no balancing influence from consumers and no process within the FDA to evaluate its recommendations (Chapter 6), is a failure of advisory committee management. Perhaps advisory committees should contain fewer topical experts and more members with expertise in principles of good decisionmaking and the evaluation of evidence. A committee so constituted might run a reduced risk of standing accused of having conflicts of interest.

Analytic Capability and Long-Range Vision

Leadership passes to the organization that has access to information and the ability to analyze it. Federal agencies should avoid exclusive reliance upon the entities which they regulate for analysis of data and modeling of decision problems. The FDA should have had some independent capacity to analyze the information presented at the July 1983 BPAC meeting that suggested that with only three or four suspect donors, an automatic recall policy would completely deplete the nation's supply of AHF concentrate (Chapter 6). In addition, there did not seem to be any focus within the Public Health Service prepared to, or charged to, analyze the options, costs, and benefits of the options for protecting the blood supply that were discussed at the January 4, 1983, meeting convened by CDC.

In addition, agencies need to monitor more systematically the long-term outcomes of blood transfusion and blood product infusion and to think far ahead to anticipate both new technologies and new threats to the safety of the blood supply. Because new pathogens can enter the blood supply and be propagated very rapidly through it, a low level of suspicion about a threat should trigger high-level consideration of how to manage and monitor the problem.

Through its fact-finding interviews and through written documents, the Committee found little evidence that the PHS agency heads and the Assistant Secretary for Health were involved in making decisions about protecting the blood supply in 1983 and 1984 when HIV was becoming increasing apparent as a threat. Most decisions and interagency communication seems to have occurred several levels below the top.

Presumptive Regulatory and Public Health Triggers

The Committee believes that the Public Health Service should prepare for future threats to the blood supply by specifying in advance the types of actions that should occur once the level of concern passes a threshold. In the face of scientific uncertainty, the PHS needs a series of criteria or triggers for taking regulatory or other public health actions to protect the safety of blood and blood products. The Committee favors a series of triggers in which the response is proportional to the magnitude of the risk and the quality of the information on which the risk estimate is based. Not all triggers should lead to drastic or irrevocable actions; some merely require careful consideration of the options or developing new information. This general principle is detailed by examples in each of the Committee's four areas of inquiry. Table 8.1 summarizes these triggers and corresponding actions.

Product Treatment

Whenever they propose new methods of protecting the safety of the blood supply, blood regulatory agencies must perform cost-utility or cost-benefit analyses to evaluate whether the intervention will advance the public health at reasonable costs. If manufacturers do not have market incentives, resources, or access to data to test promising methods, public agencies should create incentives or provide resources or access to data. In this case, the trigger is a new proposal to increase safety, and the action is for the public sector to assume responsibility for thorough analysis and development, or to create incentives for industry to do so.

Table 8.1. Triggers for Taking Actions in Response to Uncertain Risks

Trigger Risks	Action
Product Treatment	
Proposal to increase safety	Public sector to assume responsibility for thorough analysis and development
Initiation of risk-benefit or cost-benefit analysis	Ensure that the analysis takes into account possible secondary and other benefits
Donor Screening	
Identification of a high-risk population	Self-deferral and segregation of lots
Plasma fractionators' action to increase screening	All companies consider why they should not follow suit and set in motion a consensus development mechanism
Availability of a surrogate test or other partially effective interventions that have minimal risks	Use the test/intervention unless it is certain to be redundant prior to realizing its benefits
Recall	
Implementation of a new test or treatment process	Recall untested or untreated products as expeditiously as possible
Beginning of a recall action	Provide clear guidance and monitoring
Communication of Risk	
New information relevant to a public health agency's actions	Tell affected communities what they need to know to make an informed choice among listed options: the facts, the gaps in knowledge, and the implications thereof

When performing a cost-effectiveness analysis of new treatments for blood products, the potential to protect against other threats should always be a part of the analysis. Here, the trigger is the initiation of a cost-effectiveness analysis, and the action is to ensure that the analysis takes into account secondary benefits.

Donor Screening

Whenever epidemiologists identify a high-risk donor group, the FDA should immediately tell blood banks to create a way to defer that group and tell collection agencies to segregate and separately treat supplies obtained from those populations. Concerns about stigmatizing subpopulations and maintaining the supply of blood products should influence the means of taking actions, not whether to take action. In this case, the trigger to action is the identification of a high-risk population, and the action is deferral and segregation of lots.

Whenever any segment of the industry institutes a donor screening program, the FDA should require all segments of the industry to follow suit with actions that they believe will be at least as effective in promoting safety. Public regulators have a responsibility to monitor these efforts and to forge consensus or to impose the most effective methods as information concerning efficacy becomes available. Here, the trigger is one company's action to take an additional safety measure, and the response is for all companies to follow suit, or to be held accountable when they do not.

Blood banks should use a partially effective intervention that has little or no risk unless they can show that a better method will rapidly supersede it. In this case the trigger is the availability of an inherently risk-free, partially effective intervention, and the response to use that test/intervention unless it is certain to become redundant prior to realizing its full benefits.

Recall

When a test or treatment makes a product safer, manufacturers should withdraw all stocks of untested or untreated product as quickly as possible. Where immediate complete withdrawal might injure the public health, withdrawals should be partial or staged. Here, the trigger is the implementation of a new test or treatment process, and the action is to recall untested or untreated products as expeditiously as possible, given other considerations of public health.

A limited, staged, or selective recall places responsibility on public regulatory agencies to establish criteria for selecting lots for recall, to provide processes to permit effective implementation of the recall by industry, and to monitor the recall to assure that removal of the products occurs in the prescribed manner. In this case the trigger is the initiation of a recall action, and the response is to provide clear guidance and monitoring.

Communication to Patients and Providers

Whenever new information triggers inquiry into a possible threat to the blood supply, both patients and their physicians should have access to the information. Public officials should presume that candid statements and rigorous actions will enhance rather than erode public confidence and that persons using blood or blood products have the right to understand fully the risks and benefits of using these products. In this case, the trigger is new information relevant to the public health, and the action is to tell affected individuals what they need to make an informed choice: the facts, the gaps in knowledge, and the implications thereof.

RECOMMENDATIONS

The Committee's charge was to learn from the events of the early 1980s the lessons that would help the nation prepare for future threats to the blood supply. The Committee identified potential problems with the system in place at that time (as summarized earlier in this chapter) and proposes changes that, if implemented in the early 1980s, might have moderated some of the effects of the AIDS epidemic on recipients of blood and blood products. This analysis has led the Committee to the following recommendations for Public Health Service agencies, for the blood and plasma fractionation industry, and for health care providers and the public. These recommendations address both public health options and individual clinical options.

The Committee is mindful of several caveats. First, the Committee is acutely aware of the difficulties of retrospective analysis, as described in Chapter 1. Second, the Committee has not considered its recommendations from perspectives other than blood safety. Finally, the Committee tried to identify opportunities for institutional change that would respond to the problems that the Committee diagnosed. The Committee based its recommendations on the institutions as they functioned in the early 1980s, not as they exist now. The organizations responsible for blood safety and public health will have to evaluate their current policies and procedures to see if they fully address the issues raised by our recommendations.

The Public Health Service

Several federal agencies necessarily play important, often different roles in managing a public health crisis such as the contamination of blood and blood products by the AIDS virus. The National Blood Policy of 1973 charged the

Public Health Service (including the CDC, the FDA, and the NIH) with responsibility for protecting the nation's blood supply.

Leadership

The Committee has come to believe that a failure of leadership contributed to delay in taking effective action, at least during the period from 1982 to 1984. This failure led to incomplete donor screening policies, weak regulatory actions, and insufficient communication to patients about the risks of AIDS.

In the event of a threat to the blood supply, the PHS must, as in any public health crisis, insist upon coordinated action. The Secretary of Health and Human Services is responsible for all the agencies of the Public Health Service,[1] and therefore the Committee makes

> **Recommendation 1: The Secretary of Health and Human Services should designate a Blood Safety Director, at the level of a deputy assistant secretary or higher, to be responsible for the federal government's efforts to maintain the safety of the nation's blood supply.**

Choosing a "lead person" is important because it is in the nature of federal agencies and their leaders to be at once competitive and protective. This condition is healthy in reasonable measure and in normal times. However, a serious threat to public health requires that agencies communicate, cooperate, and learn to view the world through each other's lenses. Once there is an action plan, the Secretary of Health and Human Services must hold the agency leaders accountable for enforcing cooperation in implementing the plan.

To be effective in coordinating the various agencies of the PHS, the Blood Safety Director should be at the level of a deputy assistant secretary or higher, and should not be a representative of any single PHS agency. When a threat does arise, the Blood Safety Director should create a crisis management team.

One such action was to establish, in July 1982, the Committee on Opportunistic Infections in Hemophiliacs (see Chapter 3). This group seems to have been organized by the CDC, but there is no record of its operations after August of that year.

---

[1] In the 1980s and now, the PHS agencies report to the Assistant Secretary of Health. As this report was being written, theDepartment of Health and Human Services has proposed to eliminate the office of the Assistant Secretary, so that the PHSagencies would report directly to the Secretary.

Blood Safety Council

The AIDS crisis revealed that the institutions in place to ensure blood safety, both public and private, were unable to work cooperatively toward a common goal of a safe blood supply. The institutions were not accountable to anyone but themselves, and they failed to cooperate, to coordinate their activities, and to communicate effectively with physicians and the public. The Committee has become convinced that the nation needs a far more responsive and integrated process to detect, evaluate, and respond to emerging threats to the blood supply. To this end the Committee makes

Recommendation 2: The PHS should establish a Blood Safety Council to assess current and potential future threats to the blood supply, to propose strategies for overcoming these threats, to evaluate the response of the PHS to these proposals, and to monitor the implementation of these strategies. The Council should report to the Blood Safety Director (see Recommendation 1). The Council should also serve to alert scientists about the needs and opportunities for research to maximize the safety of blood and blood products. The Blood Safety Council should take the lead to ensure the education of public health officials, clinicians, and the public about the nature of threats to our nation's blood supply and the public health strategies for dealing with these threats.

Supplying safe blood and blood products to the nation—a public good—requires the cooperation of public and private institutions. The Blood Safety Council would give voice to the public's interest in having these institutions cooperate and would provide opportunities for them to do so.

The lessons of HIV transmission through blood and blood products show the need for an advisory council with a significantly greater level of diversity, responsibility, and authority than the current Blood Products Advisory Committee of the FDA. The BPAC is limited by the regulatory mission of the FDA which it advises, and there is no other body primarily concerned with blood safety as a whole. Representatives from governmental agencies, academia, the blood bank community, industry, and the public all have relevant expertise and perspectives and should be involved in the Blood Safety Council. A broad-based range of expertise in areas of hematology, infectious diseases, epidemiology, blood product manufacturing, blood collection and delivery, risk assessment, consumer advocacy, and cost-benefit analysis is essential.

The proposed Blood Safety Council would facilitate the timely transmission of information, assessment of risk, and initiation of appropriate action both during times of stability and during a crisis. The Council should report to the Blood Safety Director (see Recommendation 1). The Council would not replace the PHS agencies responsible for blood safety but would complement them by providing a forum for them to work together and with private organizations. The PHS agencies would be represented on the Council (see below and Figure 8.1). The Council would not have its own surveillance capability, but would work with CDC and FDA to interpret the information that those organizations can provide. It would not carry out or fund research itself, but would work with those at NIH and in the private sector to identify priorities for blood safety research. The Council would not have regulatory power, but would inform FDA actions from a blood safety rather than a product-specific perspective.

The organizations and groups that should be included in the Blood Safety Council, and the reasons for including them, are as follows:

- The FDA can provide a direct link between itself, the essential regulatory agency responsible for the safety of blood and blood products, and important sources of information, scientific support, and disease surveillance findings.
- The CDC can provide expertise in epidemiology, infectious diseases, and immunology as well as communicate the results of ongoing disease surveillance studies. The CDC's newly established emerging infectious disease program would also provide valuable information.

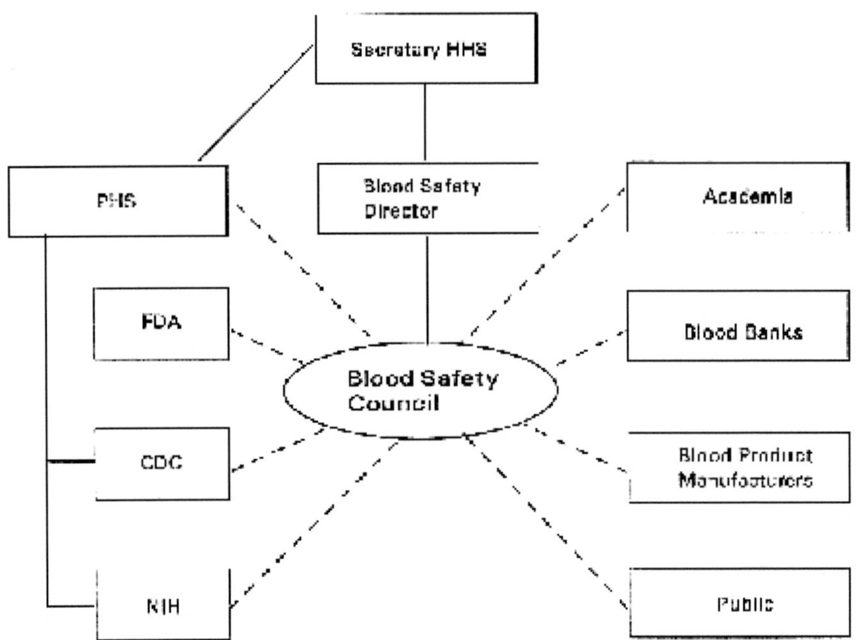

Figure 8.1. Blood Safety Council relationships.

- The NIH can provide scientific expertise and the means to communicate information about essential research needs to the appropriate institutes for support of research.
- Representatives from academia can bring independent scientific and medical expertise, especially in hematology, infectious diseases, epidemiology, risk assessment, and cost-effectiveness analysis.
- Representatives from the volunteer blood collection community can bring experience with blood safety concerns and the knowledge of blood bank operations that is necessary to evaluate proposed change.
- Representatives from the private-sector blood product manufacturers and biotechnology companies can bring both experience with blood safety concerns and knowledge of plasma fractionation operations.
- Representatives of the general public (who may in the future require blood transfusions) and individuals who currently require frequent use of blood products, such as hemophilia patients, bring important perspectives on the trade-offs that must be considered in evaluating response options.

The Blood Safety Council should consider the following activities and issues:

Surveillance. Although the FDA and the CDC keep track of events in blood and blood product recipients, their surveillance systems are passive and incomplete. The Blood Safety Council should work with the CDC to design a system of active surveillance for adverse reactions in blood recipients, as described in Recommendation 5 below. If such a system is established, the Council would benefit from its results and should participate in its governance.

Expert Panel on Best Practices. Drawing on its members' knowledge about blood and blood product safety concerns, and about clinical alternatives, the Blood Safety Council could establish a panel of experts to provide the public and providers of care with information about risks and benefits, alternatives to using blood products, and recommended best practices, as described in more detail in Recommendation 13 below.

Investigate Methods to Make Blood Products Safer. The Council should evaluate new methods to make blood and blood products safer. One promising approach is double inactivation in the preparation of blood products, which minimizes the risk of transmission of infectious pathogens in the blood of the donor pool. At present, the FDA requires only a single inactivation process (usually solvent detergent or heat treatment) for most blood products manufactured in the United States. With the goal of maximizing the safety of the blood supply at minimal added cost, the Blood Safety Council should encourage the FDA to evaluate double inactivation methods and expeditiously relicense products manufactured by the improved technologies, if appropriate. The Blood Safety Council should also consider, at least yearly, in a public forum, opportunities to maximize the safety of the blood supply.

Another promising approach is to reconsider minimum pool size requirements in plasma product manufacturing. The FDA currently requires a large number of donors to be included in plasma pools used in the manufacture of plasma products in order to ensure a wide range of antibodies in preparations of intravenous gamma globulin. Pooling of plasma obtained from numerous donors, although permitting some economy of scale, also increases the risk that a large fraction of manufactured blood products will be contaminated by a single infected donor. The Blood Safety Council should consider this issue and address the safety and efficiency trade-offs in changing the minimum pool size.

The Blood Safety Council would provide information relevant to the decisions that individuals as well as public and private decisionmakers need to make. The forum would not have direct regulatory or other authority, but would function as a forum for holding the organizations with authority responsible for blood safety. In short, the Blood Safety Council could advocate the public's need for a responsible process for decisionmaking about public health policy. The following examples illustrate how regular public discussions of blood safety issues, in the presence of representatives from the relevant organizations' perspectives, could provide an opportunity to hold the organizations with authority accountable for blood safety.

If it had existed in the 1970s, for instance, the Blood Safety Council might have called for the development of heat-treated AHF concentrate to reduce the risk of hepatitis, which would have also reduced the risk of HIV transmission. It would have been able to do so if the NIH and blood products industry representatives on the Council had been called upon to make periodic reports to the Council during the 1970s about their efforts to deal with the hepatitis problem. These representatives would have fed the discussions of the Council back into their own organizations' decisionmaking.

In 1983, the Council could have provided a forum for CDC to present its concerns about HIV in the blood supply and held the FDA, the NHF, and the blood banks and fractionators accountable for responding constructively. CDC created a forum on its own by convening the January 4, 1983, meeting in Atlanta, but as the Committee's analysis indicates, the follow-up on this meeting was insufficient. If a standing Blood Safety Council had existed, the CDC scientists who had concerns about the safety of blood and blood products would have had an opportunity to hold blood collection organizations accountable for their decisions regarding donor deferral and surrogate testing. It would also provide an opportunity to hold plasma fractionators and the FDA accountable for its decisions with regard to heat-treated AHF.

Later that year, the Council could have provided a mechanism to evaluate the claims that automatic recall of AHF would have virtually eliminated the supply of AHF. As the analysis in Chapter 6 indicates, neither the BPAC nor the FDA staff had the capacity to analyze claims that a automatic recall would have such an effect. The Blood Safety Council could have insisted that the FDA commission a formal decision analysis of the options for surrogate testing, or the Council might have performed such an analysis itself. The FDA would retain its regulatory authority, and continue to get advice from the BPAC, but the Council would have provided critical information relevant to the agency's decision.

Finally, if the Council had established an expert panel on best practices as described above and in Recommendation 13, hemophilia patients and their physicians would have had a more credible source of information about the risks of HIV infection and their clinical options than the NHF was able to provide. The operations of such a panel are described below under Recommendation 13.

Compensation Policy

When a product or service provided for the public good has inherent risks, the common law tort system fails to protect the rightful interests of patients who suffer harm resulting from the use of those products or services. Each claim requires extended, costly, and complex adjudicative procedures to establish liability. The results are erratic and unpredictable, and therefore inequitable (IOM 1985).

The doctrine of strict liability holds manufacturers accountable for injuries that are incurred from products that are inherently dangerous because diligence cannot fully eliminate their risks. The public health imperative of assuring enough vaccine for widespread use argues for limits on the strict liability doctrine for vaccine-related injuries. The chief concern is that fear of liability will discourage manufacturers from producing a vital public good. To vitate this concern, a federal compensation system has removed vaccine-related injuries from the scope of strict liability laws (Mariner 1992). The federal government established a mechanism for compensating individuals suffering harm from vaccine-related complications. Its rationale is that consent to undergo vaccination confers benefits to the entire community.

Blood-product-related injuries have also been removed from the scope of strict liability law by blood shield laws, which are in force in most states, and which protect society's interests in having an adequate blood supply. The blood shield laws serve to protect providers and manufacturers of blood and blood products from liability claims in instances where they take all due care to ensure the safety of the product. These laws, however, are unique in the manner in which they limit liability. The shield laws have made it difficult, and often impossible, to obtain compensation for HIV infection acquired from blood or blood products. To address this asymmetry between the protection that blood shield laws offer for manufacturers and adequate protection of individual rights, the Committee makes

Recommendation 3: The federal government should consider establishing a no-fault compensation system for individuals who suffer adverse consequences from the use of blood or blood products.[2]

An effective no-fault system requires prospective standards and procedures to guide its operations. In a no-fault system, individual plaintiffs would not have to prove that their adverse outcome was a result of negligence related to manufacture of a blood product. Therefore, there needs to be an objective, science-based process to establish which categories of adverse outcomes are caused by blood-borne pathogens and which individual cases deserve compensation. As with vaccines, a tax or fee paid by all manufacturers or by the recipients of blood products could finance a compensation system. Rather than attempt to allocate blame for HIV infections through blood and blood products, some countries have established such no-fault compensation programs for individuals infected with HIV as a result of their use of blood and blood products. Countries fund these programs in a variety of ways, including direct government support and joint public/private resources.

Making recommendations about compensating affected individuals for damages incurred in the past is outside the Committee's mandate. However, had there been a no-fault compensation system in the early 1980s, it could have relieved much financial hardship suffered by many who became infected with HIV through blood and blood products in the United States. The no-fault principles outlined in this recommendation might serve to guide policymakers as they consider whether to implement a compensation system for those infected in the 1980s.

The Centers for Disease Control and Prevention

The CDC has an indispensable role to play in protecting our nation's health: to detect potential public health risks and sound the alert. Because of its expertise in detecting and evaluating possible infectious disease outbreaks, the Committee believes that the CDC should take responsibility for a surveillance system to detect adverse outcomes from blood and blood products. The following two

---

[2] One Committee member (Martha Derthick) abstains from this recommendation because she believes that it falls outside of the Committee's charge.

recommendations embody an important principle: separating the assessment of risk from the management of the consequences of risk. The FDA, in its role as guarantor of the safety of the blood supply, has the responsibility for managing threats to the blood supply. The CDC should detect potential threats and assess the magnitude of the danger.

Early Warning Systems

A nation needs individuals and organizations that identify problems and raise concerns that may be difficult to confront. The CDC plays this role in the Public Health Service. The CDC appears to have been prescient in raising the possibility that the blood supply was contaminated early in the AIDS epidemic, but it was relatively ineffective in convincing other agencies of the potential gravity of the situation. In order to improve CDC's efficacy in this critical role, the Committee makes

> **Recommendation 4: Other federal agencies must understand, support, and respond to the CDC's responsibility to serve as the nation's early warning system for threats to the health of the public.**

Officials in the government, scientists, and physicians in the private sector seem to have discounted the CDC warnings about the transmissibility of AIDS through blood and blood products because the swine flu episode in the 1970s had cost the agency considerable credibility. If, in 1983, the involved public and private organizations had the attitude called for in this recommendation, CDC's recommendations regarding donor screening and surrogate testing might have led to earlier, more effective screening and donor deferral policies.

Consistent with the precept of separating risk assessment and risk management as described above, CDC's role is to characterize and assess risks, and communicate this to others. The FDA and other organizations have the responsibility to manage the risks through regulation, clinical practice guidelines, and other means. The Committee believes that CDC should be able to play its designated role without fearing loss of credibility if it sometimes proves to be wrong. Implementing this recommendation may be difficult. As a start, the Secretary of Health and Human Services should insist that an agency that wishes to disregard a CDC alert should support its position with evidence that meets the same standard as that used by the CDC in raising the alert.

Surveillance

In order to carry out its early warning responsibility effectively, the CDC needs good surveillance systems. Because blood products are derived from human beings and may contain harmful biologic agents that were present in the blood of a donor, blood products are inherently risky, a principle long recognized by blood shield laws. The Committee, believing that the degree of surveillance should be proportional to the level of risk, makes

> **Recommendation 5: The PHS should establish a surveillance system, lodged in the CDC, that will detect, monitor, and warn of adverse effects in the recipients of blood and blood products.**

If such a system had existed in 1982, data about the risks of HIV transmission through blood and blood products might have been available sooner and might have been more definitive. In dealing with newly approved pharmaceuticals, the FDA increasingly demands careful post-approval study of potential adverse effects (the so-called "Phase IV Trial"). Two existing systems for vaccine adverse events—the CDC/FDA Vaccine Adverse Event Reporting System (VAERS) and the CDC's Large-Linked Database (LLDB)—might be useful models (Institute of Medicine 1994).

The Food and Drug Administration

The FDA has legal authority to protect the safety of the nation's blood supply. Accordingly, it is the lead federal agency in regulating blood-banking practice, the handling of source plasma, and the manufacture of blood products from plasma. The Committee found cause for concern when it evaluated the FDA's actions in protecting the public from HIV in the nation's blood supply during the 1980s. The record reveals many opportunities to improve the agency's capacity to deal with crises involving the blood supply, most notably with respect to the safety of AHF concentrate. In responding to these opportunities, the Committee's recommendations focus on decisionmaking and the role of advisory committees in formulating the FDA's response to crises.

Risk Reduction

In a crisis, decisionmakers may become so preoccupied with seeking solutions that will dramatically reduce danger that they will fail to implement solutions that are less effective but are likely to improve public safety to some degree. Partially effective risk-reducing improvements, as described herein, can save lives, pending the development of more efficacious safety measures. In order that the perfect not be the enemy of the good, the Committee makes

Recommendation 6: Where uncertainties or countervailing public health concerns preclude completely eliminating potential risks, the FDA should encourage, and where necessary require, the blood industry to implement partial solutions that have little risk of causing harm.

In the event of a future threat to the blood supply, the FDA should encourage small, low-risk solutions to large, difficult problems. The FDA's actions during the early 1980s are evidence that the agency should change its attitude toward regulation in order to adopt this proactive approach. Some examples from Chapter 6 illustrate how the FDA might have encouraged practices that would have reduced the risk faced by recipients of blood or a blood product.

Example: Destroy Unscreened Blood When Possible. When hospital blood banks first started to screen donors by questioning them for risk factors, there was a period of transition during which its stocks contained two classes of blood or plasma: blood from screened donors, which was relatively safe; and blood from unscreened donors, which had a higher probability of containing HIV. Within a few weeks of starting to screen donors, blood from unscreened donors would have been either used or discarded. In the instructions contained in its letter of March 24, 1983, the FDA could have recommended that blood banks adopt a policy of using blood from screened donors whenever possible during the transition period, a policy that some blood banks may have adopted on their own. Requiring all blood banks to adopt this policy would not have compromised the nation's blood supply, and it would have prevented at least a few instances in which a patient received an infected unit of blood.

Example: Destruction of Potentially Contaminated Cryoprecipitate. Blood banks store cryoprecipitate from a single unit of donated blood in the frozen state for up to one year. The FDA could have issued a directive that required the blood banks to check their inventory of frozen cryoprecipitate and destroy possibly contaminated units whenever they learned of a previous donor who had AIDS or was strongly suspected of having AIDS.

Example: Phased Recall. In July 1983, there was considerable reluctance to recall untreated Factor VIII concentrate at a time when much of the supply was almost certainly contaminated with HIV. The FDA apparently feared that the ensuing shortage of Factor VIII would have caused more harm than the HIV virus. A phased withdrawal would have been a compromise between no withdrawal and immediate total withdrawal. This middle path might have avoided a factor concentrate shortage and still reduced the number of hemophiliacs who became infected.

Example: Lookback. The FDA formally instituted a "lookback" policy in 1991, years after it was clear that AIDS had a long incubation period during which a patient could transmit HIV through sexual contact or contact with blood. Lookback required blood banks to contact recipients of blood from infected donors and notify them that they might be a HIV carrier and should be tested for HIV antibodies. Earlier action on lookback might have reduced secondary transmission of HIV.

Decision Processes

In all fields, decisionmaking under uncertainty requires an iterative process. As the knowledge base for a decision changes, the responsible agency should reexamine the facts and be prepared to change its decision. The agency should also assign specific responsibility for monitoring conditions and identifying opportunities for change. In order to implement these principles at the FDA, the Committee makes

> **Recommendation 7: The FDA should periodically review important decisions that it made when it was uncertain about the value of key decision variables.**

An example illustrates the principle of iterative decisionmaking. During 1983, most blood bank officials opposed asking prospective male donors if they had ever had sex with a man. They were worried that regular donors might take offense and stop donating blood. They were also concerned about some gays would lie about their homosexuality and donate blood in reprisal for being singled out as the target of the questioning. Eventually, some blood collection centers began to ask questions about sexual preference. If the FDA had carefully monitored these experiments, it would have soon learned that the blood bank officials' fears were groundless. The FDA might then have revised its requirements for donor screening to include direct questions about high-risk sexual practices.

Regulatory Efforts

Although the FDA has a great deal of regulatory power over the blood products industry, the agency appears to regulate by expressing its will in subtle, understated directives. This informal approach to regulation is often necessary to permit a timely response and to preserve needed flexibility. The FDA used this approach, for example, in July 1983 when it issued recommendations to withdraw lots of AHF concentrate that plasma fractionators had identified as containing material from a donor that had AIDS. The language in the July 1983 communication failed to specify, however, whether the agency considered the recommendations to be binding on industry. While most regulated industries might have interpreted these letters as mandatory, that question should not have been left to the judgment of individual entities. Taking this into account, the Committee makes

Recommendation 8: Because regulators must rely heavily on the performance of the industry to accomplish blood safety goals, the FDA must articulate its requests or requirements in forms that are understandable and implementable by regulated entities. In particular, when issuing instructions to regulated entities, the FDA should specify clearly whether it is demanding specific compliance with legal requirements or is merely providing advice for careful consideration.

In 1983, the FDA chose a middle ground when faced with the decision to withdraw all AHF concentrate. The agency recommended that plasma fractionators withdraw individual lots of AHF concentrate when a donor was suspected of having AIDS. This decision was certainly defensible. However, the process for this "case-by-case" withdrawal was seriously compromised by the vagueness of the criteria specified for a recall. The agency failed to specify a process for deciding whether a donor may have had AIDS. The agency should have specified a process for reviewing donors who did not fully satisfy the diagnostic criteria for AIDS but who were suspected of having the disease. When deciding whether to withdraw a lot of AHF concentrate, the FDA asked plasma fractionators to take into account the time of the donation in relation to the diagnosis of AIDS and the effect of the recall on product availability. However, the FDA did not specify parameters for assessing either of these decision criteria. With greater forethought, the FDA could have avoided the potential for a seriously flawed implementation of a policy that otherwise appeared to balance benefits, risks, and harms.

Advisory Committees

The FDA made several decisions in 1983 that appear to have been influenced by the blood-industry-based (profit and nonprofit) members of the BPAC. The BPAC membership did not include individuals with expertise in the social, ethical, political, and economic aspects of the issues that BPAC was deliberating at the time. The FDA apparently did not seek independent analysis of the recommendations made by the members of the BPAC, some of whom were employed by the blood industry. In the early 1980s, the FDA appeared too reliant upon analyses provided by industry-based members of the BPAC and the BPAC. For example, see the discussion in Chapter 6 of the July 19, 1983, BPAC meeting which resulted in the decision for case-by-case rather than automatic recall of lots of AHF when one donor was suspected of having AIDs. Chapter 6 also contains a discussion of the December 15, 1983, BPAC meeting, which effectively curtailed actions on surrogate testing of blood for months. The Committee's analysis of the FDA's management of its advisory committee leads to the following three recommendations:

Recommendation 9: The FDA should ensure that the composition of the Blood Products Advisory Committee reflects a proper balance between members who are connected with the blood and blood products industry and members who are independent of industry.

The FDA should select some BPAC members because they can provide independent judgment, question the analyses provided by blood-industry-based BPAC members, and hold the FDA accountable for a high standard of public responsiveness. The BPAC should have at least one voting member who is a representative of consumer interests. BPAC members who vote to establish policy should have neither the appearance of a conflict of interest nor a true conflict of interest.

An agency that is practiced in orderly decisionmaking procedures will be able to respond to the much greater requirements of a crisis. The BPAC meetings cited before Recommendation 9 above provide examples to support this recommendation. Applying this principle to the use of advisory committees, the Committee makes

Recommendation 10: The FDA should tell its advisory committees what it expects from them and should independently evaluate their agendas and their performance.

The FDA staff and its advisory committees should structure their relationship so that they invigorate each other. The agency should hold an advisory committee accountable for its performance through periodic independent evaluation. By placing unresolved issues on future agendas, the committee can hold the FDA accountable for taking follow-up action between committee meetings. The IOM Committee to Study the Use of Advisory Committees by the Food and Drug Administration makes further recommendations to strengthen the FDA advisory committee system (IOM 1992).

Advisory committees provide scientific advice to the FDA; they do not make regulatory decisions for the agency (IOM 1992). As Chapter 6 indicates, the

FDA in 1983 did not independently verify the estimates of the risk of blood-product-related HIV infection. The FDA did not analyze the public health implications of the BPAC's recommendation against automatic recall of AHF concentrate that contained plasma from donors suspected of having AIDS. The FDA's lack of independent information and its own analytic capacity meant that it had little choice but to incorporate the advice of the BPAC into its policy recommendations. To ensure the proper degree of independence between the FDA and the blood products industry, the Committee makes

> **Recommendation 11: The FDA should develop reliable sources of the information that it needs to make decisions about the blood supply. The FDA should have its own capacity to analyze this information and to predict the effects of regulatory decisions.**

Communication to Physicians and Patients

One of the crucial elements of the system for collecting blood and distributing blood products to patients is the means by which to convey concern about the risks inherent in blood products. In today's practice of medicine, in contrast to that of the early 1980s, patients and physicians each accept a share of responsibility for making decisions. Patients' informed consent is required for risky procedures. From early 1983, it was clear that AHF concentrate was a risky product. The failure to tell hemophilia recipients of Factor VIII concentrate about the risks of this treatment and about alternative treatments seems especially serious in the light of present-day emphasis on the autonomy of patients in decisions involving their health.

Clinical Practice

One powerful lesson of the AIDS crisis is the importance of telling patients about the potential harms of the treatments that they are about to receive. The NHF dedicated itself to providing information to individuals with hemophilia and their physicians. Their strategy, however, was seriously flawed. As discussed in Chapter 7, the NHF provided treatment advice, not the information on risks and alternatives that would enable physicians and patients to decide for themselves on a course of treatment. Hemophilia patients did not have the basis for informed choice about a difficult treatment decision.

Considerable scientific and medical uncertainties characterized the early years of the AIDS epidemic. For individuals medically dependent on the use of blood and blood products, these uncertainties created complex dilemmas about clinical options for their continued care. In instances of great uncertainty, it is crucial for patients to be fully apprised of the full range of options available to them and to become active participants in the evaluation of the relative risks and benefits of alternative treatments. As the case studies in Chapter 7 indicate, the failure to communicate adequately about these options prevented many hemophiliacs from making choices in which they accepted responsibility for balancing the risk of AIDS and the risks of bleeding. Ultimately the failure to communicate led to a powerful sense of betrayal that exacerbated the tragedy of the epidemic for many patients and their families. To encourage better communication, the Committee makes

> **Recommendation 12: When faced with a decision in which the options all carry risk, especially if the amount of risk is uncertain, physicians and patients should take extra care to discuss a wide range of options.**

Medicine has many "gray areas" in which the correct course of action is not clear. Guidelines should identify these areas and spotlight the importance of full disclosure of risks, discussion of the broadest range of clinical options, and incorporation of the patient's preferences into an individualized recommendation. Given the inherent risks and uncertainties in all blood products, the public and the providers of care need expert, unbiased information about the blood supply. This information includes risks and benefits, alternatives to using blood products, and recommended best practices. As Chapter 7 indicates, the NHF (the only organization that stepped in to provide information to hemophiliacs and the physicians who were treating them) focused on practice recommendations rather than complete information on risks and options. In order to provide the public and providers of care with the information they need, the Committee makes

> **Recommendation 13: An expert panel should be created to inform the providers of care and the public about the risks associated with blood and blood products, about alternatives to using them, and about treatments that have the support of the scientific record.**

One lesson of the AIDS crisis is that a well-established, orderly decisionmaking process is important for successfully managing a crisis. This applies as much to clinical decisionmaking as to the public health decision process addressed by the earlier recommendations. As the narrative indicates, there are both public health and clinical approaches to reducing the risk of blood-borne diseases. The Blood Safety Council called for in Recommendation 2 would deal primarily with risk assessment and in the public health domain, actions that would reduce the chance that blood products could be vectors of infectious agents. The primary responsibility of the expert panel on best practices called for in Recommendation 13 would be to provide the clinical information that physicians and their patients need to guide their individual health care choices. To be most effective, this panel should be lodged in the Blood Safety Council (see Recommendation 2) so that both bodies can interact and coordinate their activities in order to share information about emerging risks and clinical options.

Any organization that supplies this information must adhere to accepted norms for documenting evidence. The Committee believes that the public's interest would be best served by creating one publicly accountable source of this information. This function would build on the experience of the Agency for Health Care Policy and Research, which has an established guideline development process and issues guidelines on topics such as the management of chronic pain, screening for AIDS, and management of urinary incontinence (El-Sadr, et al. 1994; Jacox, et al. 1994).

Experience in developing practice guidelines for hemophilia treatment and blood transfusion is an important element of preparedness for future threats to the blood supply. There are now well-established processes such as those recommended by the IOM Committee to Advise the Public Health Service on Practice Guidelines (IOM 1990, 1992) and used by the Agency for Health Care Policy and Research. The U.S. Preventive Services Task Force (1989) uses another system process. Guideline developers should perform a thorough literature search, identify well-designed studies, describe fully the evidence on harms and benefits, and explain the connection between the evidence and the recommendations. They should seek critical evaluation from a wide spectrum of individuals and organizations and should periodically reexamine the recommendations in the light of changing knowledge.

Credibility

During the early 1980s, in its role as the guardian of the interests of the hemophilia patient community, the NHF was the principal source of information about using blood products. The outcome of the NHF efforts was that individuals with hemophilia and their families lost faith in the NHF as the rightful steward of their interests. The reasons discussed in Chapter 7 include the NHF's unwavering recommendation to use AHF concentrate, its dependence on funds contributed by the plasma fractionation industry, and the composition of the NHF expert panel (MASAC) that formulated treatment recommendations (e.g., the panel's lack of infectious disease experts and decision analysts).

Toward the end of providing the highest-quality, most credible information to patients and providers, the Committee makes

Recommendation 14: Voluntary organizations that make recommendations about using commercial products must avoid conflicts

of interest, maintain independent judgment, and otherwise act so as to earn the confidence of the public and patients.

One of the difficulties with using experts to give advice is the interconnections that experts accumulate during their careers. Organizations that regulate an industry may get advice from the same experts who advise the industries. Organizations that give treatment advice may rely on experts whose employer relies upon support from industry. As a result, an expert may have a history of relationships that raise concerns about whether he or she can be truly impartial when advising a course of action in a complex situation. The Committee believes that the best way to avoid these risks is to choose some panelists who are not expert in the subject of the panel's assignment but have a reputation for expertise in evaluating evidence, sound clinical judgment, and impartiality.

Financial conflicts of interest influence organizations as well as individuals. As indicated in Chapter 7 and above, the financial relationships between the NHF and the blood products industry seriously compromised the NHF's credibility. The standards for acknowledging conflicts of interest are higher than they were 12 years ago. Public health officials and the medical professions must uphold this new standard. Failure to do so will threaten the fabric of trust that holds our society together.

REFERENCES

Douglas, M. *Risk Acceptability According to the Social Sciences*. Russell Sage Foundation, New York; 1985

El-Sadr, W., et al. *Evaluation and Management of Early HIV Infection, Clinical Practice Guideline No. 7*. AHCPR Publication No. 94-0572. Rockville, MD: Agency for Health Care Policy and Research, Public Health Service, U.S. Department of Health and Human Services; January 1994.

Fischoff, B. Treating the Public with Risk Communications: A Public Health Perspective. *Science, Technology and Human Values*, vol. 12; 1987.

Fischoff, B., et al. Acceptable Risk. 1981.

Institute of Medicine. *Clinical Practice Guidelines: Directions for a New Program*. M.J. Field and K.N. Lohr, eds. National Academy Press, 1990.

Institute of Medicine. *Guidelines for Clinical Practice: From Development to Use*. M.J. Field and K.N. Lohr, eds. National Academy Press, 1992.

Institute of Medicine. *Research Strategies for Assessing Adverse Events Associated with Vaccines*, National Academy Press, 1994.

Institute of Medicine. *Vaccine Supply and Innovation*, National Academy Press, 1985.

Institute of Medicine. The *Artificial Heart: Prototypes, Policies and Patents*. J.R. Hogness and M. VanAntwerp, eds., National Academy Press, 1991.

Jacox, A., et al. *Management of Cancer Pain, Clinical Practice Guideline No. 9*. AHCPR Publication No. 94-0592. Rockville, MD: Agency for Health Care Policy and Research, Public Health Service, U.S. Department of Health and Human Services; March 1994.

Mariner, Wendy K., "Legislative Report: The National Vaccine Injury Compensation Program," *Health Affairs*, Spring 1992 vol. II.

National Research Council. *Improving Risk Communication*. National Academy Press, Washington, D.C.; 1989.

National Research Council. *Risk Assessment in the Federal Government: Managing the Process*. National Academy Press, Washington, D.C.; 1983.

National Research Council. *Science and Judgment in Risk Assessment* . National Academy Press, Washington, D.C.; 1994.

Nelkin, D. Communicating Technological Risk: The Social Construction of Risk Perception. *Annu. Rev. Public Health*, 1989.

U.S. Preventive Services Task Force. *Guide to Clinical Preventive Services*. Williams and Wilkins, Baltimore, Maryland; 1989.

Appendixes

A

Individuals Interviewed by the Committee

Richard Aguilar, Jr., Pharm.D.
Caremark Western Medical
 Specialties

Louis M. Aledort, M.D.
Mt. Sinai Medical Center

Harvey Alter, M.D.
National Institutes of Health (NIH)

Arthur Amman, M.D.
Pediatric AIDS Foundation

David Aronson, M.D.
George Washington University
 Medical Center

Thomas M. Asher, Ph.D.
HemaCare Corporation

John Bacich, Jr.
Baxter Healthcare Corporation

Llewelys F. Barker, M.D., Ph.D.
National Institute of Allergy and
 Infectious Disease, NIH

Val D. Bias
Marc Associates, Inc.

Jonathan Botelho
National Hemophilia Foundation

Joseph Bove, M.D.
Yale University Blood Bank

Edward Brandt, Jr., M.D.
Oklahoma University Health
 Center

Charles J. Carman, M.D.
Retired

William Coenen
Council of Community Blood
 Centers

James Crispen, M.D.
Private Practitioner

James W. Curran, M.D., M.P.H.
Centers for Disease Control

Calvin Dawson
National Hemophilia Foundation

Shelby Dietrich, M.D.
Huntington Hospital Hemophilia
    Center

Dennis Donohue, M.D.
Private Consultant

Corey Dubin
Committee of Ten Thousand

Michael Dubinsky
Center for Biologics Evaluation
    and Research, Food and Drug
    Administration (FDA)

Edgar Engleman, M.D.
Stanford University Blood Center

Jay Epstein, M.D.
Center for Biologics Evaluation
    and Research, FDA

Bruce L. Evatt, M.D.
Centers for Disease Control and
    Prevention

Steve Falter
Center for Biologics Evaluation and
    Research, FDA

Frederick Feldman, M.D.
Armour Pharmaceuticals

William Foege, M.D., M.P.H.
Emory University

Boyd Foegel
Center for Biologics Evaluation and
    Research, FDA

Donald Francis, M.D.
Genentech

Joseph C. Fratantoni, M.D.
Center for Biologics Evaluation
    and Research, FDA

Bruce Furie, M.D.
New England Medical Center

Robert S. Gallo, M.D.
National Cancer Institute, NIH

James J. Goedert, M.D.
National Cancer Institute, NIH

Edward Gompert, M.D.
Baxter Healthcare Corporation

William J. Hammes
Miles, Inc.

Leon W. Hoyer, M.D.
American Red Cross

Petra Jason
Miami, Florida

Carol Kasper, M.D.
Orthopedic Hospital's Hemophilia
    Treatment Center

Dana Kuhn, M.Div., Ph.D.
Virginia Commonwealth University

Beth Leahy
Armour Pharmaceuticals

Peter H. Levine, M.D.
The Medical Center of Central
    Massachusetts

Karen Lipton, J.D.
American Association of Blood
  Banks

Jeanne M. Lusher, M.D.
Children's Hospital of Michigan

Clyde B. McAuley, M.D.
Alpha Therapeutic Corporation

Jeffrey McCullough, M.D.
University of Minnesota

Merle McPherson, M.D.
Maternal and Child Health Bureau

Harry M. Meyer, M.D.
Private Consultant

Thomas Montgomery
U.S. House of Representatives,
  Subcommittee on Oversight and
  Investigations

Carol M. Moore
Miles, Inc.

James Mosley, M.D.
University of Southern California

Milton Mozen, Ph.D.
Miles, Inc.

George Nemo, M.D.
National Heart, Lung, and Blood
  Institute, NIH

June E. Osborn, M.D.
University of Michigan

Peter Page, M.D.
American Red Cross

Paul Parkman, M.D.
Private Consultant

Herbert Perkins, M.D.
Irwin Memorial Blood Bank

Marla S. Persky
Baxter Healthcare Corporation

John Petricciani, M.D.
Genetics Institute

Kenneth R. Pina, Esquire
Rhone-Poulenc Rorer, Inc.

Johanna Pindyck, M.D.
Retired, New York Blood Center

Gerald V. Quinnan, Jr.
Uniformed Services University of the
  Health Sciences

James Reilly
American Blood Resources
  Association

Harold Roberts, M.D.
University of North Carolina

Michael Rodell, Ph.D.
Private Consultant

Donald Rosenblitt, M.D.
University of North Carolina

Jack Ryan
Miles, Inc.

S. Gerald Sandler, M.D. F.A.C.P.
Georgetown University Hospital

Edward Shanbrom, M.D.
Private Consultant

Arthur Silvergleid, M.D.
Blood Bank of San Bernadino-
    Riverside Counties

Arthur R. Thompson, M.D.
Puget Sound Blood Center

Richard Valdez, Sr.
Hemophilia/HIV Peer Association

Jonathan Wadleigh
Committee of Ten Thousand

Charles Wallas, M.D.
American Association of Blood
    Banks

Timothy M. Westmoreland
U.S. House of Representatives,
    Subcommittee on Health and the
    Environment

B

Individuals Providing Oral and Written Testimony (for a public meeting held September 12, 1994)

Christina Gudavich for Tiffany
    Althouse
Jenison, Michigan

American Blood Resources
    Association
Annapolis, MD

Robert Baldwin
Bedford, TX

Larry Bark
Iowa Falls, IA

Peter Brandon Bayer
Tampa, FL

Luis Berrios
National Hemophilia Foundation
New York

Val Bias
National Hemophilia Foundation
New York

Jonathan A. Botelho
National Hemophilia Foundation
New York

William P. Brock, III
Ft. Worth, TX

Ed Burke
Dunwoodie, GA

Regina Butler
Division of Hematology
Childrens Hospital of Philadelphia

Kristine Richardson for Beth Carew
National Hemophilia Foundation
New York

Jorge L. Casal
North Lauderdale, FL

Fred E. Cashion
Snellville, GA

Ryan and Debbie Chedester
Bunkie, LA

Donna Cialone
Fenpark, FL

Donald Colburn
National Hemophilia Foundation
New York

Mollie and Ray Dattoli
Fort Worth, TX

Calvin Dawson
Apopka, FL

James Deefillipi
Arlington, VA

Art DeMario
Prince George, VA

Larkey Sheldon De Neffe, M.S.
Portland, OR

Elaine DePrince
Cherry Hill, NJ

Jan, Ken, and Leo Dixon
Youngsville, LA

Corey Dubin
Goleta, CA

Marlys Edwardh
Toronto, Ontario
Canada

Randy and Gale Ellman
Mt. Verde, FL

William Eurto
Ft. Worth, TX

Helen R. Flowerday
Daly City, CA

Dawn Foote
Caledonia, MI

Shirley A. Gaulzetti
Birmingham, MI

Kathleen and Stephanie Gerus
National Hemophilia Foundation
New York

Margaret M. Greilick
Traverse City, MI

Edith M. Gutowski
Bloomfield Hills, MI

Paul F. Haas, Ph.D.
National Hemophilia Foundation
New York

Charles Hill
Chickamauga, GA

Michael and Courtney Hylton
Costa Mesa, CA

Queen E. and Percuial Ingram
Pageland, SC

Warren Ingram
Alpharetta, GA

Petra Jason
Miami, FL

Karen Jentzen-Nunnelly
Hudsonville, MI

Sherwin and Dorothea Jordan
Pageland, SC

Dana Kuhn, M.Div., Ph.D.
Midlothian, VA

Sanford R. Kurtz, M.D.
American Society of Clinical
   Pathologists
Washington, D.C.

James P. Kryfko
Plano, TX

Joyce Lawson
Kingsport, TN

Mark L. Leverone
Smithsburg, MD

Linda and Grant Lewis
Licking, Missouri

Beulah T. and Moses A. Louallen
Jefferson, SC

Lauraine and Ryan Lovelady
Damascus, AR

Edward and Pamela Maslak
Toledo, OH

Anthony W. McDaniel
Katy, TX

William L. and Clara A. McKinney
Richardson, TX

Emma Lee Miller
Baltimore, MD

Thomas Morabito
Alamos, CO

Aubrey Motz
Coconut Creek, FL

Rick Nagler
Manassas, VA

Ron Niederman
E. Brunswick, NJ

Luis and Deborah Noriega
Tucson, AZ

Brian O'Mahoney
World Hemophilia Federation
Montreal, Quebec
Canada

Victoria S. Ornowski
Katy, TX

Jackie Otis
Minot, ND

David and Sharon Perrigo
Conway, AR

Glenn Pierce, M.D., Ph.D.
National Hemophilia Foundation
New York

Herbert F. Polesky, M.D.
College of American Pathologists
Washington, D.C.

Karen Procopio
Chester Springs, PA

Christine and Doyle Pullum
Lafayette, LA

Oscar Ratnoff, M.D.
University Hospitals of Cleveland

Louise Ray
Orlando, FL

Ted Reumke
Arlington, VA

Edward G. Rogoff, Ph.D.
Hemophilia Association of
    New York
New York

Katherine Royer
Tigared, Oregon

Brent Runyon
Wilmington, NC

Maxine Segal
Miami, FL

Joan Carole Shipers
Mr. Pleasant, MI

Mary Lou Simpson
Pittsburgh, PA

Lisa and Brent Smith
Edwardsville, IL

Joseph M. Smith
Evans, GA

Ellis Sulser
Chantilly, VA

Mary Ann and Wayne I.
    Swindlehurst
Hudsonville, MI

Richard J. Valdez, Sr., and
    Richard J. Valdez, Jr.
Cardiff, CA

Linda D. Vining
Morgan City, Louisiana

Jonathan Wadleigh
Committee of Ten Thousand
Stoughton, MA

Sylvia and Steve Ward
Baltimore, MD

David L. White
Albany, GA

Mike Williams
Dallas, TX

Melissa Wright
Narberth, PA

C

Chronological Summary of Critical Events, National Hemophilia Foundation (NHF) Communications, Knowledge Base, Risk Assessment, Clinical Options, and NHF Actions

Table C.1 Chronological Summary of Critical Events, NHF Communications, Knowledge Base, Risk Assessment, Clinical Options, and NHF Actions

Critical Event	NHF Communication	Knowledge Base	Risk Assessment	Clinical Option	NHF Action
July 16, 1982: CDC MMWR reports immune-suppressive disorder identified in three hemophiliac patients	July 14, 1982: Patient Alert #1 sent to NHF chapters and treatment centers	Speculation that it may be transmitted similarly to hepatitis virus by blood and blood products	Risk is minimal	No change in treatment	Dr. Aledort, NHF medical co-director to serve on PHS task force Surveillance and reporting system being planned by CDC with NHF cooperation "Dear Colleague" letter sent (July 19, 1982) to physicians by Dr. Aledort asking them to report any cases to state health departments and the NHF
July 16, 1982: FDA Office of Biologics holds information exchange meeting on the three cases with NHF and CDC representatives	July 19, 1982: Chapter Advisory #2 issued	Cause of disease unknown Epidemic known by CDC in some homosexuals and recent Haitian immigrants CDC investigat-	No indication blood products are involved Risk is minimal	No change in treatment (refers to this as a CDC recommendation)	

		ing: (1) linkage between hemophiliacs and other populations; (2) whether the disease may be a virus transmitted similarly to hepatitis by blood products			
July 27, 1982: PHS meeting on opportunistic infections in hemophiliacs	July 30, 1982: NHF issues Medical Bulletin #2 and Chapter Advisory #3 (no mass mailings to chapter members required)	The cause of the dysfunction found in three hemophiliacs is unknown, now defined as AIDS	No information provided	No information provided	NHF agrees to work with CDC, FDA, and NIH to establish surveillance system of hemophiliacs with symptoms of opportunistic infections

Critical Event	NHF Communication	Knowledge Base	Risk Assessment	Clinical Option	NHF Action
December 10, 1982: CDC MMWR reports four additional cases in hemophiliacs and one suspect case in an infant who had received a blood transfusion	December 9, 1982: NHF issues Chapter Advisory #4 December 10, 1982: Medical Bulletin #3 issued December 21, 1982: NHF issues Medical Bulletin #4 and Chapter Advisory #5	Two cases are children with hemophilia Not acquired from contact with each other or other high-risk groups All cases exposed to Factor VIII, no common lots found No conclusive evidence that cryoprecipitate or fresh frozen plasma will reduce the risk of AIDS	Illness may pose a significant risk for hemophiliacs Increased concern that AIDS may be transmitted through blood products	Advisable not to introduce concentrates to patients who have never used them before (e.g., newborns, children under age 4, newly diagnosed cases, and mild hemophiliac cases) No change in treatment for those who have received factor concentrates, and one should not withhold the use of clotting factor therapy when needed	NHF sends out December 10 CDC MMWR to chapter members and emphasizes that patients and parents should be aware of potential risks NHF provides treatment alternatives to chapter members for individuals not previously exposed to concentrate
January 4, 1983: CDC meeting in Atlanta to review data	January 17, 1983: NHF issues Medical Bulletin #5 and Chapter Advisory #6	Growing incidence and increasing concern among hemophiliac		Cryoprecipitate should be used for newborns and children under age 4	MASAC meeting on January 14, 1983, issues 12 recommendations to prevent AIDS in hemophiliac

patients that AIDS may be transmitted through blood products

Benefits of using cryo-precipitate therapy vs. factor concentrate for severe hemophilia A are under review

DDAVP should be used whenever possible with mild or moderate hemophilia A

Reevaluate all elective surgical procedures

patients; the clinical options (at left) were recommendations made to physicians

Critical Event	NHF Communication	Knowledge Base	Risk Assessment	Clinical Option	NHF Action
March 4, 1983: PHS issues recommendations to reduce the risk of AIDS	March 9, 1983: NHF issues Medical Bulletin #6 and Chapter Advisory #7	Sexual contact should be avoided with persons known or suspected to have AIDS; multiple sex partners increase the probability of developing AIDS		Physicians should adhere strictly to medical indications for transfusions, and autologous blood transfusions are encouraged	NHF urges Congress to provide additional funding to support AIDS research NHF issues mental health report to orient those who treat hemophiliacs to the potential impact of AIDS and asks for medical observations, such as: the impact of the AIDS threat (e.g., number of calls from patients); behavioral or emotional problems; evidence of withholding or refusing factor replacement for acute bleeds; and the treatment center's response

May 1983: Hyland Therapeutics recalls lot—a donor was identified who developed AIDS	May 11, 1983: NHF issues Medical Bulletin #7 and Chapter Advisory #8		Risk is low (12 hemophiliacs out of 20,000 developed AIDS)	NHF and NHF AIDS Task Force recommends hemophiliacs maintain use of clotting-factor treatment
August 25–26, 1983: Hyland Therapeutics and ARC announce recall of lots (two each) from identified donors who were confirmed to have died of AIDS	September 7, 1983: NHF issues Chapter Advisory #9	Not scientifically established that AIDS is transmitted through blood products		NHF reaffirms its recommendation that patients maintain use of concentrate or cryoprecipitate as prescribed by their physicians
October 31, 1983: Cutter Laboratories announces withdrawal of 13 lots of Factor VIII and 1 lot of Factor IX, all from a donor who recently died of AIDS	November 2, 1983: NHF issues Chapter Advisory #11	Not scientifically established that AIDS is transmitted through blood products	Only a fraction of 1% of all hemophiliacs have contracted AIDS No common lots have been identified, thus suggesting the great majority of hemohiliacs are not susceptible to AIDS	Despite the concern that may be raised by the recall of plasma products, the NHF reaffirms its recomendation that patients maintain the use of concentrate or cryorecipitate as prescribed by their physicians

Critical Event	NHF Communication	Knowledge Base	Risk Assessment	Clinical Option	NHF Action
December 2, 1983: CDC MMWR update on AIDS in hemophiliac patients; results of treatment center survey show no cases occurred before September 1981; 21 hemophiliacs have been diagnosed with AIDS, additional patients have been reported with AIDS-related symptoms that do not fit the CDC criteria for an AIDS diagnosis	December 2, 1983: NHF issues Medical Bulletin #8 with attached CDC MMWR (December 10); Medical Bulletin #9 and Chapter Advisory #12 issued on December 21, 1983	Etiology remains unknown, epidemiological evidence suggests an infectious disease Possibility of transmission by blood and blood products is supported by increased incidence of AIDS in IV drug users and transfusion recipients Cryoprecipitate and factor concentrates are associated with transmission of known viral agents (i.e., cytomegalovirus, hepatitis B, and non-A, non-B hepatitis)		MASAC revises January 14, 1983, recommendations to prevent AIDS: adds modification of donor screening language; screen donors for symptoms; expedite the development of processing methods to inactivate viruses potentially present in factor concentrates	

January 16, 1984: Alpha Therapeutic recalls three lots contaminated with AIDS from a donor diagnosed with AIDS	NHF issues Medical Bulletin #10 and Chapter Advisory #13			NHF reaffirms its recommendation that patients maintain use of concentrate or cryoprecipitate as prescribed by their physicians	MASAC recommends to blood product manufacturers that any lot of concentrate be recalled if it includes material from an individual who has been identified as having AIDS, or from an individual who, in the best judgment of the manufacturers, has characteristics strongly suggestive of AIDS
January 1984: *Annals of Internal Medicine* publishes article on sexual transmission of AIDS	January 30 and February 3, 1984: NHF issues Medical Advisory #11 and Chapter Advisory #14	First case of sexually transmitted AIDS from hemophiliac to spouse: a 70-year-old hemophiliac died of AIDS in May 1983; his wife had developed symptoms in January 1982	In the medical and scientific communities there are different points of view about whether sexual partners of hemophiliacs are at increased risk for AIDS; but all agree that if sexual partners are at increased risk for AIDS, the risk is "truly remote"	Individual patients and their treaters need to consider whether or not they wish to use prophylactic methods if diagnosed with AIDS or strongly suspected of having AIDS; discuss with physician or treatment center team matters concerning sexual activity	NHF recommends open discussion between sexual partners and advice from physicians

Critical Event	NHF Communication	Knowledge Base	Risk Assessment	Clinical Option	NHF Action
April 2, 1984: core testing initiated	April 16, 1984: NHF issues Chapter Advisory #15	January–March 1984: 9 new cases of AIDS among hemophiliacs, total now is 33; fluctuations, such as an increase in the number of AIDS cases, are due to the small number base of hemophiliacs; antibody to hepatitis B core protein is found in many of the high-risk groups		DDAVP approved by FDA	
April 1984: *Lancet* publishes Montagnier's isolation of LAV; *Science* publishes Gallo's isolation of HTLV-III (September 1985)	May 9, 1984: NHF issues Chapter Advisory #16	HTLV-III may cause AIDS; both a test and a vaccine are several years away; genetic production of Factor VIII will repor-tedly also be available in several years			

July 13, 1984: CDC MMWR reported 72% of severe asymptomatic hemophiliacs had antibody to LAV antigens using the Western blot test	July 31, 1984: NHF issues Chapter Advisory #17 and Medical Bulletin #12	HTLV-III/LAV implicated as the causative agent for AIDS; too early for scientific information about the relationship between testing positive and having AIDS	Testing positive for HTLV-III/LAV does not suggest a diagnosis of AIDS	No information from NHF; CDC MMWR states that prevention measures should stress that transmission has been only from sexual contact, sharing of contaminated needles, and, less often, from transfusion of blood or blood products	
August 31, 1984: Alpha Therapeutic recalls four lots of Factor VIII and four lots of Factor IX from an identified donor who was confirmed to have AIDS	September 6, 1984: NHF issues Medical Bulletin #13 and Chapter Advisory #18			NHF reaffirms its recommendation that patients maintain use of concentrate or cryoprecipitate as recommended by their physicians	MASAC reaffirms October 23, 1983, policy on recall

Critical Event	NHF Communication	Knowledge Base	Risk Assessment	Clinical Option	NHF Action
October 5, 1984: ARC recalls AHF found to have been from a single donor who developed AIDS	October 13, 1984: NHF issues Medical Bulletin #15 and Chapter Advisory #20 containing MASAC recommendations concerning AIDS and the treatment of hemophilia	Heat-treated products appear to have no negative impact in terms of inhibitor development from heat treatment Insufficient data to know with certainty whether heat-treated products should be universally adopted; preliminary evidence suggests that HTLV-III/LAV is heat labile		On October 13, 1984, MASAC revises its recommendations: treaters using coagulation factor concentrates should strongly consider changing to heat-treated products Reevaluate all elective surgical procedures Use DDAVP for mild or moderate hemophiliacs Cryoprecipitate should be used for newborns, children under age 4, and newly diagnosed patients; continue treating bleeding episodes with clotting factor as prescribed by their physicians Provide patient education and psychosocial support	

October 26, 1984: CDC MMWR reports information on the viral inactivation success of heat treatment	November 5, 1984: NHF issues Medical Bulletin #16 and Chapter Advisory #21	MMWR provides scientific evidence on the efficacy of heat treatment		NHF reiterates MASAC recommendation that treaters should strongly consider changing to heat-treated products
November 4, 1984: the media reports that 70%–90% of hemophiliacs are infected with AIDS	November 5, 1983: NHF issues Medical Bulletin #17 and Chapter Advisory #22 in response to misleading information	58 Cases of AIDS in hemophiliacs; 32 have died	The presence of antibodies for HTLV-III/LAV does not suggest a diagnosis of AIDS	
FDA licenses three manufacturers for heat-treated Factor IX (1984)	December 11, 1984: NHF issues "sensitive" Medical Bulletin (#19) that includes a list of AIDS cases among hemophiliacs; 58 cases are listed. December 12, 1984: NHF issues Medical Bulletin #18 and Chapter Advisory #23	Not known whether heat changes effectiveness for patients with inhi-bitors		Treaters should strongly consider changing to heat-treated products; studies are under way to determine efficacy for hepatitis

Critical Event	NHF Communication	Knowledge Base	Risk Assessment	Clinical Option	NHF Action
October 1984: CDC determines that heat treatment is effective against HIV	December 4, 1985: NHF issues Medical Bulletin #32 and Chapter Advisory #37			MASAC recommends (and the NHF Executive Committee approves) that physicians prescribe only heat-treated products for patients who do not have inhibitors Heat-treated products should be used for newborns, children under age 4, and newly diagnosed hemophiliacs Hepatitis B vaccine should be administered shortly after birth because of the problem of non-A, non-B hepatitis (not eliminated with heat treatment) risks and benefits should be weighed for each individual DDAVP should be used	

for mild or moderate hemophilia A patients; when it does not work, these patients should be treated with cryoprecipitate; for newborns, children under age 4, and newly identified patients with mild or moderate factor IX deficiency, fresh frozen plasma can be used, but in many circumstances, heat-treated product Factor VIII or IX may be the more appropriate therapy

All elective surgery procedures should be evaluated with respect to their advantages and disadvantages

Patients should continue treating bleeding episodes with clotting factor as prescribed by their physicians

NOTE: ARC = American Red Cross; CDC = Centers for Disease Control; DDAVP = desmopressin acetate; FDA = Food and Drug Administration; HTLV-III = human T-cell lymphotropic virus, type III; IV = intravenous; LAV = lymphadenopathy-associated virus; MASAC = Medical and Scientific Advisory Council; MMWR = *Morbidity and Mortality Weekly Report;* NHF = National Hemophilia Foundation; NIH = National Institutes of Health; and PHS = Public Health Service.

CHRONOLOGICAL SUMMARY OF CRITICAL EVENTS, NATIONAL HEMOPHILIA
FOUNDATION (NHF) COMMUNICATIONS, KNOWLEDGE BASE, RISK
ASSESSMENT, CLINICAL OPTIONS, AND NHF ACTIONS

D

Key Documents Provided to the Committee

1. National Hemophilia Foundation, Hemophilia Patient Alert #1; July 14, 1982.
2. Foege, William H., M.D. *Summary Report on Open Meeting of PHS Committee on Opportunistic Infections in Patients with Hemophilia* ; August 6, 1982.
3. Gury, David J., Vice President, Plasma Supply, Alpha Therapeutic Corporation. Letter to all source affiliates; December 17, 1982.
4. Foege, William H., M.D. *Summary Report on Workgroup to Identify Opportunities for Prevention of Acquired Immune Deficiency Syndrome* ; January 4, 1983.
5. American Association of Blood Banks, American Red Cross, and Council of Community Blood Centers. Joint Statement on Acquired Immune Deficiency Syndrome (AIDS) Related to Transfusion; January 13, 1983.
6. National Hemophilia Foundation, Medical and Scientific Advisory Council. Recommendations to Prevent AIDS in Patients With Hemophilia; January 14, 1983.
7. Bove, Joseph, M.D., Chairman, Committee on Transfusion Transmitted Diseases, American Association of Blood Banks. *Report to the Board—Committee on Transfusion Transmitted Diseases*; January 24, 1983.
8. American Blood Resources Association. ABRA Recommendations on AIDS and Plasma Donor Deferral; January 28, 1983.
9. American Red Cross National Headquarters. Memorandum to Mr. deBeaufort from Dr. Cumming; February 5, 1983.
10. Petricciani, John, M.D., Director, Food and Drug Administration, Office of Biologics. Letter to all establishments collecting human blood for transfusion; March 24, 1983.

11. Petricciani, John, M.D., Director, Food and Drug Administration, Office of Biologics. Letter to all establishments collecting source plasma; March 24, 1983.
12. Petricciani, John, M.D., Director, Food and Drug Administration, Office of Biologics. Letter to All licensed manufacturers of plasma derivatives; March 24, 1983.
13. National Hemophilia Foundation. Medical Bulletin #7: NHF Urges Clotting Factor Use Be Maintained; May 11, 1983.
14. American Association of Blood Banks, American Red Cross, and Council of Community Blood Centers. Joint Statement on Directed Donations and AIDS; June 22, 1983.
15. Donohue, Dennis, M.D., Director, Food and Drug Administration, Division of Blood and Blood Products. Memorandum to John Petricciani, M.D., Director, Food and Drug Administration, Office of Biologics; July 21, 1983.
16. Reilly, Robert, Executive Director, American Blood Resources Association. Letter to John C. Petricciani, Director, Food and Drug Administration, Office of Biologics; July 27, 1983.

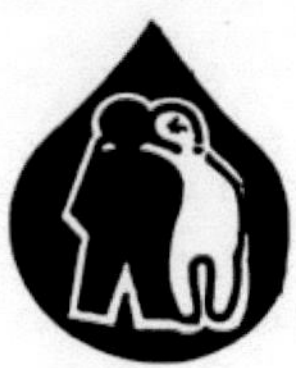

HEMOPHILIA NEWSNOTES

MEMOPHILIA PATIENT ALERT #1

The Centers for Disease Control (CDC) issued a report that three hemophiliacs had developed rare and unusual infections associated with a condition in which there is a decrease in the body's ability to combat disease. These three cases represent an unusually high rate of this disorder and may have developed as a result of an unknown potentially immuno-suppressive agent. One hypothesis that is being investigated by CDC is that the agent may be a virus transmitted similar to the hepatitis virus by blood or blood products.

It is important to note that at this time the <u>risk</u> of contracting this immuno-suppressive agent is <u>minimal</u> and CDC is not recommending any change in blood product use.

A "blue ribbon" panel of experts is being established within the United States Department of Health and Human Services for the purpose of evaluating the problem. NHF Medical Co-Director, Dr. Louis Aledort, will serve on this panel. Concurrent with the work of the panel, CDC will be working closely with NHF and hemophilia treatment centers to establish a carefully planned surveillance and reporting system, and will keep NHF posted on new developments. NHF will keep you informed, but once again, CDC is not advising a change in treatment regimen at this time.

IMPORTANT

REMEMBER, CDC IS NOT ADVISING A CHANGE IN
TREATMENT REGIMEN AT THIS TIME, IF THERE
ARE ANY QUESTIONS, CONTACT YOUR PHYSICIAN
OR HEMOPHILIA TREATMENT CENTER.

July 14, 1982

NATIONAL HEMOPHILIA FOUNDATION 19 WEST 34th STREET·SUITE 1204·NEW YORK, NEW YORK 10001 (212) 563-02

Summary Report on Open Meeting of PHS Committee on Opportunistic Infections in Patients with Hemophilia

I. The Meeting On July 27, 1982, from 8:30 a.m. to 4:30 p.m. a meeting was held to consider the significance of the occurrence of opportunistic infections (OI) with <u>Pneumocystis carinii</u> pneumonia (PCP) in three patients with hemophilia.

Invited participants included representatives of the CDC, FDA, NIH, National Hemophilia Foundation, American National Red Cross, various blood banking organizations, National Gay Task Force, New York City Health Department, and the New York Inter-Hospital Study Group on the Acquired Immune Deficiency Syndrome (AIDS) and Kaposi's Sarcoma (KS) (Attachment 1).

The morning was spent reviewing the various contributory disciplines related to the problem: the epidemiology of AIDS/KS; immunosuppression associated with AIDS/KS; the course, complications, etc. of hemophilia; description of Factor VIII concentrate and other blood products; and a description of the three hemophilia patients with opportunistic infections.

The afternoon was spent discussing the significance of the finding and the appropriate course of action.

II. Aspects of Discussion

A. AIDS (and the sequelae of KS and OI) are occurring in several populations—homosexual men, recent Haitian entrants and I.V. drug abusers. The possibility exists that it is occurring in patients with hemophilia.

B. If the PCP observed in three patients with hemophilia represents the same process as seen in other groups with AIDS, then a possible mode of transmission is via blood products, in this case Factor VIII concentrate. This finding would strengthen the existing hypothesis that AIDS is caused by a transmissible agent.

C. Other seemingly unusual disorders among hemophilia patients were mentioned at the meeting, including cases of Burkitt's Lymohoma, unexplained thrombocytopenia, and possibly other opportunistic infections; but these have not been studied sufficiently to establish their relationship to AIDS.

D. There are 11,000 to 15,000 persons with hemophilia in the United States with varying severity of condition. The morbidity and mortality from hemophilia as well as the lifestyle of hemophilia patients has changed considerably over the past 10 years. These patients are treated with either a product derived from fresh frozen plasma (cryoprecipitate) or a protein concentrate prepared from these precipitates called antihemophilic factor or Factor VIII. Such therapy has allowed the development of home treatment regimens which permit patients to live a more normal life, including sharing educational and vocational opportunities and pursuits with the rest of the population. The number of days of hospitalization annually has decreased markedly for hemophilia patients on home treatment programs. Hemorrhage (spontaneous and traumatic) remains the major cause of death in hemophilia patients.

E. Almost all patients regularly receiving Factor VIII or cryoprecipitate develop hepatitis B and non-A—non-B (NANB) infections. These products have been shown to transmit these infections. Because of the freedom and reduction of suffering permitted hemophilia patients by Factor VIII concentrate, the product's benefits are perceived by patients to vastly outweigh currently known risks.

F. The Factor VIII normally present in fresh plasma is heat labile and inactivated by many types of chemical or physical treatment. For this reason, the techniques developed for the production of Factor VIII concentrate from fresh plasma are known to have little effect on hepatitis viruses. There are five commercial producers of Factor VIII concentrate. Lots of Factor VIII concentrate are prepared from plasma pooled from 1,000 - 5,000 donors. Donors come from many parts of society. Most material is pooled from paid donors in plasmapheresis centers. Hemophilia patients use large amounts of Factor VIII (40,000 to over 65,000 factor units per year) from multiple preparations with subsequent potential exposure to material derived from thousands of donors.

G. The occurrence of PCP in three patients with hemophilia is disturbing, particularly since there is no previous evidence that this infection is common in hemophilia patients. The two patients who had immunologic studies performed demonstrated a T-cell abnormality similar to that among other patients in other high-risk groups with AIDS/KS. There is no known intrinsic immune disorder in hemophilia patients that would permit or promote such opportunistic infections.

III. Conclusions and Recommendations There was general agreement among all participants on the following:

A. Conclusions

1. The pathologic process should be termed Acquired Immune Deficiency Syndrome (AIDS). Kaposi's Sarcoma and the various opportunistic infections are sequelae of the AIDS state.

2. AIDS has characteristics which suggest an infectious etiology.
3. There is an increased risk of AIDS for homosexual men I.V. drug abusers, and among Haitians who have recently enfered the United States. The recent occurrence of PCP in three patients with hemophilia raises the question whether the underlying immunodeficiency seen in these patients has the same etiology as among other groups with PCP. High priority should be given to obtaining information that will answer this question.
4. There is need to determine if certain blood products, particularly Factor VIII, are risk factors for AIDS.

B. To this end, we make the following recommendations:

1. An active surveillance system should be instituted at once to determine if other suspicious cases of AIDS (including OI, KS, or lymphodenopathy) are occurring in hemophilia patients. The CDC, the National Hemophilia Foundation, and the Hemophilia treatment centers volunteered to work together to establish this system and have begun its development.
2. Detailed laboratory studies are needed urgently to develop data relating to the immunologic competence of patients with hemophilia who have no symptoms of opportunistic infection. In addition, it is important to identify promptly and test any patient with hemophilia exhibiting disorders that are considered suspicious (such as thrombocytopenia, Burkitt's Lymphoma, persistent lymphodenopathy, etc.).
3. There is urgent need to determine practical techniques to decrease or eliminate the infectious risks from Factor VIII. Several experimental means of accomplishing this are currently being evaluated. A meeting of the FDA's Advisory Panel on Blood and Blood Products will be held in early September to discuss and evaluate these approaches.
4. There should continue to be broad input into these issues, including representatives from the gay community, hemophilia groups, etc.
5. Concerns were raised over the adequacy of funding to support these new activities, such as active epidemiologic surveillance and intensive laboratory studies. In addition, the existing Federal grants and contracts mechanisms are not responsive to rapid funding of urgent problems. Thus the National Cancer Institute's use of contract funds for AIDS research could not be provided to investigators for at least several months. It would be helpful if the Department could identify resources quickly to assist in these studies.

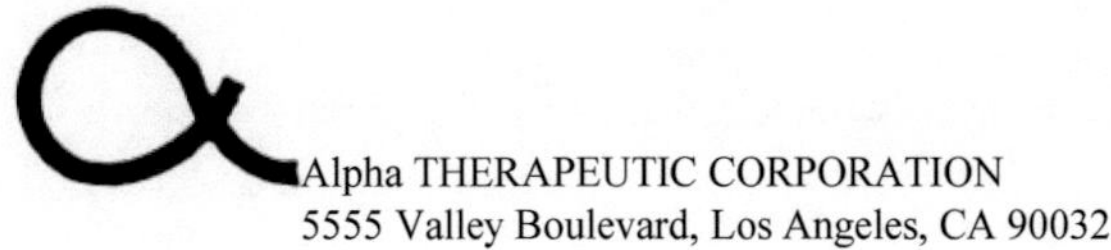

Alpha THERAPEUTIC CORPORATION
5555 Valley Boulevard, Los Angeles, CA 90032

December 17, 1982

SENT FEDERAL EXPRESS TO ALL SOURCE AFFILIATES

(Individual inside addresses and salutations on each letter)

Much attention has been focused on the incidence of Acquired Immune Deficiency Syndrome (AIDS) and the possible transmission of this disease through blood products. While there is little known about what AIDS is or how to detect its presence in its early stages, there are three groups of people that have been identified with a higher incidence of the disease, male homosexuals, intravenous drug abusers, people who have been in Haiti.

Alpha Therapeutic Corporation is concerned that we take all precautions possible to screen donors to minimize the possibility of transmitting AIDS. Therefore, we have modified our specification for plasma to ask that all donors be screened to exclude donors who may be part of any of the following groups:

— Persons who have been in Haiti
— Drug Abusers
— Male Homosexuals

This screening procedure must be in effect by December 27. Plasma collected after December 26, 1982, from donors that have not been screened for these groups should not be sent to Alpha. Please note that this restriction does not apply to donors of special Hepatitis plasma.

Enclosed please find:

1. Copy of revision to plasma specification.
2. Copy of screening history form to be included in donor record file.

3. Copy of planned deviation to operating procedures.
4. We have prepared the following information for distribution in the Alpha Therapeutic Donor Centers:
a. Copy of memorandum we have prepared for donors.
b. Copy of memorandum for donor center employees.
c. Copy of memorandum to be given to donors that may be deferred as a result of questions.

We realize this is not a complete study on AIDS but represents a good portion of the current thinking. You may wish to use this information informing your own donors and employees regarding AIDS.

While we recognize the potential for the rejection of long term donors, we strongly believe that the loss of these donors is more than offset by the protection of our patients.

We will keep you informed as new data becomes available on this extremely important subject. If you have questions, please contact your regional director or myself.

Sincerely,
ALPHA THERPEUTIC CORPORATION
David J. Gury,
Vice President
Plasma Supply
DJG: mcd

attachments
** PLEASE RETURN A COPY OF THIS AS ACKNOWLEDGMENT OF RECEIPT AND IMPLEMENTATION.
Signature
Date

Alpha THERAPEUTIC CORPORATION
5555 Valley Boulevard, Los Angeles, CA 90032

December 17, 1982

TO: ALPHA THERAPEUTIC CORPORATION SOURCE PLASMA CENTERS

The following changes to Alpha Therapeutic Corporation Commodity Specification 92-3015, Source Plasma (Human), are effective December 27, 1982.

3.　　　　REQUIREMENTS

(Add)　　3.1.6　　Donor Screening

　　　　　　　3.1.6.1　　All donors will be screened to exiled those potential donors who are from or have been in Haiti; have ever used illicit drugs intravenously; and male donors who have had sexual contact with a man.

4.　　　　PREPARATION FOR DELIVERY

(Add)　　4.1.3　　Certification

　　　　　　　4.1.3.1　　Each shipment of Source Plasma will be accompanied by the following certification statement. The document must include name and address of the location; shipping date; and signed by the Center Manager. The Certificate should be attached to ATC Plasma Shipping and Receiving Report form 0192-A-480-RI-10/80.

　　　　　　　4.1.3.2　　"I certify that all donors whose plasma is contained within this shipment have certified they are not from or have not been in Haiti; have never used illicit drugs intravenously; and that male donors have never had sexual contact with a man."

David J. Gury
Vice President, Plasma Supply

Marietta Carr
Vice President, Regulatory Affairs

President

2DR #0669

Medical Reception will ask all potential donors the following questions in addition to the Medical screening questions currently used:

1) Have you ever been to Haiti?
2) Have you ever used illicit drugs intravenously?
3) Have you ever had sexual contact with a man? (For male donors only).

If any of the above questions are answered "yes", the donor must be rejected.

Summary Report on Workgroup to Identify Opportunities for Prevention of Acquired Immune Deficiency Syndrome January 4, 1983

I. The Meeting

On January 4, 1983, from 8:30 a.m. to 4:30 p.m., a meeting was held in Atlanta to consider existing opportunities for prevention of Acquired Immune Deficiency Syndrome (AIDS), both by person-to-person transmission and by blood or blood products. This meeting was a follow-up to a meeting held July 27, 1982 in Washington, D.C. which considered the significance of the occurrence of AIDS in three patients with hemophilia.

Invited participants included representatives of the National Hemophilia Foundation, American National Red Cross, various blood banking organizations, National Gay Task Force, New York and San Francisco Health Departments, Conference of State and Territorial Epidemiologists and the Pharmaceutical Manufacturers Association as well as staff members of the CDC, FDA and NIH (Attachment 1).

The morning was devoted to reviewing recent information pertinent to AIDS, risk groups and the blood and plasma donation process: the epidemiology of AIDS, AIDS among persons with hemophilia and those receiving transfusions, potential laboratory screening tests, current recommendations and regulations for screening of blood and plasma donors, the demographics of blood donation and the separation and processing of blood and blood derivatives, including Factor VIII. Discussion was then held on various alternative opportunities for prevention.

II. Aspects of Discussion

A. AIDS continues to be a major public health problem. In addition to the previously described high risk groups (homosexual men, intravenous drug users, recently arrived Haitians, etc.), persons with hemophilia are also at increased risk of developing AIDS presumably by introduction of a transmissible agent in Factor VIII concentrate. Five cases of AIDS have been reported in persons with hemophilia since the three described in July and two to three more are considered to be possible cases.

B. One case of AIDS has occurred in an infant who received a platelet transfusion from a man who subsequently was diagnosed as an AIDS patient. Several other AIDS cases under investigation (five) have no risk factors but have received blood products within the past two years. Some participants were reluctant to accept the hypothesis that AIDS has been transmitted by whole blood in the absence of additional evidence.

C. Guidelines for prevention of AIDS cases by person-to-person-transmission were generally accepted by the workgroup (proposed guidelines are in Attachment 2).

D. A consensus was reached that it would be desirable to exclude high risk donors to reduce the risk of AIDS transmission via blood and blood products. However, no consensus was reached as to the best method of doing this. The principal strategies are:

1. voluntary restriction by potential donors within high risk groups;

2. exclusion of donors on the basis of history and/or physical examination at the time of donation, e.g., a positive response to questions such as, "Have you had sexual contact with another man?", "Are you a past or present intravenous drug user?", "Are you Haitian?" etc. On physical exam, patients with lymphadenopathy, etc. could be excluded.

3. Use of a "surrogate" laboratory test; a test which when positive is associated with high risk groups for AIDS.

4. A combination of these strategies.

    All these strategies will be difficult to evaluate for effectiveness.

E. Voluntary restriction has the advantage of enabling high risk groups to play a major and responsible role in protecting others in society. It is independent of the blood supply system. It is inexpensive, and is relatively easy to initiate. The disadvantages are that it has the limitations of not being able to influence less responsible persons and being unlikely to reach and motivate some proportion of those for whom it is intended.

F. Questioning donors for their nationality, sexual orientation or personal habits has the advantages of being an easy extension of the screening history already used in blood donation, is inexpensive, can be directed toward high risk groups and causes little disruption in the blood collection and processing routine. It has the disadvantage of being potentially intrusive into personal matters, may be viewed as unethical, might institutionalize a stigma on groups already prone to prejudice and persecution, and may be ineffective in identifying persons in these high risk groups. Concerns about record privacy have been raised. A considerable proportion of practicing homosexual males may not consider themselves high-risk for AIDS and others may be reluctant to disclose their sexual orientation. Similarly, recently emigrated Haitians and drug users may be reluctant to identify themselves. Some commercial plasmapheresis processors are already excluding by history some AIDS high risk groups.

G. Surrogate laboratory tests have the advantages of being objective and can be done on specimens already being drawn for HBsAg. They respect donor privacy and may be most effective in eliminating potential transmitters of AIDS. They have the disadvantage of adding expense to the blood collection process, both through test cost, administrative overhead, and loss of blood units already collected. Further, they may stigmatize as unsatisfactory many "normal" donors for each potential AIDS transmitter that is rejected.

For example, if the presence of hepatitis B core antibody is used as a laboratory surrogate screening test:

1. In CDC's specimen file, 90 percent of known definite AIDS cases are positive for anti-Hb_c and would be excluded as blood donors.

2. Approximately five percent of the general population of voluntary donors are positive for anti-HB_c, though this figure may vary by blood center. These results would be determined after collection, and the collected units would have to be destroyed, unless they could be safely and practically processed into other blood products.

3. The costs of the test might add to the cost of processing. The loss of each destroyed unit represents further expense and there might be additional overhead costs. The costs of preventing an unknown number of AIDS cases (and possibly non-A, non-B hepatitis cases) are unknown, but each such case is very costly in direct and indirect costs and the intangible costs of grief and suffering.

4. Concern was expressed over availability of adequate anti-HB_c test materials. However, information suggests that some companies are already planning production of large quantities of anti-HB_c and that demand would provoke an adequate supply.

5. As the epidemiology of AIDS changes, high risk groups may have lower rates of positivity for anti-Hb_c.

6. This additional laboratory test will require new training and procedures for many laboratories.

H. Alterations in blood processing could also reduce the risk of AIDS transmission. The FDA expects an improved Factor VIII concentrate to be available within 12 months. This product would be heat treated sufficiently to inactivate hepatitis B virus and presumably eliminate other transmissible agents from the finished product. Although preliminary data on such treated Factor VIII materials suggest that there is little loss in activity, detailed information on increased costs, product availability and likelihood of reducing AIDS risk are not yet available.

II. Conclusions and Recommendations

A. The workgroup participants represented various organizations, governmental agencies and constituent groups concerned with and affected by AIDS and the blood and plasma donation process. They have differing perceptions of:

1. The likelihood that AIDS is caused by a transmissible agent;

2. The risk of AIDS from blood donation (both whole blood and pooled plasma); and

3. The best approach for establishing altered guidelines for blood donation, donor screening or testing and donor restriction.

B. The workgroup meeting was successful in presenting the most recent data on AIDS and blood/blood products and as a forum for differing views to be expressed. This enabled all participants to gain further insight and appreciation of an extraordinarily complex health problem.

C. I recommend that each Public Health Service Agency (CDC, FDA, NIH) provide candidate sets of recommendations for the prevention of AIDS in patients with hemophilia and for the other recipients of blood and blood products to Dr. Jeffrey P. Koplan, Assistant Director for Public Health Practice, CDC. The three agencies should then develop a uniform set of recommendations on AIDS for your office.

January 13, 1983

JOINT STATEMENT ON ACQUIRED IMMUNE DEFICIENCY SYNDROME (AIDS) RELATED TO TRANSFUSION

American Association of Blood Banks, American Red Cross, and Council of Community Blood Centers

Recent reports of abnormal immune function, Kaposi's sarcoma, and opportunistic infections in some gay males, Haitian entrants, and intravenous drug users and in others suggest that a new disease of unknown etiology has appeared in the United States. The disease has been called Acquired Immune Deficiency Syndrome (AIDS). Over 800 cases of AIDS have been reported with a very high mortality rate. While the major foci seem to be New York, San Francisco and Los Angeles, cases have been reported from other areas of the United States.

The predominant mode of transmission seems to be from person to person, probably involving intimate contact. The possibility of blood borne transmission, still unproven, has been raised. This latter impression is reinforced by eight confirmed cases in hemophiliacs treated with antihemophilic factor (AHF) concentrate, by a case in a newborn infant who received 19 units of blood components, one of which was from a donor who later died of AIDS, and by fewer than 10 unconfirmed case reports in other transfusion recipients. No agent has been isolated and there is no test for the disease or for potential carriers. Evidence of transmission by blood transfusion is inconclusive.

The finding of cases in hemophiliacs, especially those who use antihemophilic factor concentrate, coupled with the long incubation period and the continuing increase in reported cases is of sufficient concern to warrant the following suggestions for action on the part of blood banks and transfusion services. We realize that there is no absolute evidence that AIDS is transmitted by blood or blood products, and we understand the difficulty in making recommendations based on insufficient data. There is a need for additional information about this disease. Public health authorities should allocate resources to study the etiology of AIDS, its mode of transmission, and appropriate preventative measures and therapy. Blood centers and transfusion services should continue to assist public health agencies investigating AIDS. Given the possibility that AIDS may be spread by transfusion, we are obligated to respond with measures that seem reasonable at present. The lack of a specific test means that our major effort must revolve around two areas: 1) additional caution in the use of blood and blood products and 2) reasonable attempts to limit blood donation from individuals or groups that may have an unacceptably high risk of AIDS. Our specific suggestions follow:

1. Blood banks and transfusion services should further extend educational campaigns to physicians to balance the decision to use each blood component against the risks of transfusion, be they well-established (e.g. hepatitis, cytomegalovirus, malaria) or under investigation (e.g. AIDS).

2. Autologous blood transfusions, as an alternative to allogeneic transfusion, should be considered more frequently, especially in elective surgery.

3. Blood banks should plan to deal with increased requests for cryoprecipitate. Altered T lymphocyte function, a component of AIDS, has been reported to be less

frequent in hemophilia patients who are treated with cryoprecipitate rather than AHF concentrate. Although this does not necessarily imply that cryoprecipitate is free of risks, this finding may lead to an increased demand for ryoprecipitate.

4. Donor screening should include specific questions to detect possible AIDS or exposure to patients with AIDS. In particular, all donors should be asked questions designed to elicit a history of night sweats, unexplained fevers, unexpected weight loss, lymphadenopathy or Kaposi's sarcoma. All positive or suggestive answers should be evaluated before anyone donates.

5. Persons with responsibility for donor recruitment should not target their efforts toward groups that may have a high incidence of AIDS.

6. A major area of concern is whether attempts to limit voluntary blood donation by individuals from groups with a high prevalence of AIDS are appropriate at present. This question has medical, ethical and legal implications.

a. The presently available medical and scientific evidence that AIDS can be spread by blood components remains incomplete. Fewer than 10 cases of AIDS with possible linkage to transfusion have been seen despite approximately 10 million transfusions per year. Ongoing epidemiologic studies of all cases of AIDS are being conducted at this time. Should evidence of a clearly implicated donor population become apparent, specific recommendations to the blood banking community will be made promptly.

b. There is currently considerable pressure on the blood banking community to restrict blood donation by gay males. Direct or indirect questions about a donor's sexual preference are inappropriate. Such an invasion of privacy can be justified only if it demonstrates clear-cut benefit. In fact, there is reason to believe that such questions, no matter how well-intentioned, are ineffective in eliminating those donors who may carry AIDS. Blood banks should work with the leadership of groups which include some individuals at high risk of AIDS.

7. While there is no specific test for AIDS, there are laboratory and clinical findings that are present in nearly all AIDS patients. The use of these non-specific markers, for example, lymphopenia, immune complexes, and anti-HBc, are being evaluated in those areas of the country where AIDS is prevalent. We do not advise routine implementation of any laboratory screening program for AIDS by blood banks at this time.

These recommendations are made with full realization that the cause of AIDS is unknown and that evidence for its transmission by blood is inconclusive. We believe, however, that we must respond to the possibility that a new and infectious illness has surfaced. Until more information is available, we believe that the measures outlined above are prudent and appropriate.

We will continue to monitor new developments and revise our position promptly should medical or scientific finding indicate that a different course of action is warranted.

This joint statement was developed by the American Association of Blood Banks, the American Red Cross, and the Council of Community Blood Centers, with assistance from the American Blood Commission, National Gay Task Force, and the National Hemophilia Foundation Resources Association, the Centers for Disease Control and the Food and Drug Administration.

<u>Recommendations of the Medical and Scientific Advisory Council submitted to the NHF Board of Directors</u>

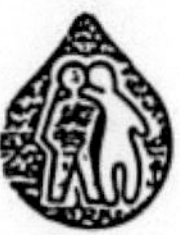

THE NATIONAL HEMOPHILIA FOUNDATION
THE NATIONAL HEMOPHILIA FOUNDATION MEDICAL AND SCIENTIFIC ADVISORY COUNCIL
January 14, 1983
<u>RECOMMENDATIONS TO PREVENT AIDS IN PATIENTS WITH HEMOPHILIA</u>

I. Recommendations for physicians treating patients with hemophilia.

A. It is recommended that cryoprecipitate be used to treat patients in the following groups except when there is an overriding medical indication:

- newborn infants and children under 4;
- newly identified patients never treated with factor VIII concentrate;
- patients with clinically mild hemophilia who require infrequent treatment.
- Similar guidelines should be applied to factor IX deficiency patients where fresh frozen plasma can be used instead of concentrate.

B. The potential advantages and disadvantages of cryoprecipitate versus factor VIII concentrate therapy for severe hemophilia A are not clear at the present time and are controversial. The Medical and Scientific Advisory Council does not offer a specific recommendation at this time, but will continue to review the data.

C. DDAVP should be used whenever possible in patients with mild or moderate hemophilia A.

D. All elective surgical procedures should be evaluated with respect to the possible advantages or disadvantages of a delay.

II. Recommendations to factor VIII concentrate manufacturers:

A. Serious efforts should be made to exclude donors that might transmit AIDS. These should include:

1. Identification, by direct questioning, individuals who belong to groups at high risk of transmitting AIDS, specifically male homosexuals; intravenous drug users; and those who have recently resided in Haiti.

2. Evaluation and implementation (if verified) of surrogate laboratory tasts that would identify individuals at high risk of AIDS transmission.

3. In addition, the manufacturers should cease using plasma obtained from donor centers that draw from population groups in which there is a significant AIDS incidence. It is clear from the epidemiologic data that the pool of individuals at risk for AIDS transmission is not uniform throughout the country and that a great deal could be achieved by excluding donors from the "hot spots".

B. Efforts should be continued to expedite the development of processing methods that will inactivate viruses potentially present in factor VIII concentrates.

over

19 WEST 34th STREET · SUITE 1204 · NEW YORK. NEW YORK 10001 · (212) 563–0211

C. There should be an evaluation of the possibility that the yield of factor VIII in pheresis donors could be increased using DDAVP or exercise to maximize yield. This would permit a reduction in the size of the donor pool and would compensate for losses in plasma that might occur due to steps noted above.

D. There should be an evaluation of the feasibility of fractionating and processing plasma so that lyophilized small pool products are available. While this will certainly be more costly, it may be the only way to break out of the present dilemma without going to an all-cryoprecipitate effort.

E. Concentrate manufacturers should immediately cease purchase of recovered plasma for factor VIII concentrate from blood centers that do not meet the criteria listed in II A above. These criteria should also apply to the production of cryoprecipitate.

F. Manufacturers should accelerate efforts towards the production of coagulation factor concentrates by recombinant DNA technology.

III. Recommendations to regional and community blood centers:

A. Those centers that are in regions in which there is a very low incidence of AIDS should increase capacity for cryoprecipitate production to be used locally and in other regions.

B. These centers should evaluate the feasibility of preparing small pool lyophilized cryoprecipitate for hemophilia treatment.

C. The production of cryoprecipitate should also adhere to criteria detailed in IIA, above.

Report to the Board Committee on Transfusion Transmitted Diseases

The major report of your Committee on Transfusion Transmitted Diseases has been issued as our recommendations to the Association. These few additional paragraphs are more my current views and concerns than a formal committee report. Nonetheless, because of my recent experiences I am anxious to share some thoughts with you.

The report that we have submitted to our members is, in my view, appropriate considering the data at hand. Since we met, however, an additional child with AIDS has been admitted to a Texas hospital. At birth the child had received seven transfusions, one of which came from a donor who now seems to have AIDS. This case increases the probability that AIDS may be spread by blood. Furthermore, the CDC continues to investigate the current cases aggressively and may even have a few more. While I believe our report reacts appropriately to the data at hand, I also believe that the most we can do in this situation is buy time. There is little doubt in my mind that additional transfusion related cases and additional cases in patients with hemophilia will surface. Should this happen, we will be obliged to review our current stance and probably to move in the same direction as the commercial fractionators. By that I mean it will be essential for us to take some active steps to screen out donor populations who are at high risk of AIDS. For practical purposes this means gay males.

The matter of arranging an appropriate screening program is delicate and difficult. We have had excellent cooperation from individuals in the gay community and our deliberations have been made easier by their knowledge and ability to help us. I have no doubt that they will continue to support us and, should we need to be more aggressive in this area, will help us do it in a way that is socially responsible.

Blood banks that wish to sell plasma for further fractionation already face the need to do something. Perhaps our Committee should prepare guidelines with suggested wording for them to use. We are reluctant to do this since we do not want anything that we do now to be interpreted by society (or by legal authorities) as agreeing with the concept - as yet unproven - that AIDS can be spread by blood.

All in all this is a knotty problem and one that we will not solve easily.

I want to make a few comments about the process by which our joint document developed. We spent a great deal of time and energy and did the best we could in attempting to reach a consensus. The difficulty was to get AABB, ARC, CCBC and all the other groups to adopt a position which was acceptable to each other. It was impossible to have a small meeting; everybody wanted to attend. When we got the group together we were able to hammer out a statement that pleased the attendees. Unfortunately, the statement had to go through several iterations with our own Board and the Boards of the other involved organizations. In all probability these modifications resulted in a better statement, but the process of getting these changes incorporated and run back and forth through the three organizations was difficult. We have had a good start at working together on this and we hope to keep it up. The mechanism was a little less smooth when it came to releasing the statements and the public relations that went with it.

I hope that we are equipped psychologically to continue to act together. I have been in contact with ARC (Dr. Katz) and CCBC (Dr. Menitove) and believe that the three of us can, together, work out whatever new problems may arise. We plan frequent conference calls to keep each other informed.

I want to comment about the Committee. They worked well together and I was particularly pleased with the input of advisory members. Having individuals who are not associated with the blood banks nor a traditional part of the blood banking community proved most useful to us. Their comments and suggestions were excellent. In a like manner, we were helped by participants from the National Gay Task Force. As we continue to react to the various challenges before us, I am sure that their help will be essential. Finally, let me acknowledge the help from the Central Office and, in particular from Lorry Rose.

No immediate end to the publicity is in sight and we will get continued calls for us to act more aggressively. We need to do whatever is medically correct. In addition, we may have to do a little more, since we are accused of burying our heads in the sand. We are not being helped by the spate of publicity about this illness, but will continue to react responsibility to whatever scientific and medical information we have.

Joseph R. Bove, M.D., Chairman
Committee on Transfusion Transmitted Diseases
American Association of Blood Banks
JRB: tmf
1/24/83

ABRA American Blood Resources Association P.O. Box 3346 • Annapolis, MD. 21403

January 28, 1983

ABRA RECOMMENDATIONS ON AIDS AND PLASMA DONOR DEFERRAL

The American Blood Resources Association (ABRA) recommends that its member firms who are involved in the collection of plasma for the manufacture of certain products used in the treatment of hemophilia, a coagulation deficiency, take the following actions to eliminate plasma donors who may be in those groups identified as having a high risk to Acquired Immune Deficiency Syndrome (AIDS).

In the past two years, over 800 cases of AIDS have been reported in the United States. The disease is of unknown etiology, resulting in abnormal immune function, Kaposi's sarcoma and opportunistic infections with a high mortality rate. It appears most frequently in homosexuals, Haitians, and intravenous drug abusers. Several recent cases of AIDS in hemophiliacs and in recipients of various blood products, suggest that AIDS may be of infectious etiology.

The American Blood Resources Association represents the United States commercial plasmapheresis industry who performs 10 million plasmapheresis procedures each year, representing one-half of all donor collections in the United States. ABRA is concerned that steps be taken as soon as possible to screen plasma donors to minimize the possibility of transmitting AIDS. After extensive discussions with various organizations representing the Public Health Services, national blood banking groups and the National Hemophilia Foundation, the leadership of ABRA believes that the most significant action which can be taken, at this time, to reduce the potential risk of AIDS in certain plasma products, is to seek either voluntary donor exclusion or to modify the donor screening procedures to eliminate individuals from the plasma donor population who are in those groups identified as having a high risk to AIDS.

ABRA recommendations focus on three areas: 1) donor education, 2) donor screening, and 3) surrogate laboratory testing.

In the area of education, the Association recommends the preparation of an information document describing AIDS, including statements on how individuals in high risk groups may reduce their risk of exposure, and statements intended to discourage high risk individuals from donating plasma. In addition, the Association recommends that plasmapheresis center management initiate staff education programs on AIDS and its symptomatology.

For donor screening, the Association recommends that donors be required to read the information about AIDS and acknowledge that they are not members of the high risk groups identified; and that individuals in high risk groups be excluded from donating plasma. Further, on a continuing basis, expand the medical history and examination to include the question, "Have you had AIDS or close contact with someone with AIDS?" All donors should be asked questions designed to elicit history of night sweats, unexpected weight loss, unexplained fevers, lymphadenopathy, or Kaposi's sarcoma. Anyone found to exhibit any of these symptoms should not be allowed to donate plasma without further medical studies.

For additional laboratory testing, the Association recommends that no large scale testing be initiated at this time. Assessment of issues such as the adequate availability of testing reagents and equipment of any of the several possible tests under consideration, their economic and logistical impact upon the plasma supply network, the efficacy of the test to exclude high risk individuals, and other potential consequences to plasma products resulting from the imposition of additional testing requirements is currently under study.

These ABRA recommendations are intended to apply to all plasma donors collected by plasmapheresis for use in the production of antihemophilic factor concentrate. The Association is forwarding these recommendations to other national and international organizations concerned with donor standards and blood and blood product quality. Each year, the blood banking community recovers plasma from several million voluntary blood donor units which are then used in the production of antihemophilic factor concentrate products used in the treatment of hemophiliacs. Therefore, it is the view of the ABRA leadership that all donors, whether they are participating on plasmapheresis programs or on voluntary blood donor programs, should be screened to eliminate individuals identified in the AIDS high risk groups.

ABRA will consider changing and updating these recommendations as more medical and scientific information becomes available. For more information, call the Association's National Office at (301) 263-8296.

American Red Cross

To Hr. de Beaufort

Date February 5, 1983

From Dr. Cumming

Subject Dr. Katz's 1/26/83 AIDS Memo

(a)   "Is AIDS transmissible by blood?"

- The available evidence strongly suggests that AIDS is transmissable.
- The available evidence strongly suggests that AIDS is transmissable via AHF concentrate to hemophiliacs.
- There is not enough evidence to draw any other scientific conclusions.

(b)   "Will elimination of donor groups that are at high risks of contacting AIDS decrease incidents of AIDS? (Note discrepency in approach to Haitian entrants and to gays.)"

Scientifically, we don't know since the transmission mechanism is unknown at present. In the future, however, it is likely to be shown that such, will be the case. In the interim it will be largely an ethical/political/marketing/legal issue. From the standpoint of product marketing we will be better off making direct and visible attempts at elimination of such groups. Ethically, I don't think sexual preference is the proper business of anyone (or any institution) other than the individuals involved in the sexual act. Legally it would seem that we are open to suit in any event i.e. by the gays if we attempt to exclude them, by patients who might contacts AIDS if we don't make every attempt to exclude gays. Haitians and any other group associated with AIDS. Setting aside the ethical issue, politically and on balance, it would seem we should make every attempt to eliminate as donors all groups associated with AIDS. However, this position leaves us vulverable from a standpoint of scientific leadership and it ignors the question of whether or not attempts to eliminate gays and other groups associated with AIDS will be successful.

(c)   "Should ARC pursue (b) above?"

- The answer to this question lies in staying focused on "the facts."
- Relevant facts are: (1) the focal group of concern is the gays, we are not likely to incur much resistance with respect to elimination of any other group; (2) as a proportion of the donor population only the gays are significant (greater than 1%); (3) homosexuals and bisexuals constitute up to 25% of the donor population; (4) it is

only <u>male</u> gays that are associated with AIDS. thus they probably equal 15% or less of the donor population; (5) the whole blood needs of the total country could be met by 9% of the population between 18 and 65 years old donating once per year (or 6% donor, 1.5 times per year); (6) eliminating all gay males (homosexuals bisexuals) would only increase the population of the population (18 to 65) required to donate once per year from about 9% to [Text incomplete in source] 11% (or 6% donating less than 2 times per year); (7) only a [Text incomplete in source] reportedly "small" subset of days are those associated with AIDS the so called "fast lane" or "bath house" gays (♀ ≈ 70 different partners and 1100 contacts per year); (8) elimination of only the "fast lane" gays from the donor pool probably would not notice increase the 9% requirement; (9) direct questioning as a means of eliminating gays could be counterproductive; (10) the scientific basis for elimination of gays does not exist at present; (11) [Text incomplete in source] incidence of AIDS is highly concentrated at present

roughly 75% of the cases involve male homosexuals
roughly 95% of the cases involve males
cases have occurred in only 32 of the 50 states
669 of 800 cases (84%) were from just 4 states (New York 51%. California 20%. Florida 7%, and New Jersey 6%)
In each state one or two cities account for the bulk of all cases reported

— New York City = 97% of cases in New York State
— San Francisco = 60% of cases in California
— Los Angeles = 28% of cases in California
— Miami = 63% of cases in Florida
— Newark = 40% of cases in New Jersey

(12) historically the incidence of AIDS has been doubling about every six months but this trend is not reflected in figures for November and December 1982.

We are currently pursing elimination of groups at risk of contact AIDS by means which are likely to eliminate all groups with the possible exception of gays (e.g. checks for IV drug use. travel questions, symptom questions, prohibitions on hemophiliacs). And we are working with gays groups on voluntary exclusion. Of those actions which have been suggested, the only things we are not [Text incomplete in source] are:

(1) asking direct questions of gays; and (2) laboratory testing of blood samples. As time goes on we are liable to get more and more pressure to utilize these means also. If AIDS continues to double every 6 months, the concentration in gay males continues, and absent evidence to the centrary, this pressure is likely to be overwhelming in 6 to 12 months. Even if the evolving evidence of an epidemic wanes CDC is likely to continue to play up AIDS-- ----it has long been noted that CDC increasingly needs 2 major epidemic to justify its existence. This is especially true in light of Federal funding cuts and fact that AIDS probably played some positive role in CDC's successful battle with OMB to fund a new $15,000.000 viralogy lab. This CDC perspective is also obvious from the general "marketing nature" of the January 4, 1983 Atlanta meeting e.g. abundent press at a "scientific" meeting, presentation without hard copy, hard selling SBA and HBC testing, etc. In short, we can _not_ depend on CDC to provide scientific, objective, unbias leadership on the topic. However because CDC will continue to push for more action from the blood banking community, the public will believe there is a scientific basis and means for eliminating gays.

As I understand it, additional scientific pressure to eliminate gays can be brought to bear from our experience with hepatitus.

In the absence of scientific evidence to the contrary and given the continuing use of direct questioning by the plasma sector, marketing pressure will build for us to use direct questioning.

The bottom line----in the absence of scientific evidence to the contrary, within 6 to 12 months we won't have any choice but to use at least direct questioning and probably laboratory tests to "attempt" to eliminate gay males. I say attempt because the efficacy of both direct questions and laboratory tests are disputable. I personally believe that direct questioning will be counterproductive in most ARC regions, given the public nature of the blood donation process. How many men in Buffalo, New York are going to step forward, out of their closet, in front of their peers and admit they are "queers"? Or even call in later to have their donation discarded?

To the extent the industry (ARC/CCBC/AABB) sticks together against CDC, it will appear to some segments of the public at least that we have a self interest which is in conflict with the public interest, unless we can clearly demonstrate that CDC is wrong. A January 1983 incidence figure which is consistent with November and December 1982 and inconsistent with CDC's hypothesis of doubling every 6 months would be helpful in this regard.

In the short run our position has all the ear marks of a lossless one. The question would seem to be how do we minimize the short run loss and hopefully gain in the long run?

(d)   &

(e)   "If ARC pursues (c), how?"

Since (c) refers to (b), this question really means elimination of donor groups at high risk which means gays and methods we are not currently employing viz. direct questions and lab tests. Furthermore (e) can be viewed as providing additional criteria for (d), which is the way I have treated the question below.

In the long term I believe the interests of the ARC and the American public are best served if the ARC Blood Services follows pathways based on science, logic and ethics. Stated another way, we should attempt to be the voice of reason where less than rationality frequently prevails. In the short run (6 to 12 months) there is little time to develop the science surrounding AIDS. We can, however, take steps in this direction. Logically we must prepare to implement more steps designed to eliminate high risk groups. Ethically we don't belong in anyones bedroom.

I suggest that we work with CCBC and the AABB to design a comprehensive research program focused on the four hot spots of New York, San Francisco. Los Angeles and Miami. Research Program <u>assumptions</u> are: (1) AIDS will continue to grow as a national epicemic; (2) AIDS will be shown to be transmitted by all blood products; (3) it will not be possible to demonstrate the AIDS safety of any blood product for at least 2 years (The incubation period for AIDS is variously estimated at 7 months to 7 years); and (4) the association of AIDS with homosexuals will continue but delate. Program purposes should be to develop specific techniques (e.g. laboratory tests, direct/ indirect questions, education) to eliminate groups at risk of transmitting AIDS and determine the relative effectiveness and efficiency of alternative techniques (e.g. demonstrate whether or not direct questions eliminate gays). This is essentially Kelner's "hot spot" approach except that it has a substantially broader scope i.e. the techniques won't be limited to HBc testing. The program should be initiated with baseline data collection within one month while design and negotiation is ongoing regarding other aspects. Also, the faster and more visibly we move, the more of a leadership position we can capture. The program should be designed to begin to yeild results in six months e.g. 3 months of baseline data collection followed by three months of technique application, with results immediately feed into previously developed computer analytic routines.

The six month time frame is critical in that I believe our current position as announced in the BSD's is a good one, but we won't be able to hold out for more than 6 to 12 conths (as discussed above) unless we have objective evidence to prove that recommended direct questions and 1ab tests don't work. This poses an interesting question on the precise statement of the null hypothesis.

The long term impact should be to enhance our scientific credibility. If we base our policies on scientific/objective information, we should not have to change frequently which I think would be disasterous to our public image (unless the weight of scientific evidence shifts accordingly).

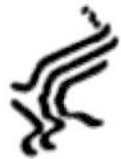

DEPARTMENT OF HEALTH & HUMAN SERVICES
Food and Drug Administration Bethesda. MD 20205

March 24, 1983

FROM: Director,
Office of Biologics
National Center for Drugs and Biologics

SUBJECT: Recommendations to Decrease the Risk of Transmitting
Acquired Immune Deficiency Syndrome (AIDS) from Blood Donors

TO: All Establishments Collecting Human Blood for Transfusion

The Acquired Immune Deficiency (AIDS) Syndrome has caused serious concern among members of the blood banking community because of the implications for transfusion recipients if this disease is proven to be transmissible by blood or blood products. The major organizations engaged in blood collection have recently reached a consensus as to steps which should be taken to decrease the risk of transmitting AIDS by blood transfusion. Consistent with the recommendations of the American Red Cross, the American Association of Blood Banks, the Council of Community Blood Centers, and the Public Health Service Interagency Committee (copy attached), the Office of Biologics is advising all establishments collecting blood for transfusion to institute additional measures designed to decrease blood collection from individual donors and donor groups known to be at increased risk for transmitting AIDS. The following steps should be included:

1. Educational programs should be instituted to inform persons at increased risk of AIDS that until the AIDS problem is resolved or definitive tests become available, they should refrain from blood donation because of the potential risk to recipients of their blood. As presently defined this group includes: persons with symptoms and signs suggestive of AIDS, sexually active homosexual or bisexual men with multiple partners, Haitian entrants to the United States, present or past abusers of intravenous drugs, *and sexual partners of individuals at increased risk of AIDS. Educational programs should include the individual donor as part of the donor screening procedure.

2. Re-education of personnel responsible for donor screening should be conducted with special attention to recognition of the early signs and symptoms of AIDS. The donor medical history should include specific questions designed to detect possible AIDS symptoms or exposure to patients with AIDS. Standard Operating Procedures (SOP) should be revised to include questions which elicit a history of night sweats, unexplained fevers, unexpected weight loss, or signs of lymphadenopathy or Kaposi's sarcoma.

---

* Such intravenous drug abusers are already excluded by existing regulations.

3.   The SOP should specifically inform ataff that all blood or blood products inadvertently collected, or collected for therapeutic purposes, from a donor known or suspected of having AIDS should be considered potentially highly infectious and must be immediately quarantined and disposed of expeditiously unless designated for investigative use related to AIDS. If not destroyed, such products must be labeled, stored and shipped in accordance with the standard procedures for handling infectious materials. Appropriate disposal procedures include autoclaving or controlled incineration; overwraps are required to protect staff in case of breakage.

Approved procedures developed by one of the major organizations such as the American Red Cross, the American Association of Blood Banks, the Council of Community Blood Centers and the American Blood Resources Association may be referenced in the licensed establishments' SOP without individual submission to the Office of Biologics. Alternatively, licensed establishments which develop their own procedures should submit them directly to the Office of Biologics for approval concurrent with implementation.

This memorandum is intended to be an interim measure to protect recipients of blood and blood products until specific laboratory tests are available.

John C. Petricciani,
M. D.

Attachment

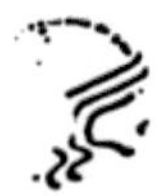

DEPARTMENT OF HEALTH & HUMAN SERVICES
Public Health Service
Food and Drug Administration Rockville MD 20857

March 24, 1983

FROM: Director,
Office of Biologics, National Center for Drugs and Biologics

SUBJECT: Recommendations to Decrease the Risk of Transmitting
Acquired Immune Deficiency Syndrome (AIDS) from Plasma Donors

TO: All establishments Collecting Source Plasma (Human)

The Acquired Immune Deficiency Syndroos (AIDS) has caused serious concein because of the implications for recipients of plasma derivatives if this disease is proven to be transmissible by blood or blood products, The major organizations involved in plasma collection have reached a consensus us to appropriate steps which should be taken to decrease the potential of blood or plasma donation by individuals who might be at increased risk of transmitting AIDS. Consistent with the recommendations of the American blood Resources Association, the American Red Cross, the American Association of Blood Banks, the Council of Community Blood Centers, and the Public Health Service Interagency Committee, (copy attached), the Office of Biologies is advising that the following steps should be taken by all establishments collecting Source Plasma (Ruman):

1. Educational programs should be instituted to inform persons at increased risk of AIDS that until the AIDS problem is resolved or definitive tests become available, they should refrain from routine plasma donation because of the potential risk to recipients of certain plasma derivatives. As presently defined, persons at increased risk include those with symptoms and signs suggestive of AIDS, sexually active homosexual or bisexual men with multiple partners, Haitian entrants to the United States, present or past abusers of intravenous drugs[*] and sexual partners of individuals at increased risk of AIDS. Each Source Plasma donor should receive information about AIDS including the need for individuals at increased risk to voluntarily exclude themselves from routine plasma programs.

2. If plasma is collected from a donor belonging to any of the groups at increased risk, a label should be affixed to each unit to restrict its use in accordance with 21 CFR 606.120(b)(6). The recommended label statements are "CAUTION: For Use in Manufacturing Albumin, PPF, or Clobulin Only" or "CAUTION: For Use in Manufacturing Noninjectable Products Only". HD-Ag positive plasma is already subject to special labeling and shipping restrictions and these programs are not affected by this memorandum.

---

[*] Such intravenous drug abusers are already excluded by existing regulations.

3. Re-education of personnel responsible for donor screening should be conducted with special attention to identifying the early signs and symptoms of AIDS in donors. The donor medical history should include specific questions designed to detect possible AIDS symptoms or exposure to patients with AIDS. <u>Standard Operating Procedures</u> (SOP) should be revised to include questions which elicit a history of night sweats, unexplained fevers, unexpected weight loss, or signs of lymphadenopathy or Kaposi's sarcoma.

4. Donors should be examined for lymphadenopathy. The initial and annual physical should provide an opportunity for an examination by the physician for generalized lymphadenopathy, while a more limited examination should be performed by an adequately trained individual on each donor on the day of plasma collection and a record made of the results of the examination.

5. An accurate record of each source plasma donor's weight prior to each donation should be made to permit ready identification of any unexplained weight loss. Any significant, unexplained decrease in weight should be considered cause for referral of the donor to a physician for complete evaluation prior to any further plasma collection. Any plasma in storage, which was previously collected from such a donor, should be quarantined until the physician's evaluation is completed.

6. The <u>SOP</u> should inform the staff that any products collected from a donor known or suspected to have AIDS should be considered potentially highly infectious and must be immediately quarantined and disposed of expeditiously and appropriately unless designated for investigative use related to AIDS. If not destroyed, such products must be labeled, stored and shipped in accordance with the standard procedures for handling infectious materials. Appropriate disposal procedures include autoclaving or controlled incineration; overwraps are required to protect staff in case of breakage.

Approved procedures developed by one of the major organizations such as the American Blood Resources Association, the American Red Cross, the American Association of Blood Banks and the Council of Community Blood Centers may be referenced in the licensed establishment's SOPs without individual submission to the Office of Biologics. Alternatively, licensed establishments which develop their own procedures should submit them to the Office of Biologics for approval concurrent with implementation. Revised labeling for plasma collected from high risk donor groups and intended for further manufacture of plasma derivatives should be submitted to the Office of Biologics (HFN-825).

This memorandum is intended to be an interim measure to protect recipients of blood and blood products until specific laboratory tests are available.

John C. Petricciani,
M.D.

Attachment

DEPARTMENT OF HEALTH & HUMAN SERVICES
Public Health Service
Food and Drug Administration Rockville MD 20857

March 24, 1983

FROM: Director,
Office of Biologics,
National Center for Drugs and Biologics

SUBJECT: Source Material Used to Manufacture Certain Plasma Derivatives

TO: All Licensed Manufacturers of Plasma Derivatives

Extensive discussions among licensed manufacturers, the Office of Biologics and concerned groups such as the <u>National Hemophilia Foundation, have led</u> to a consensus concerning an appropriate approach to decreasing the potential risk of transmitting Acquired Immune Deficiency Syndrome (AIDS) by certain plasma derivatives.

Plasma collected from <u>donors suspected</u> of being at increased risk of transmitting AIDS (as presently defined: persons with symptoms and signs suggestive of AIDS, sexually active homosexual or bisexual men with multiple partners, Haitian entrants to the United States, present or past abusers of intravenous drugs[*] and sexual partners of persons at increased risk of AIDS) should not be fractionated into derivatives already known to have a risk of transmitting infectious diseases. Plasma from donors in any of the groups identified above may be collected for use in manufacturing only albumin, plasma protein fraction (PPF), globulin or <u>in vitro</u> diagnostic products. To prevent the possible misuse of such plasma, all licensed establishments collecting Source Plasma (Human) are being advised that in accordance with 21 CFR 606.120(b)(6) each unit must be conspicuously labeled either with the statement "CAUTION: For Use in Manufacturing Albumin, PPF, or Globulin Only," or "CAUTION: For Use in Manufacturing Noninjectable Products Only". HBsAg positive plasma for use in manufacturing vaccine or <u>in vitro</u> diagnostic products is already subject to additional special labeling and shipping precautions.

We request that <u>you immediately institute procedures with your plasma</u> suppliers to assure that they have adopted appropriate donor screening practices and procedures. Copies of notices that are being sent to all establishments collecting blood or source plasma concerning measures which should be taken, are enclosed for your information along with the recent Public Health Service Interagency Recommendations.

Please advise the Office of Biologics, in writing, of the procedures you have instituted to comply with this notice. The restrictions applied by your establishment on source plasma received for manufacturing high risk plasma derivatives should be effective immediately.

John C. Petricciani,
M.D.

Enclosures
RETURN – RECEIPT REQUESTED

---

[*] Such intravenous drug abusers are already excluded by existing regulations.

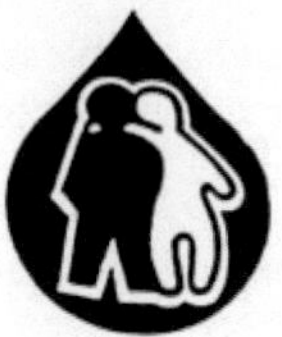

HEMOPHILIA NEWS NOTES
May 11, 1983
<u>MEDICAL BULLETIN #7</u>
<u>CHAPTER ADVISORY #8</u>
NHF URGES CLOTTING FACTOR USE BE MAINTAINED

<u>Chapters</u>—Please distribute this information to all chapter members.

<u>Physicians</u>—Please distribute this information to all providers who treath patients with hemophilia in your area.

<u>NOTE</u>: Any questions concerning the following information should be referred to your treating physician and/or NHF.

The NHF has recently recognized, and is concerned about, the fact that public media coverage of AIDS is causing some patients to abandon appropriate use of blood products because they fear contracting AIDS. The NHF AIDS Task Force considers this to be an inappropriate response and urges hemophiliacs to maintain the use of clotting factor in their treatment of hemorrhagic episodes.

In order to reduce the possible transmission of AIDS through blood products, the FDA has issued recommendations regarding the screening of potential donors for blood and plasma fractionation collection agencies. The guidelines have been developed from the screening criteria recommended by The NHF's Medical and Scientific Advisory Council in January of 1983.

A recent event emphasizes the need for careful screening of donors and the maintenance of careful medical records. You should be aware that Hyland Therapeutics Division of Travenol Laboratories, Inc. has judged it prudent for patient safety to recall a lot of AUTOPLEX. The need for such an action is not surprising, since a blood collection agency or plasma fractionation company may recognize the need to recall a product prepared from plasma of a high risk donoz who later developed symptoms of AIDS during the period of plasma fractionation and distribution.

AIDS BULLETIN

It is rot the role of The NHF to judge the appropriateness of corporate decisions made by individual pharmaceutical companies. However, we urge that patients and treaters recognize the need for careful evaluation of blood products and note that such a recall action should not cause anxiety or changes in treatment programs.

We emphasize that the incidence of AIDS in hemophiliacs is very low (12 patients out of nearly 20,000) and that the life and health of hemophiliacs depends upon blood products.

The NHF recommends that patients maintain the use of concentrates or cryoprecipitate as prescribed by their physicians. If you have any questions regarding this matter, they should be directed to your treating physician and/or The NHF.

JOINT STATEMENT ON DIRECTED DONATIONS AND AIDS

The current epidemic of acquired immune deficiency syndrome (AIDS) and attendant publicity has led to concerns that AIDS may be transmitted by blood transfusion to persons not in one of the recognized high risk groups. Of 1,601 cases of AIDS reported to the CDC, 94 percent have occurred in people belonging to four groups: homosexual or bisexual males with multiple sex-partners; intravenous drug abusers, recent entrants from Haiti, and persons with bemophilia. Only one newborn infant and 14 adult recipients of blood transfusions have been identified as cases of possible transfusion-associated. AIDS. More than 10 million persons were transfused in the United States during the three-year period that these cases were reported and, therefore, it appears at this time that the risk of possible transfusion-associated AIDS is on the order of one case per million patients transfused.

On March 25, 1983, in response to the potential risk of transfusion-associated AIDS, we pledged compliance with the Recommendations on AIDS by the Office of Biologics, FDA, and jointly implemented a nationwide program to inform all blood donors of AIDS risk groups and provided means for individuals in high risk groups to be excluded as blood donors. We concur with Secretary of Health and Human Services Margaret M. Heckler's statement of June 14, 1983, that "...all of us might also be confronted with an unnecessary and unjustified level of fear, if misunderstanding of AIDS is allowed to grow. Such a level of fear could actually impede us in our real tasks...."

One consequence of the understandable, but excessive, concern for transfusion-associated AIDS has been requests by patients and their physicians to have blood donors selected from family members, friends, coworkers, and even newly formed private donor clubs. There is no evidence to support this notion that these "directed donations" are safer than those available through the community blood bank.

The concept that family members, friends, coworkers, church members or other selected groups are sure to provide safer blood is unrealistic. These same individuals are and have been the nation's volunteer blood donors who have, in the past, given freely for all patients rather than for a particular individual. There is no reason to think that segregating these individuals into selected donor panels will provide safety over and above the level provided by current arrangements. In addition, a system of directed donation may create intense pressures on family and friends who may therefore be untruthful about their ability to meet donor requirements. It is possible that the administrative and operational complexity that will be part of any widespread application of directed donations may lead to a significant increase in clerical errors and, in this way, reduce the safety of transfusion.

Finally, there is the risk that widespread attempts to direct donations, while not increasing the safety of transfusions, will seriously disrupt the nation's blood donor system. Voluntary donation is essential for meeting our nation's needs for blood and blood products. There is a real concern that donors may refrain from routine blood donations while awaiting requests to provide directed donations and, thereby, could disrupt the blood supply to the point that routine and even some emergency needs for transfusions may go unmet.

Given these considerations, we strongly recommend that "directed donation" programs not be conducted. We reaffirm our commitment to a safe blood supply for all recipients, to maintaining the highest standards possible for selecting volunteer donors, and to strict compliance with pertinent recommendations by the United States Public Health Service and other federal regulatory bodies.

American Red Cross
American Association of Blood Banks
Council of Community Blood Centers
June 22, 1983

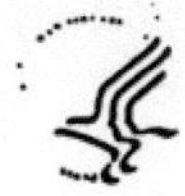

DEPARTMENT OF HEALTH & HUMAN SERVICES

Memorandum

Date July 21, 1983

From Dennis M. Donohue,
M.D. Director, D35P

Subject Results of the Blood Product Advisory Committee Meeting Related to the
Safety of Plasma Derivatives

To John C. Petriceiani,
M.D. Director, OOB, HFN-800

My interpretation of the Advisory Committee review of the Safety of Factor VIII in
relation to Acquired Immunodeficiency Syndrome (AIDS) is as follows:

The risk of transmitting AIDS to an individual hemophiliac from a specific lot of
Factor VIII is very, very small if it exists. Therefore, disposition of Factor VIII from a
pool which contains plasma collected from a donor who may have the acquired
immunodeficiency syndrome should be considered as a discrete incident. A conclusion
as to the distribution or destruction of the final product should consider such variables as:
the degree of specificity of the diagnosis, the time of onset of symptoms in relation to the
time of donation, the potential effect upon immediate supply of factor VIII and the long-
term production of this essential plasma derivative. It is emphasized that all aspects of
AIDS including the cause, method of transmission, predisposing factors and definition of
the syndrome itself, are incompletely understood inspite of the extensive and intensive
research activity focused upon these issues and the benefit from life-threatening or
disabling hemorrhage far exceeds the risk of acquiring AIDS.

Dennts M. Donohue,
M.D.

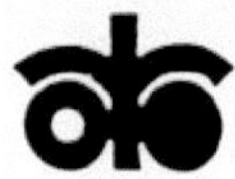

AMERICAN BLOOD RESOURCES ASSOCIATION
P.O. Box 3346 Annapolis, Maryland 21403 (301) 263-8296

July 27, 1983

Reference No. A1901

John C. Petricciani,
M.D.
Department of Health and He
Public Health Service
Food and Drug Administration 8800 Rockville Pike Bethesda, MD 20205

Dear Doctor Petricciani:

The American Blood Resources Association (ABRA) is the trade association for the collectors of source plasma (human). ABRA represents approximately 80 companies which own or operate more than one-half of all the source plasma facilities in the United States. ABRA has worked very closely with members of your staff, members of the Centers for Disease Control staff, and others in attempting to develop a responsible policy aimed at reducing the risk of transmitting acquired immune deficiency syndrome (AIDS) through blood and blood products. We recognize that the etiology of AIDS is far from clear, that blood and blood products are merely suspect as a source of transmission of AIDS, and that even if blood and blood products were directly linked to AIDS, the mechanism for the causative factor is now unknown.

On the whole, we believe that the recommendations promulgated by you on March 24, 1983 to deal with donor screening for AIDS are sound and, in general, workable.

In our opinion, however, the March 24, 1983 recommendations contain one serious flaw. The problem arises out of the differences between the requirements applicable to establishments collecting human blood for transfusion and those applicable to source plasma facilities. We note that the last sentence of paragraph one of each of the memoranda is different. It seems to impose a higher standard of donor education on source plasma collectors that upon establishments collecting human blood for transfusion. We do not understand the basis for this difference.

A more significant difference is in the omission of paragraphs four and five of the source plasma recommendations from the whole blood collectors. These two paragraphs impose specific medical requirements aimed at ascertaining the health status of particular donors. As explained below, if the recommendations are based on the theory that AIDS is transmissible by blood and blood products, they should be equally applicable to whole blood facilities. It is troublesome to the source plasma collectors that whole blood facilities are not required to perform the same screening. Indeed, the argument can be made that since plasma donors are more closely monitored over time than whole blood donors, whole blood donors should be more carefully screened, rather than the other way around.

Because of the number of apparent AIDS cases among hemophiliacs, AHF concentrate is suspected to be a source of transmission of AIDS. This is consistent with an assumption that a still unknown and unidentified virus causes AIDS. As you know, the fractionation process for AHF cannot assure that any viral matter will be inactivated, as the proteins which induce or support clotting are heat labile. (A new manufacturing process may solve this problem, but full data are not yet available.)

AFH concentrates have two principal sources—source plasma and recovered plasma (frozen plasma derived from whole blood collections). Some recovered plasma is derived from hospitals which transfuse red cells or platelets and retain the plasma for sale to a fractionator. Other recovered plasma is custom fractionated for the Red Cross. (Recovered plasma constitutes more than 1,000,000 liters of plasma for fractionation or more than 20Z of the total plasma supply.) As the fractionation process uses "pools" of plasma, a batch of AHF concentrate may be fractionated from a pool containing both source and recovered plasma. Red Cross recovered plasma is also pooled for fractionation. Thus, the safety of AHF concentrate will depend on the quality of both source and recovered plasma. Since it is known that persons who may be at-risk AIDS may donate to plasma and whole blood facilities alike, it is difficult to say with any certainty that recovered plasma is of different or better quality than source plasma. Moreover, a whole blood collection facility cannot and does not know at the time it collects a unit of whole blood whether the plasma therefrom will be put into the fractionation pipeline.

There may be justification for regarding the risk of AIDS transmission from whole blood as less than the risk from AHF concentrate because of the difficulty of documenting transfusion-related AIDS. The difference may justify requiring different screening standards for whole blood facilities and source plasma facilities but only if the products derived from whole blood facilities are used solely for transfusion. Since this is not in fact the case, we believe that establishments collecting human blood for transfusion and source plasma establishments should be subject to the same rules. Otherwise, it will be difficult for FDA to assure the public that products being furnished to the American people are safe.

We would be happy to discuss this matter with you at your convenience. Plasma call me if you have any questions or if you wish to have a meeting with us.

Sincerely yours,
Robert W. Reilly
Executive Director
RWR/cei

E

Glossary of Acronyms and Terms

Acronyms

AABB	American Association of Blood Banks	HBIG	Hepatitis B immune globulin
ABC	American Blood Commission	HBcAg	Hepatitis B Core Antigen
ABRA	American Blood Resources Association	HBsAg	Hepatitis B surface antigen
		HCFA	Health Care Financing Administration
AHF	Antihemophilic factor	HTLV	Human T-cell lymphotropic virus
AIDS	Acquired immunodeficiency syndrome	IATC	Interagency Technical Committee
		IVGG	Intravenous Gamma Globulin
ALT	Alanine aminotransferase	KS	Kaposi's sarcoma
AMA	American Medical Association	LAS	Lymphadenopathy associated syndrome
ARC	American Red Cross		
ARC	AIDS-related complex	NANB	Non-A, Non-B Hepatitis
ASCP	American Society of Clinical Pathologists	NBP	National Blood Policy
		NCI	National Cancer Institute
CBC	Canadian Blood Committee	NHF	National Hemophilia Foundation
CCBC	Council of Community Blood Centers	NHLBI	National Heart, Lung, and Blood Institute
CDC	Centers for Disease Control	NIAID	National Institute of Allergy and Infectious Diseases
C.F.R.	Code of Federal Regulations		
CMV	Cytomegalovirus	NIH	National Institutes of Health
DBDR	Division of Blood Diseases and Resources (Division of NHLBI)	NTIS	National Technical Information Service
DHEW	U.S. Department of Health, Education and Welfare	NYBC	New York Blood Center
		OoB	Office of Biologics Research and Review
DHHS	U.S. Department of Health and Human Services	OTA	Office of Technology Assessment
EBV	Epstein-Barr virus	PCP	*Pneumocystis carinii* pneumonia
ELISA	Enzyme-linked immunosorbent assay	PPF	Plasma protein fraction
		PTC	Prothrombin complex
FDA	Food and Drug Administration	RBC	Red blood cells
FFP	Fresh frozen plasma	WHO	World health organization
GAO	General Accounting Office		

Terms

ABO blood group: The major human blood type determined by the presence or absence of two antigenic structures, A and B, on red blood cells, consisting of four blood types (A, B, AB, and O).

Acquired immunodeficiency syndrome (AIDS): An acquired, as opposed to inherited (congenital), disease characterized by the progressive deterioration of host immune defenses that renders the affected individual susceptible to an array of infectious and malignant disorders that do not normally afflict persons with intact immune systems. AIDS results from infection with human immunodeficiency virus (either type 1 or type 2), and is formally defined by a case definition issued by the Centers for Disease Control and Prevention (CDC).

Active immunity: Protection against an infectious disease that results from induction of host immune defense mechanisms including antibodies (humoral immunity) and cytotoxic T-lymphocytes (cellular immunity). These host immune effectors are specifically induced by exposure to constituents of the infectious pathogen as a result of prior infection or immunization (compare with "passive immunity").

AIDS-related complex (ARC): A term formally used to describe the various signs and symptoms including lymphadenopathy, unexplained fevers, weight loss, and specific infections that characterized the early stages of AIDS. Initially it was not known whether ARC represented a prodrome to full-blown AIDS or a separate, less severe, form of the disease. With the recognition that persons who manifest these early signs and symptoms will ultimately progress to AIDS, HIV-associated disease is now recognized as a continuum spanning asymptomatic infection, mild to moderate symptomatology and, ultimately, the profound immunodeficiency of AIDS.

AIDS-related retrovirus (ARV): A retrovirus isolated from an individual with AIDS by Dr. Jay Levy's laboratory at the University of California, San Francisco. Subsequent studies demonstrated that ARV is a representative of the HIV-1 group of retroviruses.

Albumin: A small protein, synthesized in the liver, which is the principal protein in plasma and is important in maintaining plasma volume through maintenance of an osmotic gradient between plasma in the blood vessels and fluids in the surrounding tissues. Albumin also serves as the carrier molecule for fatty acids and other small molecules in plasma.

Antibody: A protein produced by immune system cells termed B-lymphocytes that is released into the tissues and bloodstream. Specific antibodies recognize and bind to specific molecules referred to as antigens and facilitate their elimination from the host.

Antigen: A molecule or component thereof that when introduced into the body stimulates the production of humoral (antibodies) of cellular (helper or cytotoxic T-lymphocytes) that specifically recognize and react to it Antigens are typically proteins or carbohydrates, but can also be nucleic acids.

Antihemophilic factor (AHF or Factor VIII): A plasma coagulation factor whose congenital deficiency results in the bleeding disorder known as hemophilia A.

Anti-inhibitor complex: An "activated" form of Factor IX concentrate, which is used in the treatment of hemophilia A patients with inhibitors to Factor VIII. (See also "Factors I-XII" and "Concentrates.")

Apheresis: A method of collection individual components of blood instead of whole blood from the donor (e.g., plasmapheresis, plateletapheresis).

Autologous: Derived from the same organism or one of its parts.

Autologous donation: A blood donation that is stored and reserved for return to the donor as needed, usually in elective surgery.

AZT (Zidovudine, ZDV): The Burroughs Wellcome trade name is Retrovir. This antiretroviral is a nucleoside analog and was the first anti-HIV agent approved in the U.S.

Biologics: Vaccines, therapeutic serums, toxodis, antitoxins, and analogous biological products used against the agents of infectious diseases or their harmful byproducts.

Blood: A complex liquid mixture of specialized cells (white cells, red cells, and platelets), proteins, and other molecules, among whose functions are the transport of oxygen and nutrients to body tissues, removal of carbon dioxide and other wastes, transfer of hormonal messages between organs, prevention of bleeding, and transport of antibodies and infection-fighting cells to sites of infection.

Blood bank: General name for a facility or part of a facility (e.g., a hospital) that stores blood and blood components and which also may collect and process blood.

Blood cells: Erythrocytes (red blood cells), leukocytes (white blood cells), or thrombocytes (platelets).

Blood center: A facility that provides a full range of blood services, including the collection, testing, processing, and distribution of blood and blood products, to a particular geographic area (e.g., community or region).

Blood components: Products separated from whole blood (i.e., red cells, white cells, platelets and plasma.) (Compare with "Plasma derivatives.")

B-Lymphocytes (B cells): White blood cells, associated with the humoral immune response, which produce antibodies. Each B cell produces a specific antibody for a specific antigen, much like a specific key is made for a specific lock. When an antibody locks with an antigen it essentially renders the antigen harmless and marks it for destruction. B-lymphocytes proliferate under stimulation from factors released by T-lymphocytes.

CD4: A molecule on the surface of macrophages and a subset of T-lymphocytes referred to as helper T cells (see "Helper T cells"). CD4 plays an essential role in the process by which helper T cells recognize and respond to their cognate antigens presented by class II major histocompatibility complex (MHC) components found on the surface of antigen presenting cells. In addition to this essential role in the normal function of the immune system, the CD4 molecule also serves as the receptor utilized by HIV to bind helper T cells and macrophages.

CD8: A molecule on the surface of a subset of T-lymphocytes referred to as cytotoxic T cells. CD8 plays an essential role in the process by which cytotoxic T cells recognize and respond to their cognate antigens presented by class I major histocompatibility complex (MHC) components present on the surface of host cells.

Coagulation: The process of blood clotting, in which the plasma protein prothrombin (Factor II) is converted to thrombin, which in turn converts the soluble plasma fibrinogen (Factor I) to insoluble fibrin.

Coagulation concentrates or complexes: Products obtained through selective precipitation of the proteins in plasma, resulting in concentrated forms of the plasma proteins that are needed for blood to coagulate (clot). Immune globulins and albumin are also obtained in this manner. (See also "Cold ethanol precipitation technique.")

Coagulation factors or proteins: Naturally occurring proteins in plasma (e.g., Factor VIII, Factor IX) that aid in the coagulation of blood. (See also "Factors I-XII")

Cofactor: Factors or agents that are necessary or that increase the probability of the development of disease in the presence of the basic etiologic agent of that disease.

Cold ethanol precipitation technique: The principal method used to separate plasma into its major protein groups. A three-variable system (temperature, ionic strength, and ethanol concentration) is used to precipitate different proteins in the following order: Fraction I (chiefly Factor VIII and fibrinogen); Fraction II (the immune globulins); Fractions III and IV (other coagulation proteins and trace components); Fraction V (the albumins); and Fraction VI (the remaining residue).

Components: See "Blood components."

Concentrates: In general, refers to blood cells or proteins that have been separated from the rest of blood or plasma in concentrated form. For example, preparations of platelets that are separated from whole blood after donation are called "platelet concentrates" (see also "Coagulation concentrates").

Core protein: Proteins that make up the internal structure or "core" of a virus. The integral protein of HIV is composed of three units: p24, p15, and p18.

Cross-matching: Testing to determine compatibility of blood types between donor and recipient.

Cryoprecip-itate: A precipitate that remains after blood plasma has been frozen and then thawed. This precipitate is rich in Factor VIII (antihemophilic factor), fibrinogen, and fibronectin.

Cytomegalovirus (CMV): A virus related to the herpes family, CMV infections may occur without causing any symptoms or may result in mild flu-like symptoms of aching, fever, mild sore throat, or enlarged lymph nodes. Severe CMV infections can result in retinitis, hepatitis, mononucleosis, or pneumonia, especially in immune-suppressed persons. CMV is shed in body fluids such as urine, semen, saliva, feces, and sweat. One of a group of highly host-specific herpes virus that infect man, monkeys, or rodents, with the production of unique large cells bearing intranuclear inclusions.

Directed donations: Donations from identified individuals, such as family and friends, intended to be used as the sole source of blood for the patient for whom the donations were made.

Envelope: Proteins present on the surface of a virus particle that play an essential role in the initiation of virus infection of host target cells. The envelope proteins of HIV are composed of two subunits: gp120, which specifically binds to CD4 on the surface of target T cells and macrophages, and gp41, which is embedded in the membrane of HIV and facilitates fusion with the cell surface membrane of the target cell during the earliest stages of the virus infection cycle.

Enzyme: Any of a group of catalytic proteins that are produced by living cells and that mediate and promote the chemical processes of life without themselves being altered or destroyed.

Erythrocytes: Red blood cells.

Etiologic agent: Causative agent.

Factors I-XII: Refers to a classification of the multiple factors involved in coagulation. For example, hemophilia A is a result of a deficiency in Factor VII, while hemophilia B is a deficiency in Factor IX.

Fibrinogen: Factor I; a plasma protein, synthesized in the liver, which is involved in coagulation as the precursor of fibrin.

Fractiona-tion: See "Plasma fractionation."

Fresh frozen plasma (FFP): Plasma that has been frozen soon after collection to preserve the activity of the coagulation proteins.

Gamma globulin: A fraction of proteins present in blood-derived serum defined by their mobility during electrophoretic separation. The gamma globulin fraction includes many types of antibodies that are present in the circulation.

Gene: The basic unit of heredity; an ordered sequence of nucleotide bases, comprising a segment of DNA. A gene contains the sequence of DNA that encodes one polypeptide chain (via RNA).

Globulins: Simple proteins in the blood serum which contain molecules central to immune system functioning.

Granulocytes: White blood cells (leukocytes) containing neutrophilic, basophilic, or eosinophilic granules in their cytoplasm; a term used to identify a particular subset of white blood cells in one of several methods of classification.

HIV-1: The retrovirus, human immunodeficiency virus type 1, that is responsible for most cases of AIDS worldwide. HIV-1 was first discovered in 1983 by investigators at the Pasteur Institute, and was demonstrated to be the etiologic agent of AIDS by investigators at the National Institutes of Health in 1984. HIV-1 is a member of the lentivirus subfamily of retroviruses. The related virus, HIV-2 (see below), is responsible for the remainder of cases of AIDS.

HIV-2: A retrovirus, human immunodeficiency virus type 2, that is distantly related to HIV-1. HIV-2 infections result in a clinical syndrome of immunodeficiency that is indistinguishable from HIV-1 induced AIDS, but may do so over a longer time period. HIV-2 infection is most common in West Africa, but is seen with increasing frequency in regions of India and Asia.

Helper T cells (T4, CD4+ T cells): Lymphocytes bearing the CD4 marker that are responsible for many immune system functions, including turning antibody production on and off.

Hematocrit: The volume occupied by the cellular elements of blood in relation to the total volume.

Hematology: The science of blood, its nature, function, and diseases.

Hemoglobin: The protein in red blood cells that carries oxygen to cells and carries carbon dioxide away from them.

Hemolytic transfusion reaction: An antigen-antibody reaction in the recipient of a blood transfusion that results in the destruction of red blood cells.

Hemophilia: A rare, hereditary bleeding disorder caused by a deficiency in the ability to synthesize one or more of the coagulation proteins; e.g., Factor VIII (hemophilia A) or Factor IX (hemophilia B).

Hemorrhage: The escape of blood from the vascular system.

Hepatitis: Inflammation of the liver; may be due to many causes, including viruses, several of which are transmissible through blood transfusions.

Hepatitis B (HBV): Viral liver disease that can be acute or chronic and even life threatening, especially in people with poor immune response. Like HIV, HBV can be transmitted by sexual contact, contaminated needles, or blood products. Unlike HIV it can also be transmitted through close casual contact.

Hepatitis C (HCV): A viral liver disease that can be acute, chronic or even life-threatening. Alpha interferon has been FDA approved for treatment.

Histocompatibility: The extent to which individuals or their tissues are immunologically similar.

HTLV-III: Former name for HIV.

Hyperimmune globulins: Immune globulin products derived from the plasma of donors with high titers of antibodies specific for a given antigen, such as anti-Rh globulin used for the prevention of hemolytic disease of the newborn.

Human T-cell lymphotropic virus, type III (HTLV-III): A name used to describe certain isolates of HIV-1 shortly after the identification of the etiologic agents of AIDS. This terminology has been abandoned in favor of the term, HIV-1, to refer to all related virus isolates.

Immune complexes: Combinations of antibodies and antigens that may either circulate in the blood or be deposited in the tissues. Immune complexes are found in certain infectious and autoimmune diseases.

Immune deficiency: Breakdown or inability of certain parts of the immune system to function, thus making a person more susceptible to certain diseases they would not normally get.

Immune globulin (immunoglobulin): A type of plasma protein that comprises the antibodies.

Immune response: The activity of the immune system when confronted with an infection.

Immune system: The complicated and highly integrated system of cells and cellular products that produce a host from infectious diseases or toxic substances. The immune response consists of both so-called cellular and humoral components. Cellular immune responses are initiated by interaction of host immune system cells with foreign antigens. Cytotoxic T cells recognize and kill host cells that display foreign antigens, such as virus-infected cells. Helper T cells recognize foreign antigens displayed by specific host cells termed antigen-presenting cells, and then help to initiate and propagate the responses of B-lymphocytes and other T-lymphocytes that are specific for the same antigen. Humoral immune responses refer to those mediated by antibodies that are produced by B-lymphocytes, but that can travel to and act at distant sites in the body.

Immunity: A natural or acquired resistance to a specific disease. Immunity may be partial or complete, long lasting or temporary.

Immunogen: A preparation such as a vaccine (typically composed of protein or carbohydrate) that is administered to generate a specific immune response against that substance.

Immunoglobulin: Serum proteins manufactured by B-lymphocytes in response to antigens. Elevated levels of immunoglobulins have been seen in HIV + persons. Why this occurs is not fully understood but is believed to by caused by faulty regulation of the B cells.

Im-munotherapy: Therapy that attempts to reconstruct or enhance a damaged immune system.

Interferon: A class of glycoproteins (proteins with carbohydrate groups attached at specific locations) important in immune function and thought to inhibit viral infections.

Kaposi's sarcoma (KS): A type of malignancy (cancer) that is commonly seen in persons with AIDS. Kaposi's sarcoma results from the abnormal proliferation of the endothelial cells that line blood vessel walls. Although the disease is also seen in individuals not infected with HIV, it is much more severe in the setting of HIV infection. Recent studies suggest that Kaposi's sarcoma may be caused by a virus of the Herpesvirus family.

Leukocytes: White blood cells. Lymphocytes and granulocytes are particular types of leukocytes.

Lym-phadenopa-thy syndrome (LAS): A condition that follows HIV infection that is characterized by lymphadenopathy (swollen lymph nodes) at multiple locations in the body. This syndrome was identified as one of the components of the AIDS-related complex (ARC), and was used as a marker for persons at risk of developing AIDS before HIV was identified. Like the term ARC, the term "lymphadenopathy syndrome" is now considered antiquated and no longer used.

Lym-phadenopa-thy-associ-ated virus (LAV): The name used by investigators at the Pasteur Institute to describe a retrovirus they isolated in 1983 from an individual with lymphadenopathy syndrome. This virus is now known to be a member of the HIV-1 group of viruses.

Lympho-cytes: Specialized white blood cells involved in the immune response.

Lym-phosarcoma: A subset of malignant diseases of lymphocytes known as lymphoma.

Lyophilized: Freeze-dried.

Monoclonal antibodies: Homogeneous antibodies derived from clones of a single cell. Monoclonal antibodies recognize only one chemical structure and thus have remarkable specificity. They are easily produced in large quantities and have a variety of industrial and medical uses.

Nonre-placement fee: An additional fee that may be charged to users of whole blood or red cells if no replacement donations are made.

Normal serum al-bumin: Concentrates of albumin obtained through plasma fractionation and used to maintain or restore plasma volume. The appropriateness of using albumin preparations instead of other fluids is under examination (see also "Plasma protein fraction.")

Opportunis- A disease or infection caused by a microorganism that does not ordinarily
tic infection: cause disease but which, under certain conditions (e.g., impaired immune
responses), becomes pathologic.

p24 anti- Antibodies that are produced following HIV infection that recognize a
body: protein component of the virus core known as p24. The presence of
antibodies that recognize this and other constitutents of the HIV virus
particle are used to diagnose the presence of active HIV infection.

p24 antigen: A protein component of the core of the HIV virus particle. A p24 antigen
test detects the presence of this protein in the serum of infected persons.
The presence of p24 in the serum is indicative of active HIV replication in
an infected person. Due to insensitivity of the test, it is being supplanted by
more sensitive tests based on the detection of HIV RNA.

Passive im- Disease resistance in a person or animal due to the injection of antibodies
munity: from another person or animal. Passive immunity is usually short-lasting.
(Compare with "Active immunity.")

Pathogen: Any microorganism capable of causing disease.

Perfluro- Organic compounds in which all the hydrogen atoms have been replaced by
chemicals fluorine atoms and which are chemically inert and not metabolized by the
(PFCs): body.

Plasma: The liquid portion of blood, which contains nutrients, electrolytes
(dissolved salts), gases, albumin, clotting factors, wastes, and hormones
(about 10 percent of the blood).

Plasma cells derived from B cells that produce antibodies.
cells:

Plasma Products derived from the fractionation of plasma to concentrate selected
derivatives: proteins. (Compare with "Blood components.")

Plasma The separation of plasma into its major proteins. (See also "Cold ethanol
fractiona- precipitation technique.")
tion:

Plasma pro- A product of plasma fractionation that is at least 85 percent albumin and
tein frac- used interchangeably with albumin preparations. (See also "Normal serum
tion (PPF): albumin.")

Plasma- Collection of plasma. (See also "Apheresis.")
pheresis:

Platelets Cells (minute protoplasmic disks) in blood which are involved in blood
(thrombo- clotting.
cytes):

Prothrom- Factor II; an inactive plasma protein precursor of thrombin.
bin:

Prothrom- A product of plasma fractionation consisting of Factors II, VII, IX, and X,
bin com- but mostly Factor IX; also known as Factor IX complex (concentrate). Used
plex (PTC): in the treatment of hemophilia B. An "activated" form of this concentrate is
used in the treatment of hemophilia A patients with inhibitor to Factor VIII.
(See also "Anti-inhibitor complex."

Recombi- Techniques that allow specific segments of DNA to be isolated and inserted
nant DNA into a bacterium or other host (e.g., yeast, mammalian cells) in a form that
techniques: will allow the DNA segment to be replicated

and expressed as the cellular host multiplies. The DNA segment is said to be "cloned" because it exists free of the rest of the DNA of the organism from which it was derived.

Recovered plasma: Plasma removed from outdated blood or remaining after the cells have been removed but not frozen in time to preserve the coagulation proteins; it is fractionated for the remaining proteins.

Red blood cells: The oxygen-carbon dioxide transporting cells of blood; erythrocytes.

Retrovirus: A diverse family of viruses that share a common strategy for replicating that depends on an enzyme known as reverse transcriptase. Retroviruses contain genetic information consisting of RNA which must first be copies by reverse transcriptase into a DNA copy during the early stages of the viral life cycle. The DNA copy of the retrovirus then integrates into the chromosomes of the host cell and produces the requisite RNA and protein constituents of additional virus particles.

Rh blood group: A major blood group consisting of genetically determined substances present on the red blood cells of most persons and of higher animals and capable of inducing intense antigenic reactions. (See also "ABO blood group.")

Seroconversion: The point at which antibodies become detectable. When a person's HIV anti-body status changes from negative to positive.

Seropositive: Test HIV positive.

Serum: The clear portion of any animal liquid separated from its more solid elements, especially in clear liquid (blood serum) which separates in the clotting blood.

Source plasma: Plasma collected directly by plasmapheresis for fractionation into plasma derivatives.

Surrogate markers: Laboratory tests which may predict clinical outcomes or indicate whether a drug is effective without having to wait for clinical endpoints. Surrogate markers under study in HIV disease include CD4 counts, p24 antigen, beta-2 microglobulin, plasma viremia, and quantitative PCR. Sometime surrogate markers are used instead of clinical changes as the endpoints for a clinical trial.

T4 (helper) cell (CD4): A subset of T-lymphocytes that play a critical regulatory role in the immune system, and whose deficiency is responsible for the immunodeficiency characteristic of AIDS. Helper T-lymphocytes are defined by expression of the CD4 (previously known as T4) cell surface molecule, and are responsible via their production of specific cytokines for the induction of humoral and cellular immune responses.

T8 (suppressor) cells (CD8): A subset of T-lymphocytes that play an essential role in the host's immune response to intracellular pathogens such as viruses or parasites. Cytotoxic T cells express the CD8 (previously known as T8) molecule on their surfaces which facilitates their ability to recognize and kill host cells that display evidence of infection by foreign pathogens.

T-lympho-cytes: T-lymphocytes are the primary effector cells for the host cellular immune response. They are derived from progenitor (precursor) cells that are produced in the bone marrow. These progenitor cells migrate to the thymus where they mature into functional effector cells. Mature T cells leave the thymus, and migrate to many areas of the body to provide protection from infectious pathogens or other foreign substances.

Thrombin: An enzyme that induces clotting by converting fibrinogen to fibrin; precursor form in blood is prothrombin.

Typing and screening (T&S): Determining ABO and Rh blood groups and screening of blood for unexpected antibodies prior to transfusion.

Vaccine: A preparation of killed organisms, living attenuated organisms, living fully virulent organisms, or parts of microorganisms, that is administered to produce or artificially increase immunity to a particular disease.

Viral proteins: The main components of a virus. The core of HIV includes the proteins p24 and p18. Its envelope includes the proteins gp141 and gp120.

Virus: A subcellular organism composed of genetic material and protein; able to reproduce only within a living cell. When viruses infect a cell they can cause disease, often ultimately killing the host cell. Though they vary greatly, all viruses have genetic material surrounded by at least one protein shell. Viruses may subvert the host cell's normal functions, causing the cell to behave in a manner determined by the virus.

White blood cells: General description of specialized cells involved in defending the body against invasion by organisms and chemical substances and including the circulating white blood cells and the cells of the reticuloendothelial system; defenses mediated through phagocytosis and immune responses; leukocytes.

SOURCES

Blood Policy and Technology (Washington, D.C.; U.S. Congress, Office of Technology Assessment, OTA-H-260, January 1985).

The Common Factor, Newsletter for the Committee of Ten Thousand. Issues: No. 3 (December 1992), No. 4 (April 1993), No. 5 (June 1993), and No. 6 (October 1993).

Review of the Public Health Service's Response to AIDS: A Technical Memorandum (Washington, D.C.; U.S. Congress Office of Technology Assessment, February 1985).

F

Committee and Staff Biographies

COMMITTEE

Harold C. Sox, Jr., M.D. (Chair), graduated from Stanford University (B.S. physics) and Harvard Medical School. After serving as a medical intern and resident at Massachusetts General Hospital, he spent two years doing research in immunology at the National Institutes of Health and three years at Dartmouth Medical School, where he served as Chief Medical Resident and began his studies of medical decisionmaking. He then spent 15 years on the faculty of Stanford University School of Medicine, where he served as Chief of the Division of General Internal Medicine and Director of Ambulatory Care at the Palo Alto VA Medical Center. In 1988, he returned to Dartmouth as a Joseph M. Huber Professor of Medicine and Chair of the Department of Medicine. Dr. Sox directs the Robert Wood Johnson Foundation Generalist Physician Initiative at Dartmouth. He is a Regent of the American College of Physicians and chairs its Educational Policy Committee. He chairs the U.S. Preventive Service Task Force and the Institute of Medicine Committee to Study HIV Transmission Through Blood and Blood Products. He was elected to the Institute of Medicine of the National Academy of Sciences in 1993. His books include *Medical Decision Making*, and *Common Diagnostic Tests: Selection and Interpretation*. He is a member of the editorial board of the *New England Journal of Medicine* and is an Associate Editor of *Scientific American Medicine*.

Shulamith Bar-Shany, M.D., graduated from Haddassah-Hebrew University Medical School, and trained in hematology and transfusion medicine at Mt. Sinai Hospital in New York City. From 1969 to 1980, she held the position of Medical Director of Magen David Adom (MDA) Blood Banks in Tel Aviv,

Israel. From 1980 through 1991, she served as Director of MDA Blood Services. Since retiring in 1991, she continues her work as an ARMDI Fellow, pursuing medical and scientific activities in the field of viral hepatitis.

David Blumenthal, M.D., M.P.P., is Chief, Health Policy Research and Development Unit, and Associate Physician at Massachusetts General Hospital in Boston, Massachusetts. He is also an Associate Professor of Medicine and Associate Professor of Health Care Policy at Harvard Medical School. From 1987 to 1991, he was Senior Vice President at Boston's Brigham and Women's Hospital, a 720-bed Harvard teaching hospital. From 1981 to 1987, he was Executive Director of the Center for Health Policy and Management and Lecturer on Public Policy at the John F. Kennedy School of Government at Harvard. During the late 1970s, Dr. Blumenthal was a professional staff member on Senator Edward Kennedy's Senate Subcommittee on Health and Scientific Research. He is a member of several editorial boards, including *The New England Journal of Medicine, Inquiry, Quality Management in Health Care*, the *American Journal of Medicine*, and the *Bulletin of the New York Academy of Medicine*. He serves on advisory committees to the National Academy of Sciences, the Institute of Medicine, the U.S. Office of Technology Assessment, and several foundations. His research interests include quality management in health care, the determinants of physician behavior, access to health services, and the extent and consequences of academic-industrial relationships in the health sciences.

Allan M. Brandt, Ph.D., is the Amalie Moses Kass Professor of the History of Medicine at Harvard Medical School. He holds a joint appointment in the Department of the History of Science at Harvard University. Dr. Brandt earned his undergraduate degree at Brandeis University and a Ph.D. in American History from Columbia University in 1983. His work focuses on social and ethical aspects of health, disease, and medical practices in the twentieth century United States. Brandt is the author of *No Magic Bullet: A Social History of Venereal Disease in the United States since 1880*. He has written on the social history of epidemic disease, the history of public health, and the history of human subject research, among other topics. He is currently writing a book on the social and cultural history of cigarette smoking in the United States.

Barbara A. DeBuono, M.D., M.P.H., began her affiliation with the Rhode Island Department of Health as a medical epidemiologist in July 1986. In October 1986, she was promoted to the position of State Epidemiologist and Medical Director for the office of Disease Control where she administered the divisions of AIDS/Sexually Transmitted Diseases, Chronic Diseases, Epidemiology/Communicable Diseases, Vital Records and Health Promotion.

On June 11, 1991, she was named Director of Health for the State of Rhode Island. She is responsible for a department that oversees maternal and child health activities, environmental health, disease control, the Board of Medical Licensure and Discipline, the Office of the Medical Examiner, among other public health programs. Prior to joining the Health Department, Dr. DeBuono completed a fellowship in infectious diseases at Brown University Medical School's Affiliated Hospitals Program in Providence. She completed her medical residency at the New England Deaconess Hospital in Boston. She holds a degree in English and biology from the University of Rochester, New York, where she subsequently received her M.D., followed by an M.P.H. from Harvard University. Since 1987, Dr. DeBuono has served as first Clinical Instructor in medicine, then Clinical Assistant Professor in medicine at Brown University Medical School.

Martha Derthick, Ph.D., is the Julia Allen Cooper Professor of Government and Foreign Affairs at the University of Virginia, where she teaches courses on American political institutions and public policy. She is the author of numerous books on American public policymaking and administration, including *Agency under Stress: The Social Security Administration in American Government* (Brookings, 1990), *The Politics of Deregulation* (coauthor, 1986), which won the Louis Brownlow Award from the National Academy of Public Administration (NAPA), and *Policymaking for Social Security* (1979), which was also awarded prizes by NAPA and the American Political Science Association.

Roger Detels, M.D., M.S., received his training at Harvard College, New York University, University of California, San Francisco, and the University of Washington. He began his research career at the U.S. Naval Medical Research Unit in Taipei, Taiwan in 1966. In 1969, he joined the research staff at the National Institute of Communicable Diseases and Stroke. In 1971 he moved to the University of California, Los Angeles (UCLA), where he served as Chair of Epidemiology (1971–1980) and as the Dean of the School of Public Health (1980–1985). Professor Detels began his research in HIV/AIDS in 1981 when he initiated a natural history study of young homosexual men in Los Angeles. In 1984 he became the principal investigator of the Los Angeles Center of the Multicenter AIDS Cohort Study, one of the largest natural history studies of HIV/AIDS in the world. He has published 59 papers on the epidemiology, natural history, immunology and biology of HIV-1 infection out of a total of more than 150 research papers. In 1988, Professor Detels initiated the UCLA/ Fogarty International Training Program in Epidemiology Related to HIV/AIDS with funding from the Fogarty International Center. The program has trained a total of 54 health professionals at UCLA from Thailand, the

Philippines, Indonesia, Singapore, Myanmar, India, China, Vietnam, Hungary, and Brazil.

William B. Dulany, J.D., is an attorney engaged in the general practice of law as a partner in the law firm of Dulany & Leahy in Westminster, Maryland. He also serves as Chair of the Board on Mason-Dixon Bancshares, Inc., Episcopal Health Ministries, Inc., and Episcopal Ministries to the Aging, Inc. He is a former Chair of the American Heart Association (National Center) and currently serves as Chair of its Public Affairs and Policy Committee. Mr. Dulany is a graduate of Western Maryland College, which awarded him an honorary degree of Doctor of Law in 1989. He attended law school at the University of Michigan and University of Maryland, where he received his J.D. in 1953. He is former President of the Maryland Bar Foundation and has been an active member of sections and committees of bar associations. He is a native of Maryland, having served in the state legislature and also as a member of Maryland's Constitutional Convention. He has served on numerous governmental agencies and committees and is a Trustee of the Maryland Historical Society.

Mark Feinberg, M.D., Ph.D., is an Assistant Professor of Medicine and Microbiology & Immunology at the University of California, San Francisco, and an Assistant Investigator at the Gladstone Institute of Virology and Immunology. He directs the Virology Research Laboratory at San Francisco General Hospital and is the Associate Director of the UCSF Center for AIDS Research. Dr. Feinberg also serves as an Attending Physician on the Medicine and AIDS/Oncology Services at San Francisco General Hospital. His basic research activities focus on the regulation of HIV gene expression, and the application of contemporary methods in molecular biology to the study of the pathogenesis of HIV disease.

Jerry Mashaw, Ph.D., received his B.A. and LL.B. degrees from Tulane University in New Orleans. He spent two years as a Marshall Scholar at the University of Edinburgh where he worked on issues of European integration and received a Ph.D. in modern European governmental studies. Dr. Mashaw returned to Tulane and joined the law faculty there in 1966 where he taught for two years before migrating to the University of Virginia. It was at Virginia that he developed his major specialty in American administrative law and authored, with Richard Merrill, one of the leading course books in that field. Dr. Mashaw joined the Yale faculty in 1976 where he is currently Sterling Professor of Law. Professor Mashaw has done extensive work on bureaucracy and the administration of federal programs. He has a particular interest in combining the fields of law, economics, and organization theory in the analysis of bureaucratic functioning. In pursuit of that interest, he founded along with Oliver Williamson, the *Journal of Law, Economics and Organization* . Professor Mashaw has been a particular student of the administration of the Social Security Disability Program, the Federal Aid Highways Program, programs of public assistance and most recently the regulation of motor vehicle safety. His books include: *Due Process in the Administrative State, Bureaucratic Justice, America's Misunderstood Welfare State, and The Struggle for Auto Safety*. Professor Mashaw is a member of the National Academy of Arts and Sciences, the National Academy of Social Insurance and various professional organizations. He is a sometime consultant to the U.S. Government and to certain private foundations.

Dorothy Nelkin holds a university professorship at New York University where she is also Professor of Sociology and Affiliate Professor in the School of Law. She was formally a professor at Cornell University. Her research focuses on controversial areas of science, technology, and medicine as a means to understand their social and political implications and the relationship of science to the public. This work includes studies of anti-science movements, the impact of new technologies, public policies concerning science, and media communication of science and risk. She has recently examined the institutional uses of the diagnostic tests emerging from research in genetics and neuroscience, and is presently working on a study of hereditarian themes in popular culture. She has served on the Board of Directors of the American Association for the Advancement of Science and on the National Academy of Sciences Committee on a National Strategy for AIDS. She has been a Guggenheim Fellow, a Visiting Scholar at the Russell Sage Foundation, and the Clare Boothe Luce Visiting Professor at NYU. She is currently on the National Institutes of Health Working Group on the Ethics, Legal, and Social Implication of the Human Genome Project. Her books include: *Controversy: The Politics of Technical Decisions; Science as Intellectual Property; The Creation Controversy; Workers at Risk; Selling Science: How the Press Covers Science and Technology; Dangerous Diagnostics* (with L. Tancredi); and *The DNA Mystique* (with S. Lindee).

Madison Powers, Ph.D., J.D., is a Senior Research Scholar at Georgetown University's Kennedy Institute of Ethics and an Assistant Professor of philosophy at Georgetown University. He received his B.A. in history/ political science from Vanderbilt University, his J.D. from the University of Tennessee, and a Ph.D. in philosophy from University College, Oxford. Professor Power's main research interests include moral and legal philosophy; medical ethics; and law, ethics, and health policy. He is currently a member of the Office of Technology Assessment's Advisory Panel on Information and Technology and the Health Care System and has served as a consultant to the President's Health Care Reform Task Force in 1993. He has published numerous articles in the areas of ethics, philosophy and health policy. In addition, Dr. Powers has taught many graduate courses in health policy analysis, ethics and health care, and law, morality and health care at Georgetown University.

Irwin M. Weinstein, M.D., is a practitioner of medicine in Los Angeles, California. He is the senior partner of an eight-person hematology/oncology group. Dr. Weinstein received his medical degree from the University of Colorado Medical School in 1949. In 1954, he joined the medical faculty at the University of Chicago as an instructor and then Assistant Professor of Medicine. During that time, Dr. Weinstein served with the U.S. Malaria Project. In 1955, Dr. Weinstein moved to the UCLA School of Medicine as an Associate Professor of Medicine and Head of Hematology at the Wadsworth General Hospital, Veterns Administration Center. Dr. Weinstein entered full-time practice of hematology and internal medicine in Los Angeles in 1959. He was appointed Clinical Professor of Medicine at the UCLA School of Medicine in 1970. Since 1982, he has been a member of the Medical School Admissions Committee. Dr. Weinstein has been a prominent member of the Cedars-Sinai Medical Center in Los Angeles since 1959, including Chief of Hematology from 1960 to 1970, and Chief of the Medical Staff from 1972 to 1974. Presently, he is an attending physician in the Department of Medicine and a member of the Board of Governors. Dr. Weinstein has been a leader in the American Society of Hematology, founding the forum on the Practice of Medicine, and serving on the Executive Committee. He has also been very active in the American College of Physicians. He served as Governor for Southern California from 1989 to 1993. In 1984, he was elevated to a Mastership in the American College of Physicians for his contributions as a practicing clinician and his contributions to the understanding of hematology and to medical education.

Carol O'Boyle Williams, R.N., is a registered nurse with a M.S. degree in public health from the University of Minnesota. She is currently a doctoral student at the University of Minnesota. Her research interests include identification of variables influencing health care worker compliance with infection prevention and control strategies. Ms. O'Boyle Williams has served in both clinical and administrative positions in nursing and infection control in acute and outpatient settings and schools. She served as a board member and chairperson of the National Association for Professionals in Infection Control (APIC) and chaired APIC's Bloodborne Pathogen Committee. She served as a member of the American Hospital Association's HIV/HBV Infected Health Care Worker Task Force. Most recently she served as an invited infection control researcher to hospitals in Costa Rica, Thailand, and Hungary. As the chairperson of APIC's Bloodborne Pathogen Committee, she also served as an invited consultant to the Centers for Disease Control and Prevention to discuss development of guidelines for prevention of HIV infection. Ms. O'Boyle Williams is currently the Clinical Nurse Specialist in Infection Control at the Minnesota Department of Health, operating the program to evaluate and monitor the practices of health care workers infected with the human immunodeficiency virus or the hepatitis B virus.

STAFF BIOGRAPHIES

Michael Stoto, Ph.D., is the Director of the Division of Health Promotion and Disease Prevention of the Institute of Medicine (IOM). He received an A.B. in statistics from Princeton University and a Ph.D. in statistics and demography from Harvard University, and was formerly an associate professor of public policy at Harvard's John F. Kennedy School of Government. A member of the professional staff since 1987, Dr. Stoto directed the IOM's effort in support of the Public Health Service's *Healthy People 2000* project and has worked on IOM projects addressing a number of issues in public health, health statistics, health promotion and disease prevention, vaccine safety and policy, and AIDS. Most recently, Dr. Stoto served as study director for the IOM committee that produced *Veterans and Agent Orange: Health Effects of Herbicides Used in Vietnam*. Dr. Stoto is co-author of *Data for Decisions: Information Strategies for PolicyMakers* and numerous articles in statistics, demography, health policy, and other fields. He is a member of the American Public Health Association, the American Statistical Association, the International Union for the Scientific Study of Population, the Population Association of America, and other organizations.

Lauren Leveton, Ph.D., is Study Director for the *Committee to Study HIV Transmission Through Blood and Blood Products*. She received a B.S. in psychology from Clark University and a Ph.D. from Pennsylvania State University College of Human Development. Dr. Leveton has a research background in behavioral health, social science, and human factors engineering. More recently, she has conducted activities in program evaluation, strategic planning, and policy development for federal agencies including the U.S. Army and the National Aeronautics and Space Administration. She worked with several NASA advisory committees, including the Advisory Committee for the Future of the U.S. Civil Space Program, the Aerospace Medical Advisory Committee, and others that reviewed priorities for space life sciences and biomedical research programs.

Cynthia Abel is a Program Officer in the Division of Health Promotion and Disease Prevention of the Institute of Medicine. She received a B.A. in government and political sciences from the University of Maryland and is working on a masters in public policy. Most recently, she worked with the IOM committee that produced *Veterans and Agent Orange: Health Effects of Herbicides Used in Vietnam* and with several other IOM committees in the area of health promotion and disease prevention. She also worked with the National Research Council's committee that produced the report *Safety Issues at the Defense Production Reactors: A Report to the U.S. Department of Energy.*

Laura Colosi, M.P.A., is the Research Assistant for the *Committee to Study HIV Transmission Through Blood and Blood Products* in the Division of Health Promotion and Disease Prevention of the Institute of Medicine. She received a B.S. in human service studies from Cornell University and a masters in public administration from Cornell's Institute for Public Affairs, with a specialization in families and social policy. Her work experience includes serving as a Research Assistant with the Office of the Assistant Secretary for Personnel Administration at the Department of Health and Human Services and also with the Office of the Deputy Attorney General at the Department of Justice.

Kristina Becker is the Project Assistant for the *Committee to Study HIV Transmission Through Blood and Blood Products.* She received a B.A. in journalism from Ohio University with a specialization in public relations and business administration. She has served as a consultant for the public affairs office of Bank One, Cleveland, and has completed several internships in the communications field.

Index

A

AABB, *see* American Association of
    Blood Banks
ABRA, *see* American Blood Resources
    Association
Acquired immunodeficiency syndrome,
    see AIDS
Advisory committees, 10, 213
    FDA, 10, 15, 45-46, 213, 231
    see also Blood Products Advisory
    Committee, FDA
Africa, 128, 129
Agency for Health Care Policy and
    Research, 233
AHF, *see* Antihemophilic factor
AIDS, 2, 67, 304
    death rate, 61-65, 116
    incubation period, 67, 68-69, 70, 73,
        115-116
    as a notifiable disease, 151-152
    see also HIV testing;
    HIV transmission
Albumin, 31, 32, 304
Aledort, Louis, 75, 147, 248
Alpha Therapeutic
    donor deferral policy, 72, 109, 110, 143
    heat treatment, 88, 91, 92, 156-157
    recalls, 162, 254, 257
American Association of Blood Banks
        (AABB), 26, 36-37, 54, 71, 104 -105
    and directed donation, 74
    Inspection and Accreditation (I&A) pro-
        gram, 37
American Blood Commission (ABC), 41
American Blood Resources Association
        (ABRA), 26, 38, 66, 67
    and donor screening and deferral, 72,
        107, 142, 143
    and surrogate testing, 72, 107
American College of Surgeons, 36
American Medical Association, 36
American Red Cross (ARC), 9, 26, 29, 30,
        34, 35, 66, 71, 115, 208
    and directed donation, 74
    recalls, 180, 252
American Society of Anesthesiologists, 36
Amyl nitrates, *see* "Poppers"
Annals of Internal Medicine, 255
Anti-HBc test, *see* Hepatitis B core anti-
    gen test
Antihemophilic factor (AHF), 1, 8, 19, 31,
        170-171, 303
    children treated, 85, 188-190
    FDA licensing, 81-82, 86-97, 91, 92,
        151, 177
    heat treatment licensing, 73, 91, 92,
        95-96, 177, 259
    and hepatitis, 5, 73, 78, 85, 155, 157-158
    home infusion, 20, 171
    immune suppression theory, 69

implicated in HIV transmission, 2, 68,
208
and plasma pooling, 1, 19, 31
recalls, 7, 58, 148, 149, 164
reducing use of, 182-185, 200, 202
risk disclosure, 8, 231
substitution with cryoprecipitate, 4, 71,
175, 176, 177, 181-182, 250, 251
surveillance programs, 67
viral inactivation, 4, 5, 57, 76, 81-82,
86-97, 154-158, 177
Anti-inhibitor complex, 32, 303
Armor Pharmaceutical, 87, 92, 96
Assistant Secretary for Health, 3, 11*n*, 42,
58, 77, 212, 218*n*
leadership changes and failures, 59, 213,
214
Autologous donation, 53, 106, 108, 177,
303

B

Baxter Healthcare, 30, 88, 92
recalls, 58, 180
Behringwerke, A.G., 86, 87-88, 93
Best practices, 12, 16, 221, 232-234
Biologics, 43-44, 303
Biologics Act, 43, 44, 47-48
Blood and plasma products, 25-34, 303
distribution and shortages, 33-34
regulation and licensing, 30, 47-48, 50
see also terms listed under Plasma
derivatives *and* Whole blood products
Blood banks and centers, 1, 9, 19, 27, 29,
34-35, 78, 208, 221, 303
community, 19, 26, 29, 35, 36, 37-38,
53-54
denial of risk, 9, 211-212
and directed donation, 74-75
donor screening policies, 6, 78, 102,
106, 162, 208, 211
hospital, 26, 29, 35, 36
licensure and registration, 49-51, 52
marginal interventions, 215, 216,
227-228
standard operating procedures, 73, 108,
142
and surrogate testing, 6, 107
Blood Products Advisory Committee
(BPAC), FDA, 3, 7, 26, 45-46, 94 ,
135, 212, 213, 219
AHF recall meeting and recommendations, 58, 75, 137, 152-153, 210, 213
donor screening policies, 71, 77

and lookback tracing, 159
panel composition and expertise, 15, 46,
121, 126, 213, 229-230
and surrogate testing, 75, 119-121
Blood Safety Director, 11-12, 218-219
Blood shield laws, 2, 48-49, 139, 223-224
Blood transfusion, 1, 9, 19, 20, 21, 27, 51,
131, 208
early AIDS cases, 58, 63, 64, 65, 68-69
Glaser case, 190-191
HIV incidence among recipients, 1, 19,
21, 169
PHS recommendations, 73, 177
Bove, Joseph, 121, 148
Brandt, Edward, 77, 148, 149, 154
Bureau of Biologics, FDA, 44, 51
1982 meeting, 66, 248
and swine flu episode, 140, 153

C

Canterbury v. Spence, 198
Case reporting, 67
chronologies, 61-65
MMWR reports, 58, 59, 68, 248, 250
CCBC, *see* Council of Community Blood
Centers
CDC, *see* Centers for Disease Control and
Prevention
CD4:CD8 ratios, 68, 76, 117-118

Center for Biologics Evaluation and
Research (CBER), FDA, 26, 44-45,
46, 52
Center for Drugs and Biologics (CDB),
FDA, 44
Centers for Disease Control and Prevention (CDC), 2, 9, 20, 26, 42 , 161,
208, 220-221
challenges to credibility of, 114,
115-116, 125-126
changes of directors, 59, 213
donor screening and deferral recommendations, 6, 71, 102, 105-117
donor screening research, 77
Emerging Infections Program, 221
initial evidence of blood-borne transmission, 2, 66, 70-71, 101, 208
interagency agreements, 77
interagency support and rivalry, 13,
116-117, 125-126, 212, 225
January 4, 1983 public meeting and outcomes, 3, 58, 70-71, 89, 102 ,
105-117, 213, 251
opportunistic disease epidemiology studies, 60, 66
risk group exclusion recommendations,
106
surrogate testing recommendations, 6,
71, 102, 106
surveillance and reporting systems,
13-14, 67, 76, 79, 221, 226, 248, 249
and swine flu episode, 59-60, 126-127,
140, 225
see also MMWR reports
Children,
see also Infants
AHF concentrate treatment of, 85,
188-190
cryoprecipitate treatment of, 71, 176, 251
early cases among, 62, 63, 64, 65, 68, 250
hemophiliac, 68, 250
Chronologies
case reporting, 61-65
critical events, 58-59, 247-259
Clinical Laboratories Improvement Act, 50
Clinical options
chronology of, 176-177, 248-259
risk communication, 8, 16, 72, 170,
175-181, 201-203, 232-233
College of American Pathologists, 36
Communication, *see* Risk communication
Community blood centers, 19, 26, 29, 35,
36, 37-38, 53-54
Compensation system, 13, 224

Competitiveness, 94-95
Confidential unit exclusion, 130
Conflicts of interest, 16-17, 213, 233-234
Cost-effectiveness analyses, 214-215
Council of Community Blood Centers
(CCBC), 27, 37-38, 54
and directed donation, 74
and initial evidence of blood-borne
transmission, 71
Creutzfeldt-Jakob disease (CJD), 128, 131
Critical events, 58-59, 247-259
Cryoprecipitate, 27, 29, 107, 305
destruction of units from AIDS patients,
164
infants treated, 71, 176, 189-190, 251
poor plasma, 27, 29
substitution for AHF concentrate, 4, 71,
175, 176, 177, 181-182, 250, 251
Curran, James, 60
Cutter Laboratories, 155, 253.
see also Miles Inc.
Cytomegalovirus (CMV), 1, 32, 120, 305

D

DDAVP (desmopressin acetate)
FDA licensing, 176
National Hemophilia Foundation

recommendation, 72, 176, 178
substitution for AHF concentrate, 251
Deaths
  from AIDS, 61-65, 116
  among hemophiliacs, 258
Delta hepatitis virus (HDV), 84
Directed donations, 74-75, 176, 305
Division of Blood Diseases and Resources
    (DBDR), 43, 90
Donation of blood, *see* Autologous dona-
    tion; Blood banks and centers;
    Directed donations; Donor screening
    and deferral; Paid donors; Plasma
    collection centers; Plasmapheresis;
    Volunteer donors
Donohue, Dennis, 71, 119, 150-151
Donor screening and deferral, 5-6, 71,
    101-103, 122
  ABRA policies, 72, 107, 142, 143
  blood industry opposition, 124
  CDC 1983 meeting and outcomes, 6, 71,
    102, 105-117
  early practices, 104-105
  education and information programs,
    72, 73, 108, 142
  gay groups influence on policy, 71,
    109-112, 122, 124, 228
  hepatitis, 103-105, 111, 129
  HIV antibody tests, 129
  HTLV I and HTLV II, 130, 131
  information deficit impacts, 3, 6, 103,
    115-116, 210
  lack of consensus regarding, 3, 70-71,
    102, 103, 105, 123-124
  lack of leadership on, 116-117, 125-128
  PHS exclusion recommendations, 6,
    107-108
  pilot and local studies, 76-77
  plasma industry policies, 72, 78, 107,
    109-110, 151-152, 162
  questioning about risk factors, 3, 6, 71,
    102, 106, 107, 109-112, 130
  regulatory triggers and actions, 215, 216
  self-deferral, 77, 101, 110, 130, 215, 216
  see also Lookback tracing

E

Elective surgery
  autologous donations, 106
  delay, 71, 177, 178, 251
ELISA (enzyme-linked immunosorbent
    assay) test, 78, 128
Emerging Infections Program, CDC, 221

Engleman, Edgar, 115, 118
Epstein, Jay, 159-160
Erythrocytes, *see* Red blood cells
Ethnic groups, anti-HBc testing, 75, 118,
    120
Exported plasma, 31, 33

F

Factor VIII concentrate, *see* Antihe-
    mophilic factor
Fatalities, *see* Deaths
FDA, *see* Food and Drug Administration
Federal Food, Drug, and Cosmetic Act,
    44, 51
Fibrinogen, 32, 305
Foege, William, 67
Food, Drug, and Cosmetics Act, 44, 48
Food and Drug Act of 1906, 43
Food and Drug Administration (FDA), 7,
    9, 14-15, 43-46, 51, 67, 70 , 71,
    135-136, 208, 221, 226-231
  advisory committees, 10, 15, 45-46,
    213, 230-231
  blood product licensing and registration,
    49-50, 139
  Center for Biologics Evaluation and
    Research (CBER), 26, 44-45, 46 , 52
  changes of administrators, 59, 212
  DDAVP licensing, 176

and donor screening policies, 6, 7, 77,
    108-109, 228
heat treatment licensing, 73, 91, 92, 96,
    177, 259
HIV tests licensing, 59, 78
and industry self-regulation, 51,
    139-140, 162-163
leadership failures, 212
and lookback tracing, 7, 136, 137-138,
    158-160, 163-164, 228
March 1983 letters to blood industry, 3,
    7, 58, 73, 108, 136-137, 142-146, 164
marginal and partial interventions, 14,
    163-166, 227
policy analyses and review, 14, 15, 228,
    230-231
recall policy, 3, 7, 52-53, 135, 137,
    138-139, 142-158, 164, 208, 211,
    228, 229-230
regulatory authority, 1-2, 7, 19-20, 47,
    138-141
relationship with blood industry, 7, 14,
    14-15, 51, 135, 138-140, 162-163,
    227, 230
rivalry with CDC, 125-126, 210
viral inactivation approval and licens-
    ing, 4, 12, 91-92, 221-222, 259
see also Blood Products Advisory
    Committee;
Bureau of Biologics, FDA
Fractionation, *see* Plasma processing and
    fractionation
Francis, Donald, 70-71, 106, 116-117
Fresh frozen plasma (FFP), 27, 29, 175,
    177, 305
substitution for AHF concentrate, 250

G

Gay activists, 71, 109-112, 122, 124, 228
Gay Related Immunodeficiency Disease
    (GRID), 66
General Accounting Office, 44
Glaser, Elizabeth, 190-191
Granulocytes, 29
Greater New York Blood Program, 110
Growth hormone, 128

H

Haitian immigrants, 61-64, 66, 69, 248
donor screening and deferral, 106, 122
HBV, *see* Hepatitis B virus

HDV, *see* Delta hepatitis virus
Health Care Financing Agency (HCFA), 51
Heat treatment, 59, 81, 86-88, 95,
    154-158, 258
FDA licensing, 73, 91, 92, 96, 177, 259
for hepatitis, 5, 73, 78
and inhibitor formation, 87, 88-89, 95,
    96, 259
Hemophilia, 1, 19, 38-39, 306,
    see also National Hemophilia Foundation
Hemophiliacs, 221
children, 68, 250
confidence in AHF concentrate, 195, 196
early AIDS cases among, 58, 62-65, 67,
    68, 89, 102, 197, 249, 250
epidemiological surveillance of, 67, 249
and hepatitis as acceptable risk, 195,
    196-197
HIV incidence among, 1, 19, 21, 64, 68,
    169, 252, 253, 258
opportunistic diseases, 58, 66-67
and risk communication, 195-200, 201,
    202-204
and sexual transmission, 178-179, 255
Hemophilia Treatment Centers, 39, 76,
    171, 173-174
Hepatitis, 1, 19, 30, 103-104, 306

as acceptable medical risk, 8, 48-49, 82,
    93, 172-173
Hepatitis A virus, 83, 84, 85
Hepatitis B core antigen (anti-HBc) test,
    76, 118
  BPAC recommendations for, 59, 75, 119
  CDC recommendations for, 6, 102, 106,
    112, 116-117
and ethnic groups, 75, 118, 120
  and homosexuals, 118, 120, 121
  as NANB virus marker, 114, 129
  objections to, 75, 113-114, 120-121
  reliability as AIDS marker, 75, 106,
    112-113, 114, 118, 119-120, 123
Hepatitis B surface antigen test, 83, 85, 105
Hepatitis B virus (HBV), 41, 43, 83-85,
    103, 131, 306-307
  and AHF heat treatment, 5, 73, 78
  inactivation methods, 4, 76, 78, 79,
    81-82, 93-95
  similarity to HIV transmission, 2, 68,
    72-73, 102, 123, 150, 208, 248, 249
Hepatitis C virus (HCV, NANB virus), 5,
    84, 85-86, 93, 129, 131, 307
HIV disease, see AIDS
HIV-1, 4, 306.
  see also Human T-cell lymphotropic
    virus
HIV testing, 78, 101, 128, 129, 131, 256
  FDA licensing, 59, 78
  positive result, relation to AIDS diagno-
    sis, 257, 258
  previously untested units, 165
  window period, 78, 129
  see also ELISA test;
  Western Blot test
HIV transmission
  AHF implicated in, 2, 68, 208
  by asymptomatic carriers, 62, 73, 116,
    137, 208
  hepatitis analogy, 2, 68, 72-73, 102,
    123, 150, 208, 248, 249
  initial evidence of blood-borne, 3, 9,
    66-70, 73, 102, 137, 148-149, 250-253
  see also Blood transfusion;
  Intravenous drug users; Maternal trans-
    mission;
  Risk groups;
  Sexual transmission
HIV-2, 129, 306
HIV-0, 129
Homosexual men, 6, 20, 102, 104, 111
  anti-HBc testing, 118, 120, 121
  behavioral hypothesis for disease, 66

differentiating higher risk, 75
and donor questioning, 3, 6, 105-106,
    109-112, 122
early cases among, 2, 20, 60, 61-65, 66,
    67, 248
opportunistic diseases among, 60, 66
see also Gay activists
Hospital blood banks, 26, 29, 35, 36
HTLV, see Human T-cell lymphotropic
    virus
Human immunodeficiency virus, see
    HIV-1;
  HIV testing;
  HIV transmission;
  HIV-2
Human T-cell lymphotropic virus
    (HTLV), 129-130, 158, 159
  HTLV III, 65, 77, 256, 257, 258, 307
  see also HIV-1
Hygienic Laboratory, NIH, 44
Hyland Therapeutics, 74, 252

I

Immune globulin, 31, 32, 33, 97, 307-308
Imported blood, 29, 33-34
Incentives to industry, 5, 95, 214-215
Incubation period, 67, 68-69, 70, 73,
    115-116

Infants
  blood transfusion cases, 58, 68, 102, 250
  cryoprecipitate treatment of, 71, 176,
      189-190, 251
  early cases among, 58, 62, 68-69, 250
Information, *see* Knowledge base and
      information deficits
Informed consent, 8, 197-199, 231
Institutional and organizational factors, 8,
      9-10, 12, 208-209, 219 , 220
Institutionalized persons, 104
Interstate commerce, 30, 47, 49-50
Intravenous drug users (IVDUs)
  donor screening and deferral of,
      104-105, 106
  early cases, 61-65, 66, 67, 69-70, 102
  maternal transmission by, 69
  opportunistic infections, 66
Irwin Memorial Blood Bank, 76, 112, 118
IV drug use, *see* Intravenous drug users

K

Kaposi's sarcoma, 60, 61, 67, 77, 308
Knowledge base and information deficits
  chronologies, 61-65, 248-259
  donor screening and deferral, 3, 6, 103,
      115-116, 210
  and regulatory actions, 3, 7, 9, 136, 141,
      208, 209
  and reliance on regulated industries, 10,
      139-140, 213
  and risk communication, 8, 197, 199,
      200, 202, 209
Koplan, Jeffrey, 116

L

Lancet, 256
Large-Linked Database (LLDB), 226
Leadership failures, 9-10, 208-209,
      212-214
  donor screening and deferral, 116-117,
      125-128
Legislation, *see names of specific statutes
      (listed under* "Regulation" *in this
      index*)
Leukocytes, see White blood cells
Liability, 223-224,
    see also Blood shield laws
  no-fault compensation system, 13, 224
Licensing and registration
blood banks, 49-51, 52

blood products, 30, 50
interstate commerce, 30, 47, 49-50
Lookback tracing, 128
  FDA policy, 7, 136, 137-138, 158-160,
      163-164, 228
  presidential directive for, 158, 159
Lymphadenopathy-associated virus
      (LAV), 77, 256, 257, 258, 308
Lymphocytes, 131, 308,
    see also CD4:CD8 ratios

M

Malaria, 1, 128
MASAC, *see* Medical and Scientific Advi-
      sory Council
Maternal transmission, 62, 69
  Glaser case, 190-191
Media, 199-200, 258
Medical and Scientific Advisory Council
      (MASAC), NHF, 27, 40, 71-72, 172,
      173, 174, 192-194, 251
  and cryoprecipitate substitution, 71,
      175, 176, 177, 200
  DDAVP recommendation, 72, 176
  and directed donation, 176
  donor screening recommendations, 72,
      143
  heat-treated product recommendation,
      177, 258
  1983 meeting, 251

recall recommendation, 75, 147, 254, 257
and sexual transmission, 178-179
Medical World News, 115
Miles Inc., 92, 157
MMWR reports
  AIDS cases, 58, 59, 68, 248, 250
  hemophiliac infection rate, 257
  opportunistic infection cases, 2, 60, 66
  transmission theories, 69-70, 257
  viral inactivation, 59, 258
Morbidity and Mortality Weekly Report,
    see MMWR reports
Multiple sex partners, 58, 73, 106

N

NANB hepatitis, *see* Hepatitis C virus
National Blood Exchange, 36
National Blood Foundation, 36
National Blood Policy of 1973, 41
National Blood Resources Program, 43
National Cancer Institute (NCI), 4, 59, 77,
    79
National Gay Task Force, 112
National Heart, Lung, and Blood
  Institute (NHLBI), 41, 43, 90
  AIDS conferences, 77
  donor screening research, 77, 118
  immunologic change study, 77
National Hemophilia Foundation (NHF),
    9, 27, 39-40, 66, 67, 172-173, 208, 210,
  see also Medical and Scientific Advi-
      sory Council
  AIDS Task Force, 173, 176, 252
  chronology of actions, 248-259
  clinical advisories and bulletins, 72, 74,
      173-174, 175-181, 212, 248-259
  and cryoprecipitate substitution, 175,
      176, 177
  DDAVP recommendation, 72, 176, 178
  experience and expertise, 192-194
  heat-treated product recommendation,
      96, 258
  initial recommendations, 3, 71-72
  and recalls, 74, 253
  and sexual transmission, 177, 178-179
  and surveillance and reporting system,
      76, 248, 249
  ties with plasma industry, 8-9, 173, 194,
      212, 234
  treatment maintenance recommenda-
      tions, 74, 252, 253, 254, 257
National Institute of Allergy and Infec-
    tious Diseases (NIAID), 43

National Institutes of Health (NIH), 2, 9,
    20, 26, 42-43, 44, 66, 67, 77, 78,
    161, 208, 221
  changes of directors, 59, 213
  research funding and priorities, 77, 90,
    161
  see also National Cancer Institute;
    National Institute of Allergy and Infec-
      tious Diseases
National Marrow Donor Program, 36
National Microbiology Institute, NIH, 44
Neoantigenicity, 87, 95
News media, 199-200, 258
New York Blood Center, 77
NHF, *see* National Hemophilia Foundation
No-fault compensation system, 13, 224
Non-A, non-B (NANB) hepatitis, *see* Hep-
    atitis C virus
Nongovernmental organizations, *see*
    Blood banks and centers;
  National Hemophilia Foundation;
   Plasma industry

O

Office of Maternal and Child Health,
    172-174
Opportunistic diseases, 308-309,
  see also Kaposi's sarcoma;
  Pneumocystis carinii pneumonia
  among hemophiliacs, 58, 66-67

among homosexuals, 60, 66
early cases, 60, 61, 66-67

P

Paid donors, 30, 31, 41, 43, 51, 104
Pasteur Institute, 4, 77
PCP, *see Pneumocystis carinii* pneumonia
Pediatric cases, *see* Children;
   Infants
Pentamidine, 60
Petricciani, John, 142, 145
Pharmaceutical companies, 31
Pharmaceutical Manufacturers Associa-
      tion (PMA), 75, 147, 149, 153
Physicians
   and blood transfusion, 177
   case reporting, 67
   communication to patients, 8, 9, 180,
      195-200, 208
   concern over patient AHF reduction, 9,
      200
   confidence in AHF concentrate, 195, 196
   counteracting media attention, 199-200
   denial and downplaying of risk, 8,
      195-196, 199-200, 202
   and hepatitis as acceptable risk, 195,
      196-197
   and informed consent, 8, 197-199
   reduction of AHF use, 178
Plasma collection centers, 9, 30, 31, 108,
      208
   donor screening, 6, 78, 108-109
   in prisons, 30
   standard operating procedures, 73, 108,
      142
Plasma derivatives, 27, 28, 29-33, 41, 43,
      50, 54, 309.
   see also Albumin;
   Antihemophilic factor (AHF);
   Anti-inhibitor complex;
   Fibrinogen;
   Immune globulin;
   Plasma protein fraction
Plasma industry, 1, 9, 19, 26, 28, 30-31, 210
   donor screening and deferral policies,
      72, 78, 107, 109-110, 151-152, 162
   heat treatment licensing, 5, 91, 92
   and NHF, 8-9, 173, 194, 212, 234
   self-regulation, 51, 139-140, 162-163
   viral inactivation research activities, 4,
      5, 79, 82, 86-88, 88, 90-91, 93
   see also Plasma collection centers;
   Plasma processing and fractionation

Plasmapheresis, *29, 30, 309*
Plasma processing and fractionation, 5,
      31, 91, 92, 309
Plasma protein fraction (PPF), 33, 309
Platelets, 27, 29, 43, 131, 309
Pneumocystis carinii pneumonia (PCP),
      60, 61, 66, 67
Political environment
   impact on regulatory actions, 7, 20, 57,
      125, 140, 141, 145-146
   insensitivity to AIDS epidemic,
      124-125, 140, 146, 161
   see also Gay activists
Pooling of plasma, 1, 19, 31
   reduction in pool size, 12, 153-154, 165,
      222
"Poppers,"; 66, 69
Practice guidelines, 12, 16, 221-222,
      232-234
Presidential Commission on the Human
      Immunodeficiency Virus, 138, 159
Prison inmates, 62, 69-70
   as donors, 30, 104, 122
Product treatment, *see* Heat treatment;
   Viral inactivation
Professional associations, 3, 26-27, 36, 71.
   see also American Association of Blood
      Banks;
   American Blood Resources Association;
   Council of Community Blood Centers
p24 antigen test, 129, 309

Public Health Service Act, 42, 44, 48, 51,
    52, 138
Public Health Service (PHS), 9, 19, 20,
    26, 41-42, 77, 208
  Blood Safety Council, 12, 219-223, 232
  Committee on Opportunistic Infections
    in Patients with Hemophilia 1982
    meeting, 58, 67, 76-77, 89, 218, 249
  initial prevention recommendations, 3,
    58, 72-73, 89, 108
  leadership failures, 11, 212-214, 218
  personnel changes, 59, 212-213
  regulatory triggers and actions, 10,
    214-217
  research activities and funding, 76-77
  risk group exclusion recommendations,
    6, 107-108
  sexual transmission prevention recom-
    mendations, 58, 73
  transfusion recommendations, 73, 177
  see also Assistant Secretary for Health;
  Centers for Disease Control and Preven-
    tion;
  Food and Drug Administration;
  National Institutes of Health
Public opinion and concern, 19, 57, 128
  impacts on blood donation, 34, 78, 111,
    121

regulatory triggers and actions, 215, 216
Recipient tracing, *see* Lookback tracing
Recombinant DNA techniques, 97,
    309-310
Red blood cells (RBCs), 25, 27, 29, 131,
    310
Red Cross, *see* American Red Cross
Regional centers, *see* Hemophilia Treat-
    ment Centers
Regulation, 47-49
  advisory committees' role, 10, 213
  industry self-regulation, 51, 139-140,
    162-163
  under Reagan Administration, 20, 57,
    125, 140
  see also Biologics Act;
    Blood shield laws;
    Clinical Laboratories Improvement Act;
    Donor screening and deferral;
    Federal Food, Drug, and Cosmetic Act;
    Food and Drug Administration;
    Licensing and registration;
    National Blood Policy of 1973;
    Public Health Service Act
Research activities, 4, 59
  and industry competitiveness, 94-95
  isolation of virus, 4, 57, 59, 71, 77-78,
    256
  NIH, 77, 90, 161

Q

Questioning of donors, 3, 6, 71, 102, 106,
    107, 109-112, 130
  opposition to, 109-112, 122, 228

R

Ratnoff, Oscar, 71
Reagan Administration
  insensitivity to AIDS epidemic,
    124-125, 140, 146, 161
  and regulation issues, 20, 57, 125, 140
Recalls
  ARC, 180, 252
  automatic, 4, 7, 75, 147, 153, 210
  delays in implementation, 7, 137,
    154-158, 164, 208
  FDA policy, 3, 7, 52-53, 135, 137,
    138-139, 142-154, 211, 228, 229
  manufacturers, 58, 74, 162, 180, 252,
    253, 254, 257
  NHF position, 74, 253
  phased and staged, 144-145, 227

PHS, 76-77
  risk group similarities, 58, 61, 62, 67, 249
  screening tests, 57, 73, 78, 79, 108
  viral inactivation methods, 57, 76, 78,
    79, 88, 89, 90-96
Resource limitations, 7, 59, 141 NHF,
    172, 192-194
Risk assessment, 209-211
  CDC role, 225
  chronology of, 248-259
  and early information deficit, 3-4, 9, 75,
    115-116, 208
Risk communication, 8-9, 15-17, 169-172,
    201-204, 211, 231-234
  CDC role, 225-226
  clinical options, 8, 16, 72, 170, 175-181,
    201-203, 232-233
  and information deficits, 8, 197, 199,
    200, 202, 209
  by National Hemophilia Foundation, 8,
    72, 172-174, 193-195, 201, 202-203,
    208, 212, 232-233
  regulatory triggers and actions, 215, 217
  sexual transmission, 178-179
Risk groups, 5, 101-102, 104, 215, 216
  case reports, 61-65
  hepatitis markers present across, 66,
    113, 118
  PHS exclusion recommendations, 6,
    107-108
  research on similarities among, 58, 61,
    62, 67, 249
  sexual contact with members of, 63,
    106, 108, 255
  see also Blood transfusion;
   Haitian immigrants;
  Hemophiliacs;
  Homosexual men;
  Intravenous drug users

S

Science, 256
  Secondary transmission, 177, 178-179
Secretary of Health and Human Services,
    11, 13, 218, 225
Self-deferral, 101, 110, 130, 215, 216
Serum hepatitis, *see* Hepatitis B virus
Sexual transmission, 2, 9, 63, 69, 101,
    178-179, 255
  and hemophiliacs, 178-179, 255
  multiple partners, 58, 73, 106
  to partners of risk group members, 63,
    106, 108, 255

PHS prevention recommendations
    regarding, 58, 73
Shanbrom, Edward, 86-87, 93
Stanford University Blood Bank, 76-77,
    118
State government
  blood bank licensing, 50-51
  blood shield laws, 2, 48-49, 224
  and case reporting, 67
Statutes, *see names of specific statutes
    (listed under* "Regulation" *in this
    index)*
Surrogate marker testing, 3, 4, 101, 310
  accuracy and reliability, 112-113, 119
  BPAC industry task force, 75, 119-121
  BPAC meeting and outcomes, 59, 75,
    103, 119-122
  CDC recommendations, 6, 71, 102, 106
  CD4/CD8 ratios, 76, 117-118
  opposition to, 72, 113-114, 120-121
  see also Hepatitis B core antigen test
Surveillance programs
  Blood Safety Council, 12, 220, 221
  CDC, 13-14, 67, 76, 79, 221, 226, 248,
    249
Swine flu episode, 59-60, 126, 127, 140,
    146, 225

T

Thrombocytes, *see* Platelets

Tort system, 12, 223-224
Trade associations, *see* American Blood
        Resources Association; Professional
        associations
Transfusion, *see* Blood transfusion
Truman v. Thomas, 198

V

Vaccine Adverse Event Reporting
  System (VAERS), 226
Vaccines, 256, 311
  liability, 223-224
  swine flu, 59, 126-127
Viral inactivation, 81, 91
  double inactivation methods, 12, 222
  FDA approval and licensing, 4, 12,
      91-92, 221-222, 259
  for hepatitis, 4, 76, 78, 79, 81-82, 93-95
  research activities, 57, 76, 78, 79, 88,
      89, 90-96
  see also Heat treatment
Volunteer donors, 1, 19, 31, 37, 41, 51,
        104, 111

W

Western Blot test, 78, 257
White blood cells (WBCs), 25, 27, 311.
  see also CD4:CD8 ratios;
    Granulocytes;
    Lymphocytes
Whole blood products, 20, 25, 27, 29, 53,
        104, 164,
  see also Cryoprecipitate;
    Fresh frozen plasma;
    Granulocytes;
    Platelets;
    Red blood cells
  Women, 61, 63, 64, 65, 69
Wyngaarden, James, 77

Z

Zero-risk approaches, 211